D0596964

Pediatric Hospital Medicine

Editor
MARY C. OTTOLINI

Pediatric Palliative Care

Editors
CHRISTINA K. ULLRICH
JOANNE WOLFE

PEDIATRIC CLINICS OF NORTH AMERICA

www.pediatric.theclinics.com

Consulting Editor
BONITA F. STANTON

August 2014 • Volume 61 • Number 4

ELSEVIER

1600 John F. Kennedy Boulevard • Suite 1800 • Philadelphia, Pennsylvania, 19103-2899

http://www.theclinics.com

THE PEDIATRIC CLINICS OF NORTH AMERICA Volume 61, Number 4
August 2014 ISSN 0031-3955, ISBN-13: 978-0-323-32022-1

Editor: Kerry Holland
Developmental Editor: Casey Jackson

The Pediatric Clinics of North America (ISSN 0031-3955) is published bimonthly by Elsevier Inc., 360 Park Avenue South, New York, NY 10010-1710. Months of issue are February, April, June, August, October, and December. Periodicals postage paid at New York, NY and additional mailing offices. Subscription prices are $200.00 per year (US individuals), $493.00 per year (US institutions), $270.00 per year (Canadian individuals), $657.00 per year (Canadian institutions), $325.00 per year (international individuals), $657.00 per year (international institutions), $100.00 per year (US students and residents), and $165.00 per year (international and Canadian residents and students). To receive students/resident rare, orders must be accompanied by name of affiliated institution, date of term, and the signature of program/residency coordinator on institution letterhead. Orders will be billed at individual rate until proof of status is received. Foreign air speed delivery is included in all *Clinics* subscription prices. All prices are subject to change without notice. **POSTMASTER:** Send address changes to *The Pediatric Clinics of North America*, Elsevier Health Sciences Division, Subscription Customer Service, 3251 Riverport Lane, Maryland Heights, MO 63043. **Customer Service: 1-800-654-2452 (US and Canada). From outside of the US and Canada: 1-314-447-8871. Fax: 1-314-447-8029. For print support, E-mail: JournalsCustomerService-usa@elsevier.com. For online support, E-mail: JournalsOnlineSupport-usa@elsevier.com.**

Reprints. For copies of 100 or more, of articles in this publication, please contact the Commercial Reprints Department, Elsevier Inc., 360 Park Avenue South, New York, NY 10010-1710. Tel.: 212-633-3874; Fax: 212-633-3820; E-mail: reprints@elsevier.com.

The Pediatric Clinics of North America is also published in Spanish by McGraw-Hill Inter-americana Editores S.A., Mexico City, Mexico; in Portuguese by Riechmann and Affonso Editores, Rua Comandante Coelho 1085, CEP 21250, Rio de Janeiro, Brazil; and in Greek by Althayia SA, Athens, Greece.

The Pediatric Clinics of North America is covered in *MEDLINE/PubMed (Index Medicus), Excerpta Medica, Current Contents, Current Contents/Clinical Medicine, Science Citation Index, ASCA, ISI/BIOMED*, and *BIOSIS*.

Printed in the United States of America.

PROGRAM OBJECTIVE
The goal of the *Pediatric Clinics of North America* is to keep practicing physicians and residents up to date with current clinical practice in pediatrics by providing timely articles reviewing the state-of-the-art in patient care.

TARGET AUDIENCE
All practicing pediatricians, physicians and healthcare professionals who provide patient care to pediatric patients.

LEARNING OBJECTIVES
Upon completion of this activity, participants will be able to:
1. Review the role of end of life care for hospitalized children, adolescents and young adults.
2. Recognize the special considerations, transitions and roles in the relationship between pediatric hospital medicine and palliative care.
3. Discuss care settings for children with life threatening illnesses.

ACCREDITATION
The Elsevier Office of Continuing Medical Education (EOCME) is accredited by the Accreditation Council for Continuing Medical Education (ACCME) to provide continuing medical education for physicians.

The EOCME designates this enduring material for a maximum of 15 *AMA PRA Category 1 Credit*(s)™. Physicians should claim only the credit commensurate with the extent of their participation in the activity.

All other health care professionals requesting continuing education credit for this enduring material will be issued a certificate of participation.

DISCLOSURE OF CONFLICTS OF INTEREST
The EOCME assesses conflict of interest with its instructors, faculty, planners, and other individuals who are in a position to control the content of CME activities. All relevant conflicts of interest that are identified are thoroughly vetted by EOCME for fair balance, scientific objectivity, and patient care recommendations. EOCME is committed to providing its learners with CME activities that promote improvements or quality in healthcare and not a specific proprietary business or a commercial interest.

The planning committee, staff, authors and editors listed below have identified no financial relationships or relationships to products or devices they or their spouse/life partner have with commercial interest related to the content of this CME activity:
Toluwalase Ajayi, MD; Aura Anania, MSW, BSW; Justin N. Baker, MD; Jimmy Beck, MD; Jay Berry; Jori F. Bogetz, MD; Douglas W. Carlson; Margaret C. Cupit; Yasmeen Daud, MD; Richard D. Goldstein, MD; Kerry Holland; Brynne Hunter; Liza-Marie Johnson, MD, MPH; Barbara Jones, MSW, PhD; Indu Kumari; Sandy Lavery; Jennifer Linebarger, MD, MPH; Sanjay Mahant, MD, MSc, FRCPC; Paul Manicone, MD; Jill McNair; Vineeta Mittal; Dominic Moore, MD; Katherine Nelson, MD, FRCPC; Monica Ogelby, MSN, CPNP; Mary Ottolinii, MD, MPH; Lindsay Parnell; Andrea Radulovic, RN, BSN, MPH; Adam Rapoport, MD, FRCPC, MHSc; Joshua Schaffzin; Scott Schwantes, MD, FAAP; Joan Sheetz, MD; Tamara Simon; Karen Smith, MD; Jennifer Snaman, MD; Bonita F. Stanton, MD; Christina K. Ullrich, MD, MPH; Kevin Weingarten, MD; Helen Wells O'Brien, MDiv, MEd, BCC; Joanne Wolfe, MD, MPH.

The planning committee, staff, authors and editors listed below have identified financial relationships or relationships to products or devices they or their spouse/life partner have with commercial interest related to the content of this CME activity:
Savithri Nageswaran, MBBS, MPH has research grants from Health Resources & Services Administration and National Palliative Care Research Center.
Jack M. Percelay, MD, MPH is a consultant/advisor for Expert Witness Services- Thomson Reuters and RelayHealth.

UNAPPROVED/OFF-LABEL USE DISCLOSURE
The EOCME requires CME faculty to disclose to the participants:
1. When products or procedures being discussed are off-label, unlabelled, experimental, and/or investigational (not US Food and Drug Administration (FDA) approved); and
2. Any limitations on the information presented, such as data that are preliminary or that represent ongoing research, interim analyses, and/or unsupported opinions. Faculty may discuss information about pharmaceutical agents that is outside of FDA-approved labelling. This information is intended solely

for CME and is not intended to promote off-label use of these medications. If you have any questions, contact the medical affairs department of the manufacturer for the most recent prescribing information.

TO ENROLL
To enroll in the *Pediatric Clinics of North America* Continuing Medical Education program, call customer service at 1-800-654-2452 or sign up online at http://www.theclinics.com/home/cme. The CME program is available to subscribers for an additional annual fee of USD 290.

METHOD OF PARTICIPATION
In order to claim credit, participants must complete the following:
1. Complete enrolment as indicated above.
2. Read the activity.
3. Complete the CME Test and Evaluation. Participants must achieve a score of 70% on the test. All CME Tests and Evaluations must be completed online.

CME INQUIRIES/SPECIAL NEEDS
For all CME inquiries or special needs, please contact elsevierCME@elsevier.com.

Contributors

CONSULTING EDITOR

BONITA F. STANTON, MD
Vice Dean for Research and Professor of Pediatrics, School of Medicine, Wayne State University, Detroit, Michigan

EDITORS

MARY C. OTTOLINI, MD, MPH
Vice Chair of Education and Professor of Pediatrics, George Washington University School of Medicine and Children's National Medical Center, Washington, DC

CHRISTINA K. ULLRICH, MD, MPH
Assistant Professor of Pediatrics, Division of Pediatric Palliative Care, Department of Psychosocial Oncology and Palliative Care; Department of Pediatric Hematology/ Oncology, Dana-Farber Cancer Institute and Boston Children's Hospital, Harvard Medical School, Boston, Massachusetts

JOANNE WOLFE, MD, MPH
Division of Pediatric Palliative Care, Department of Psychosocial Oncology and Palliative Care, Dana-Farber Cancer Institute, Boston, Massachusetts

AUTHORS

TOLUWALASE A. AJAYI, MD
Associate Medical Director, Palliative Care, Scripps Mercy Hospital San Diego; Pediatric Hospital Medicine, Rady Children's Hospital, San Diego, California

AURA ANANIA, MSW, BSW
Care Coordinator, Community Pediatric Enhanced Care Program, Brenner Children's Hospital; Department of Pediatrics, Wake Forest School of Medicine, Winston-Salem, North Carolina

JUSTIN N. BAKER, MD
Chief, Division of Quality of Life and Palliative Care; Associate Member, Department of Oncology, St. Jude Children's Research Hospital, Memphis, Tennessee

JIMMY BECK, MD
Hospitalist Division, Children's National Health System - Sheikh Zayed Campus for Advanced Children's Medicine; Adjunct Instructor of Pediatrics, The George Washington University Medical Center, Washington, DC

JAY G. BERRY, MD, MPH
Assistant Professor, Division of General Pediatrics, Department of Pediatrics, Boston Children's Hospital, Harvard Medical School, Boston, Massachusetts

JORI F. BOGETZ, MD
Postdoctoral Fellow and Clinical Instructor of Pediatrics, Division of General Pediatrics, Department of Pediatrics, Lucile Packard Children's Hospital, Stanford University School of Medicine, Palo Alto, California

DOUGLAS W. CARLSON, MD
Professor of Pediatrics and Director, Division of Pediatric Hospital Medicine, St. Louis Children's Hospital, Washington University School of Medicine, St Louis, Missouri

MARGARET C. CUPIT, BA
St. Jude Children's Research Hospital, Memphis, Tennessee

YASMEEN N. DAUD, MD
Assistant Professor of Pediatrics, Division of Pediatric Hospital Medicine, St. Louis Children's Hospital, Washington University School of Medicine, St Louis, Missouri

RICHARD D. GOLDSTEIN, MD
Assistant Professor of Pediatrics, Pediatric Advanced Care Team, Boston Children's Hospital, Dana-Farber Cancer Institute, Harvard Medical School, Boston, Massachusetts

LIZA-MARIE JOHNSON, MD, MPH, MSB
Department of Pediatrics, St. Jude Children's Research Hospital, Memphis, Tennessee; Bioethics Program, Adjunct Professor, Department of Bioethics, The Center for Bioethics & Clinical Leadership, Union Graduate College-Icahn Mt Sinai, Schenectady, New York

BARBARA L. JONES, MSW, PhD
Assistant Dean For Health Affairs and Associate Professor; Co-Director, The Institute for Grief, Loss and Family Survival, School of Social Work, University of Texas at Austin, Austin, Texas; Clinical Associate Professor of Pediatrics, University of Texas Galveston Medical School, Galveston, Texas

JENNIFER S. LINEBARGER, MD, MPH, FAAP
Medical Director, Pediatric Palliative Care Team, The Children's Mercy Hospital, Kansas City, Missouri

SANJAY MAHANT, MD, MSc, FRCPC
Pediatric Outcomes Research Team (PORT), Division of Pediatric Medicine, Department of Pediatrics, University of Toronto, Hospital for Sick Children; Institute for Health Policy, Management and Evaluation, University of Toronto; Child Health Evaluation Sciences, Research Institute, Hospital for Sick Children, Toronto, Ontario, Canada; CanChild Centre for Disability Research, Hamilton, Ontario, Canada

PAUL E. MANICONE, MD
Hospitalist Division, Children's National Health System - Sheikh Zayed Campus for Advanced Children's Medicine; Assistant Professor of Pediatrics, The George Washington University Medical Center, Washington, DC

VINEETA MITTAL, MD
Pediatric Hospitalist and Associate Professor of Pediatrics, Division of General Pediatrics, Department of Pediatrics, UT Southwestern Medical Center and Children's Medical Center, Dallas, Texas

DOMINIC MOORE, MD, FAAP
Instructor and Associate Medical Director, Rainbow Kids Palliative Care Program; Division of In-Patient Medicine, Pediatrics, Primary Children's Hospital, University of Utah, Salt Lake City, Utah

SAVITHRI NAGESWARAN, MBBS, MPH
Associate Professor, Department of Pediatrics, Wake Forest School of Medicine, Winston-Salem, North Carolina

KATHERINE E. NELSON, MD, FRCPC
Pediatric Outcomes Research Team (PORT), Division of Pediatric Medicine, Department of Pediatrics, University of Toronto, Hospital for Sick Children; Institute for Health Policy, Management and Evaluation, University of Toronto; Pediatric Advanced Care Team (PACT) and Janice Rotman Fellowship in Home Care Innovation, Division of Pediatric Medicine, Hospital for Sick Children, Toronto, Ontario, Canada

MONICA OGELBY, MSN, APRN, CPNP
Pediatric Palliative Care Program Nurse Case Manager, Pediatric Palliative Care Program, Department of Vermont Health Access, State of Vermont, Williston, Vermont

JACK M. PERCELAY, MD, MPH, FAAP, MHM
Adjunct Clinical Professor, Department of Physician Assistant Studies, Pace University College of Health Professions, New York, New York

ANDREA RADULOVIC, RN, BSN, MPH
Nurse Coordinator, The Pediatric Enhanced Care Program, Brenner Children's Hospital, Wake Forest Baptist Health, Winston-Salem, North Carolina

ADAM RAPOPORT, MD, FRCPC, MHSc
Medical Director, Paediatric Advanced Care Team (PACT), The Hospital for Sick Children; Medical Director, Emily's House Children's Hospice; Pediatric Palliative Care Consultant, The Temmy Latner Centre for Palliative Care, Mount Sinai Hospital; Assistant Professor, Departments of Paediatrics and Family & Community Medicine, University of Toronto, Toronto, Ontario, Canada

JOSHUA K. SCHAFFZIN, MD, PhD
Assistant Professor, Division of Hospital Medicine, Cincinnati Children's Hospital Medical Center, Cincinnati, Ohio

SCOTT SCHWANTES, MD, FAAP
Department of Pediatrics, Gillette Children's Specialty Healthcare, Regions Hospital, St Paul, Minnesota

JOAN SHEETZ, MD
Division of In-Patient Medicine, Pediatrics, Primary Children's Hospital, University of Utah, Salt Lake City, Utah

TAMARA D. SIMON, MD, MSPH
Assistant Professor of Pediatrics, Division of Hospital Medicine, Department of Pediatrics, Seattle Children's Hospital, University of Washington, Seattle, Washington

KAREN SMITH, MD, MEd
Division of Hospitalist Medicine, Children's National Medical Center; Assistant Professor of Pediatrics, The George Washington School of Medicine, Washington, DC

JENNIFER M. SNAMAN, MD
Fellow, Division of Oncology, Department of Pediatric Oncology, St. Jude Children's Research Hospital, Memphis, Tennessee

CHRISTINA K. ULLRICH, MD, MPH
Assistant Professor of Pediatrics, Division of Pediatric Palliative Care, Department
of Psychosocial Oncology and Palliative Care; Department of Pediatric Hematology/
Oncology, Dana-Farber Cancer Institute and Boston Children's Hospital, Harvard Medical
School, Boston, Massachusetts

KEVIN WEINGARTEN, MD, FRCPC, MHSc
Staff Physician, Paediatric Advanced Care Team (PACT), The Hospital for Sick Children,
Toronto, Ontario, Canada

HELEN WELLS O'BRIEN, MDiv, MEd, BCC
Department of Pediatrics, Gillette Children's Specialty Healthcare, Regions Hospital,
St Paul, Minnesota

Contents

> Shared decision-making is a process that helps frame conversations about value-sensitive decisions, such as introduction of assistive technology for children with neurologic impairment. In the shared decision-making model, the health care provider elicits family values relevant to the decision, provides applicable evidence in the context of those values, and collaborates with the family to identify the preferred option. This article outlines clinical, quality of life, and ethical considerations for shared decision-making discussions with families of children with neurologic impairment about gastrostomy tube and tracheostomy tube placement.

> Medical comanagement of surgical patients by pediatric hospital medicine providers has become increasingly common. Subjectively, the comanagement model is superior to more traditional consultative models because of the anticipatory preventive care and coordination hospitalists provide to patients and hospital colleagues. Although some studies have demonstrated the value of the comanagement model in adults and children, others have failed to do so. The coming years are both exciting and challenging for this emerging field as it attempts to sustain its early progress and define its future in pediatric hospital medicine.

> Family-centered rounds (FCRs) are multidisciplinary rounds that involve medical teams partnering with patients and families in daily medical decision-making. Multiple FCR benefits have been identified including improving patient satisfaction, communication, discharge planning, medical education, and patient safety. Main barriers to FCRs are variability in attending rounding, duration of rounds, physical constrains of large teams and small rooms, specific and sensitive patient conditions, and lack of

training of residents, students, and faculty on how to conduct effective and effecient FCRs. In the last decade, many programs have incorporated FCRs into daily practice due to their multiple perceived benefits. Future FCRs should focus on better operationalizing of FCRs and reporting on objective outcomes measures such as improved communication, coordination, and patient satisfaction that are crucial for healthcare.

Effective communication requires direct interaction between the hospitalist and the primary care provider using a standardized method of information exchange with the opportunity to ask questions and assign accountability for follow-up roles. The discharge summary is part of the process but does not provide the important aspects of handoff, such as closed loop communication and role assignments. Hospital discharge is a significant safety risk for patients, with more than half of discharged patients experiencing at least one error. Hospitalist and primary care providers need to collaborate to develop a standardized system to communicate about shared patients that meets handoff requirements.

Pediatric hospitalists are increasingly common in community hospitals and are playing increasingly important roles. Scope of practice and staffing models vary significantly by program. Unique aspects of small pediatric hospital medicine programs in hospitals with limited pediatric subspecialty and surgical support are discussed, including clinical and logistic considerations, training needs, and advocacy roles.

Quality improvement (QI) and comparative effectiveness research (CER) are increasingly important areas of study for the pediatric hospitalist. The focus of this article is to provide the relevant background, definitions, framework, infrastructure, and resources needed to both inform and engage the pediatric hospital medicine (PHM) community on QI and CER. In mastering these activities, PHM physicians will have a key role in shaping the health care transformation expected over the next decade and beyond.

Pediatric sedation is an evolving field performed by an extensive list of specialties. Well-defined sedation systems within pediatric facilities are paramount to providing consistent, safe sedation. Pediatric sedation providers should be trained in the principles and practice of sedation, which include patient selection, pre-sedation assessment to determine risks during sedation, selection of optimal sedation medication, monitoring requirements, and post-sedation care. Training, credentialing, and continuing sedation education must be incorporated into sedation systems to verify and monitor the practice of safe sedation. Pediatric hospitalists represent a group of providers with extensive pediatric knowledge and skills who can safely provide pediatric sedation.

Contents

for clinical practice that integrates clinical, psychosocial, and ethical concerns at the end of life (EOL) into a standard operating procedure specifically focused on inpatient deaths. Palliative care for children at EOL in the hospital setting should encompass the personal, cultural, and spiritual needs of the child and family members and aim to minimize suffering and increase support for all who are involved, including hospital staff.

PEDIATRIC CLINICS OF NORTH AMERICA

Foreword

Hospital Medicine and Pediatric Palliative Care

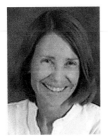

Bonita F. Stanton, MD
Consulting Editor

Most pediatricians practice in the outpatient setting. The familiarity with hospital-based practices most pediatricians acquire through their residencies rapidly ebbs as policies and activities change. Therefore, this issue of *Pediatric Clinics of North America*, focusing on two emerging pediatric specialties with strong hospital foci—pediatric hospital medicine and pediatric palliative care (PPC)—should be of great interest and importance to all practicing pediatricians.

"Born" in 2003, Pediatric Hospital Medicine (PHM) is the cornerstone of inpatient management in many pediatric wards and hospitals—and has a presence in most. In this issue, Mary Ottolini and colleagues clearly describe the range of clinical roles and activities conducted and overseen by today's PHM specialists, including communication and coordinating with primary care physicians and other specialists, facilitating shared decision-making with families, and carrying out hospital-based procedures, such as pediatric sedation. PHM specialists provide care to all hospitalized children, including children with chronic life-threatening illnesses. In their care of these children, they form close partnerships with PPC specialists.

The discipline of PPC medicine has emerged with the growth of a bewildering array of clinical options and technologies that can extend life for children with life-threatening diseases. PPC specialists help the PHM specialists and primary care pediatric providers, and the families of children with life-threatening illnesses (as well as the children themselves), navigate through these options to assure that the child's needs and the families' desires are being met. In this issue, Ullrich and colleagues artfully describe their approach to optimizing the care and well-being of these children and their families, while prolonging life and providing end-of-life support. The PPC provider achieves these goals through continual learning of new advances, communication with and education of the family, child and hospital-based and community-based providers, and frequent reassessment of child and family. PPC specialists function inside and outside

Pediatr Clin N Am 61 (2014) xvii–xviii
http://dx.doi.org/10.1016/j.pcl.2014.05.006
0031-3955/14/$ – see front matter © 2014 Published by Elsevier Inc.

pediatric.theclinics.com

of the hospital setting, although often the family and primary care pediatric provider meet the PPC provider in the hospital setting.

PHM and PPC specialists are critical members of the family of pediatric care providers. These articles provide a clear description of the great value they bring to our profession and to the children under our care.

Bonita F. Stanton, MD
School of Medicine
Wayne State University
1261 Scott Hall
540 East Canfield, Suite 1261
Detroit, MI 48201, USA

E-mail address:
bstanton@med.wayne.edu

Preface

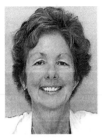

Mary C. Ottolini, MD, MPH
Editor

Pediatric Hospital Medicine (PHM) is a new and evolving specialty, with plans to petition the American Board of Pediatrics for specialty accreditation within the next year. Although Hospital Medicine is said to have started in 1996 with the definition of a hospitalist by Wachter and Goldman,[1] PHM dates its formal inception to the first Pediatric Hospital Medicine Meeting sponsored by the Academic Pediatric Association in 2003.[2,3] The roles, career path, and scope of practice for pediatric hospitalists were then ill-defined.

Over the past 11 years, PHM core competencies were published to define the scope of practice, and PHM has become a desirable career path for many. There are currently an estimated 3000 Pediatric Hospitalists in practice. As the field evolves, the need for additional training beyond residency has led to the creation of PHM-specific continuing medical education programs and fellowships. There are over 30 existing PHM fellowship programs. For the first time this year, PHM fellowship program applicants will enter the MATCH (National Resident Matching Program).

Although hospitalists are significantly involved in nonclinical pursuits, such as education, and research, the focus of this *Pediatric Clinics of North America* is on important clinical aspects of PHM practice. Authors of this issue describe the Pediatric Hospitalist's role in the community hospital setting, in providing sedation and analgesia, and in shared decision-making for medically complex, technology-dependent patients. Two articles in this issue describe processes of care that are critical to high-quality safe practice: family-centered rounds and communication with primary care providers. Hospitalists are also taking a lead role in quality improvement, working to define and implement best practices to reduce costs and improve care. Read this edition of *Pediatric Clinics of North America* to learn more about the evolution of the dynamic field of PHM and the important role Pediatric Hospitalists play in the continuum of care for infants, children, and adolescents.

Mary C. Ottolini, MD, MPH
Children's National Medical Center
111 Michigan Avenue, Northwest
Washington, DC 20010, USA

E-mail address:
MOTTOLIN@childrensnational.org

Pediatr Clin N Am 61 (2014) xix–xx
http://dx.doi.org/10.1016/j.pcl.2014.05.005
0031-3955/14/$ – see front matter © 2014 Published by Elsevier Inc.

pediatric.theclinics.com

REFERENCES

1. Wachter RM, Goldman L. The emerging role of "hospitalists" in the American health care system. N Engl J Med 1996;335:514–7.
2. Lye PS, Rauch DA, Ottolini MC, et al. Pediatric hospitalists: report of a leadership conference. Pediatrics 2006;117:1122–30.
3. Fisher ES, Rauch DA, Quinonz R, et al. Growing strong: findings from the American Academy of Pediatrics Hospital Medicine Workforce Survey 2012-13. Pediatric Academic Society Meeting, Vancouver, Canada, May 6, 2014.

Shared Decision-Making About Assistive Technology for the Child with Severe Neurologic Impairment

Katherine E. Nelson, MD, FRCPC[a,b,c,d],
Sanjay Mahant, MD, MSc, FRCPC[a,b,e,f],*

KEYWORDS

- Gastrostomy • Tracheostomy • Neurologic impairment
- Children with medical complexity • Technology dependence
- Shared decision-making

KEY POINTS

- Introduction of assistive technology, such as gastrostomy and tracheostomy tubes, for children with severe neurologic impairment is a value-sensitive decision.
- Value-sensitive decisions benefit from a shared decision-making model approach.
- Pediatric hospitalists can use a shared decision-making model to further discussions with families about assistive technology for children with neurologic impairment.

INTRODUCTION

Children with severe neurologic impairment, a growing population with high resource utilization, are frequently admitted to inpatient pediatric medicine wards with acute

Disclosure: Neither author has a relationship with a commercial company that has a direct financial interest in the subject matter or materials discussed in the article or that is making a competing product.
[a] Pediatric Outcomes Research Team (PORT), Division of Pediatric Medicine, Department of Pediatrics, University of Toronto, Hospital for Sick Children, 555 University Avenue, Toronto, Ontario M5G 1X8, Canada; [b] Institute for Health Policy, Management and Evaluation, University of Toronto, 155 College Street, Toronto, Ontario M5T 3M6, Canada; [c] Pediatric Advanced Care Team (PACT), Division of Pediatric Medicine, Hospital for Sick Children, 555 University Avenue, Toronto, Ontario M5G 1X8, Canada; [d] Janice Rotaman Fellowship in Home Care Innovation, Division of Pediatric Medicine, Hospital for Sick Children, 555 University Avenue, Toronto, Ontario M5G 1X8, Canada; [e] Child Health Evaluation Sciences, Research Institute, Hospital for Sick Children, 555 University Avenue, Toronto, Ontario M5G 1X8, Canada; [f] CanChild Centre for Disability Research, 1280 Main Street West, Hamilton, Ontario L8S 4L8, Canada
* Corresponding author. Division of Paediatric Medicine, Hospital for Sick Children, 555 University Avenue, Toronto, Ontario M5G 1X8, Canada.
E-mail address: sanjay.mahant@sickkids.ca

Pediatr Clin N Am 61 (2014) 641–652
http://dx.doi.org/10.1016/j.pcl.2014.04.001
0031-3955/14/$ – see front matter © 2014 Elsevier Inc. All rights reserved.

pediatric.theclinics.com

issues. Conversations about the introduction of life-sustaining technology often arise during admissions, and pediatric hospitalists are asked to help families navigate these complicated issues. This article discusses shared decision-making (SDM) as a strategy that can be used to help families make decisions and applies concepts from SDM to clinical cases about the introduction of technology for children with severe neurologic impairment.

SHARED DECISION-MAKING
Definition and Potential Resources

In the past 2 decades, SDM has become an accepted model for collaborative communication between providers and patients or families to determine a treatment plan when multiple options exist, each with its own slate of risks and benefits.[1] In SDM, family members express their goals and values related to the decision, the provider discusses the risks and benefits of each option, and the plan is negotiated jointly as the best of the available options within the context of those values (**Fig. 1**).[2,3] SDM differs from "paternalistic" (provider-based) and "informed" (patient or family-based) decision-making because neither the provider nor the family bears independent responsibility for the decision; instead, all sides listen to input from each other and decide together which options to pursue.[4,5] **Box 1** lists some practical tips for engaging with families in SDM conversations. **Box 2** provides some example questions for eliciting family values. Pediatric palliative care teams often have experience with elicitation of family values and can be a resource for shared decision-making. Similarly, decision aids, which present neutral evidence about various treatment options in paper or electronic form, may help facilitate the SDM process.

Importance of SDM in Decisions About Introduction of Technology

Introduction of technology has a substantial impact on families, often influencing their daily routines, as well as the frequency and intensity of their interactions with the health care system.[6,7] Technology also may have implications that are harder to measure, as they potentially affect a child's social interactions and influence parents' perceptions of their efficacy as parents.[8] The evidence about the utility of these interventions is limited; there are no randomized controlled trials demonstrating clear efficacy in this population to guide decision-making. Therefore, for decisions about technology in this population, utilization of SDM, which formally incorporates inclusion of family values in the decisional process, helps enrich the conversation and ensure that the family and provider have confidence in the resulting decision. This article

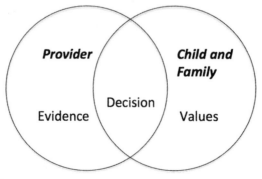

Fig. 1. SDM model.

> **Box 1**
> **Practical considerations for supporting parental decision-making**
>
> Be aware that these important decisions may require repeated discussions over time, and allow adequate time for families to absorb information between conversations. Consider a trial of shorter-term interventions (eg, nasogastric tube feeding) while more permanent options are under consideration.
>
> Explore family hopes and concerns, both around changes to daily life (eg, socialization, siblings) and influences on the big picture (eg, survival and prognosis).
>
> Understand family context, structure, external supports, and finances, as they may significantly impact the decision-making process, sometimes in nonexplicit ways. Offer opportunity for extended family (eg, grandparents) to be part of discussions.
>
> Engage and solicit opinions from health care providers the family trusts (eg, the primary care pediatrician) to help support decision-making.
>
> Provide opportunities for discussion with other parents in similar situations about their decisional processes and experiences with technology.

outlines potentially relevant evidence about the use of 2 technological devices in this population by using the process of SDM as a framework.

Role of the Hospitalist

Although many families and providers believe that a long-standing relationship is invaluable for goal-based conversations with families,[9] decisions to implement new technology may happen in the context of an acute hospitalization. When this situation occurs, the responsibility for guiding the decision-making process falls to the pediatric hospitalist. Although the hospitalist may not have a long history with the family, the use of a shared decision-making model can lead to important and meaningful conversations.

GASTROSTOMY
Case 1

Sara is an 18-month-old girl with spastic quadriplegic cerebral palsy who was admitted to the pediatrics ward with her third episode of pneumonia this winter, thought possibly related to aspiration, as she frequently chokes with feeding.

Available Options

For children who are unable to take adequate nutrition by mouth safely, several options exist for providing enteral feeds directly into the gastrointestinal (GI) system. Nasal tubes extending into the stomach (nasogastric), duodenum (nasoduodenal), or jejunum (nasojejunal) are frequently used for short-term (up to 8 weeks) feeding,[10]

> **Box 2**
> **Example questions for elicitation of values**
>
> What activities does your child particularly enjoy?
>
> Is your child currently feeling well? If not, what symptoms are most bothersome to him or her?
>
> When you think about your child's health in the future, what are you most hopeful for?
>
> When you think about your child's health in the future, what worries you the most?

and are occasionally used longer.[11] Gastrostomy tube placement, which can be performed either surgically or percutaneously with endoscopic or radiographic visualization, involves creation of a permanent tract and installation of a tube through the abdominal wall into the stomach.[12] If access to the jejunum is required, a gastrojejunostomy can be performed, which involves passing a longer tube from the gastrostomy opening through the pylorus and into the jejunum.[13] Surgical or percutaneous jejunostomy, with direct passage of a tube through the abdominal wall into the jejunum, is another, less commonly used option.[10] In general, the choice about which part of the GI tract is used (stomach, duodenum, or jejunum) depends on the child's feeding tolerance and need for tube permanency. The stomach is typically the preferred target unless reflux or stomach content aspiration risk (eg, when combined with noninvasive ventilation) precludes its use.[14] As surgical jejunostomy is uncommon and gastrostomy is often trialed before transition to gastrojejunostomy, this review focuses primarily on gastrostomy tube placement. Depending on clinical context, the continuation of oral feeding, even if clinically suboptimal because of poor nutrition or aspiration, also may be an option. **Table 1** outlines the evidence, including quality of life and ethical considerations, for each feeding option.

Evidence: Clinical Benefits

The benefit of gastrostomy tube feeding on nutritional status in patients with cerebral palsy has been established by multiple observational studies[15–17] and is acknowledged in 2 clinical guidelines.[18,19] The relationship between oromotor dysfunction and poor nutritional status in children with severe neurologic impairment is posited to be from a combination of inability to signal satiety combined with the prolonged meal times required for intake, together leading to unintentional underfeeding.[18] Transition to enteral feeding reduces meal times[20,21] and makes provision of appropriate nutrition easier.[22]

Decreased aspiration of oral feeds, although a common goal of gastrostomy tube feeding, is more difficult to study. Aspiration into the lungs can occur from feeds taken orally, but also from feeds refluxed from the stomach to the oropharynx.[23] Gastrostomy tube feeding is associated with decreased choking episodes during feeding,[20] but it also is associated with increased rates of gastroesophageal reflux.[20,24,25] An important clinical sequelae of aspiration is aspiration pneumonia,[11] which is a substantial cause of morbidity and mortality in this population.[26,27] The impact of gastrostomy tube placement on aspiration pneumonia is unclear; one observational study demonstrated decreased admissions for respiratory illnesses[28] and another reported decreased chest infection frequency after gastrostomy tube feeding.[20] Two studies also have demonstrated an association between the presence of a gastrostomy tube and increased mortality,[29,30] which is thought potentially to be related to increased risk of aspiration. However, because substantial methodological challenges are associated with these studies (including confounding by indication), and subsequent studies demonstrate a broad range of outcomes, the actual impact of gastrostomy tube feeding on respiratory morbidity and mortality is not clear.[31,32]

Clinical benefits associated with nasogastric tube feeding are similar to those for gastrostomy tube feeding. In the context of oromotor dysfunction, there are no specific clinical benefits associated with continued oral feeding, except the absence of potential complications associated with nonoral feeding methods.

Evidence: Clinical Challenges

Clinical challenges associated with initiation of gastrostomy tube feeds include increased gastroesophageal reflux and potential association with increased mortality,

Table 1
Evidence associated with various feeding methods

	Oral	Nasogastric Tube	Gastrostomy Tube
Clinical benefits	Absence of potential complications associated with other methods	Presumed similar to gastrostomy tube, but minimal data specific to nasogastric tube delivery	Improved nutrition (shorter mealtimes, easier feeding) Decreased aspiration from above (unclear effect on aspiration pneumonia) Improved comfort, alertness, and mood
Clinical risks	Risk of aspiration of feeds Potential for suboptimal nutrition	Tube misplacement Tube dislodgement Nasal ulceration from long-term use	Procedural complications including peritonitis, abscess, septicemia, death Ongoing potential complications, including site infection, tube migration/ dislodgement, stomal leakage, site infection, tube blockage Potential increase in reflux symptoms
Quality-of-life considerations	Important sensory experience Mealtime struggles to maintain adequate nutrition "Normal" life skill	No specific data	Improved caregiver quality of life Decreased caregiver stress Challenges obtaining respite care Stigma Sense of "failure" at important parental task of oral feeding Increased family costs
Ethical considerations	No specific data	No specific data	Potential tradeoffs in type of discomfort (choking vs reflux symptoms) Potential future prolongation of life in state with very poor quality

Data from Refs.[11,12,14,17–22,31,34,36,38–41,52–54]

as described previously, as well as complications related to the procedure and problems related to the tube itself. Specific procedural complications are related to the method of tube placement (surgical, endoscopic, or image-guided) and whether or not general anesthesia is required. Patient characteristics (eg, anatomy)[12] and institutional preference may impact the methodology chosen.[11] In a retrospective cohort study of image-guided gastrostomy tube placement, 5% of patients had major complications, including peritonitis (3%), subcutaneous abscess (2%), septicemia (1%), GI bleed (0.4%), and death (0.4%).[12]

Important possible ongoing complications related to a gastrostomy tube include tube migration, site infection, leakage from the stoma, development of granulation tissue around the stoma, tube blockage, and dislodgement.[14] Most patients with long-term use of a gastrostomy tube will likely encounter one or more of these complications; one prospective study of 74 children found that 82% had at least one minor complication during the 6-month follow-up period.[16] Many of these issues exist on a continuum from mild types amenable to home interventions (eg, use of cola to unclog blockage) to more serious issues requiring hospital-level evaluation and care (eg, tube dislodgement before mature development of the tract).[14]

Challenges related to nasogastric tube use include risk of tube misplacement (eg, accidental insertion into the lung), easy tube dislodgement, and nasal ulceration from long-term use.[11,12] Challenges related to continued oral feeding with oromotor dysfunction include risk of aspiration and suboptimal nutrition.

Values: Quality-of-Life Considerations

One study evaluating parental-reported quality of life (QOL) in children with neurologic impairment before and after gastrostomy tube placement did not demonstrate improvement in child QOL as assessed before and 1 year after.[17] However, another study found that the QOL of caregivers did improve following tube placement.[21] Parents also describe decreased levels of stress[20,22] and decreased worries about their child's nutritional state.[21]

In qualitative studies, parents report that gastrostomy tube placement has both positive and negative impacts on their home life.[33] Many families described challenges obtaining home and respite care because of the technical skill required to give gastrostomy tube feeds,[34] and this issue was sometimes associated with decreased parental employment.[35] Some parents also commented on increased financial burdens associated with gastrostomy tube feeds.[20,33,36] Another common theme involved changes in socialization: parents often felt stigmatized when feeding in public, perceiving that strangers were staring and judging and felt less able to go on outings because of equipment needed for feeding or discomfort feeding in public.[34,37] Finally, many parents discussed the symbolic importance of permanent gastrostomy tube feeding, framing the impact of stopping of oral feeding both in terms of their child's experience of the world and in creating a sense of failure about their inability to carry out an important task of parenthood.[36,38]

We were unable to identify studies explicitly exploring the impact of nasogastric feeding, typically a short-term intervention, on family life of children with neurologic impairment. However, the importance and meaning of oral feeding were discussed extensively in the qualitative interviews as the reference point for many families. When attempting to meet nutritional goals with oral feeds in the context of oromotor dysfunction, families often used negative language, describing feeding as "torture" or "a battle."[39] However, other parents described the value of oral feedings as representing a "normal" life skill[38,40] and as an important enjoyable sensory experience for their child.[41]

Values: Ethical Considerations

Gastrostomy tube placement represents a life-sustaining technology, and conversations about it invite consideration of big-picture goals, especially when the child's medical condition is progressive rather than static. For example, if the primary goal of gastrostomy tube placement is to maximize comfort by decreasing choking, parents may benefit from hearing that gastrostomy tubes can worsen reflux, leading to a different kind of discomfort. Also, for children with progressive underlying diagnoses, provision of artificial nutrition might in the future prolong life in a state with very poor quality. Some families may not want to potentially face a decision about forgoing artificial nutrition, and may appreciate knowing the possible impact of gastrostomy tube on end-of-life decisions before they make the decision to place one. Families struggling with the decision about gastrostomy tube feeding might benefit from the support of a pediatric palliative care team.

TRACHEOTOMY
Case 2

Jay is a 5-year-old boy with severe neurologic impairment from an unidentified source. He has intractable aspiration and has spent most of the past 6 months in hospital with respiratory infections, often requiring intubation. His father asks if a permanent breathing tube might help.

Available Options

Tracheotomy, a procedure used to create a conduit from the neck directly into the trachea allowing ventilation, can be performed to bypass an upper airway obstruction (fixed or mechanical, acquired or congenital) or to facilitate safer long-term ventilation.[42,43] In one series, tracheotomy was performed in children with neurologic impairment (12% of cohort) for airway hypotonia, recurrent pneumonia, and sleep apnea.[44] Noninvasive ventilation is a potential alternative strategy when the reason for tracheotomy is a mechanical obstruction (hypotonia, sleep apnea), recurrent apneas, or respiratory muscle weakness.[45] Aggressive symptom management without ventilation is another potential option.

Evidence: Clinical Benefits

Tracheotomy placement in children with neurologic impairment is difficult to study systematically, given the varying reasons for its use and the heterogeneity of underlying diagnoses associated with neurologic impairment. In general, a tracheotomy is performed as a last resort, when it has the potential to mitigate a specific serious problem and the family and team agree that it aligns with the goals of care. Tracheotomy may prolong a child's life; however, the potential risks must carefully be considered.

Evidence: Clinical Challenges

Clinical challenges associated with tracheotomy include procedural complications, which are outlined in **Box 3**. The rate of complication associated with tracheotomy markedly varies in different studies, ranging from 22% to 77% in one literature review.[46] Children with neurologic impairment seem to have higher mortality rates and lower rates of decannulation than children with other diagnoses: in a series of 204 children (27.5% with neurologic impairment), children with neurologic impairment had higher mortality rates (27% vs 19%) and were less likely to successfully decannulate (12.5% vs 41%) than the cohort as a whole.[47] Whether or not mechanical ventilator support through the tracheotomy is required also contributes to the severity of potential outcomes; children who are ventilator-dependent may be more fragile.

Careful tracheotomy maintenance is necessary to reduce the risk of complications and mortality. Children with tracheotomies require close supervision by a caregiver trained in tracheotomy care, as emergent situations can develop within very short periods of time and require immediate response.[48] Home care and maintenance of

Box 3
Complications after tracheotomy

Bleeding (intraoperative, early, late)

   Excessive intraoperative bleeding

   Early postoperative hemorrhage

   Late arterial erosion with hemorrhage

Loss of airway/ability to ventilate (intraoperative, early, late)

   Intraoperative inability to ventilate

   Decannulation before first tube change

   Accidental decannulation

   Inability to recannulate

   Tube occlusion

   Tube disconnection/ventilator failure

   Tube leak causing ventilator failure

   Respiratory arrest

Interstitial air (intraoperative, early, late)

   Pneumothorax

   Pneumomediastinum

Infection (early, late)

   Aspiration pneumonia

   Tracheitis

Stomal issues (early, late)

   Skin erosion

   Stomal breakdown

   Stomal bleeding

   Stomal infection

   Stomal granulation tissue

   Stomal keloid formation

Tracheal problems (late)

   Tracheomalacia

   Tracheocutaneous fistula

   Tracheal/subglottal stenosis

Other

   Esophageal injury (intraoperative)

   False passage creation (intraoperative, early, late)

   Death (intraoperative, early, late)

Data from Refs.[42,46,48,55–57]

the tube generally include air humidification to decrease mucous plugging,[48] routine tube changes,[49] and suctioning of secretions,[48] among other tasks.

Given the range and complexity of possible clinical challenges associated with tracheotomy, pediatric hospitalists may wish to involve more specialized teams with experience in tracheotomy (eg, otolaryngology, intensivists, respiratory medicine, palliative care) to provide additional information and support to families.

Values: QOL Considerations

Tracheostomy tube placement for children with neurologic impairment has a tremendous impact on families, affecting caregiving demands, financial burdens, socialization, and stress levels.[50] Many studies focus predominantly on children receiving home mechanical ventilator support, which has possibly more intense implications for daily life than tracheotomy alone. Qualitative studies suggest that families struggle with a sometimes "overwhelming" sense of responsibility for providing care,[51] as well as resentment by healthy siblings who receive less parental attention.[50] Financial concerns and social isolation are common, and are another source of stress.[50] Families worry about the constant risk of their child's unexpected death from sudden-onset complications, such as unwitnessed ventilator detachment.[50] However, despite many challenges, families find meaning and value in their children's lives.[50]

Values: Ethical Considerations

The ethics of tracheostomy tube placement for children with neurologic impairment are often complex and case-specific, and full discussion of potential issues is outside the scope of this review. However, the implications of tracheotomy on future end-of-life decisions are particularly relevant in this population because of the higher mortality rate and lower rate of successful decannulation, which mean that many children with neurologic impairment will die with their tracheostomy tubes in place. As such, it is critical for families and teams to carefully consider how a tracheostomy tube may impact the child's prognosis, including both the potential of acute mortality from tube-related complications and the risk of prolongation of life with very poor quality.

SUMMARY

SDM is a helpful communication model to engage families in the process of decision-making when the best clinical option is not clear. In SDM, the clinician explores the family's values relating to a decision, uses those values to frame the evidence about available options, and collaborates with the family to determine which option is the best fit for their child. Given the broad-reaching implications of these decisions, the SDM model is helpful to clinicians when discussing utilization of life-sustaining technology with families of children with severe neurologic impairment.

REFERENCES

1. Bauchner H. Shared decision making in pediatrics. Arch Dis Child 2001;84:246.
2. Towle A, Godolphin W. Framework for teaching and learning informed shared decision making. BMJ 1999;319(7212):766–71.
3. Godolphin W. Shared decision-making. Healthc Q 2009;12:e186–90.
4. Charles C, Whelan T, Gafni A. What do we mean by partnership in making decisions about treatment? BMJ 1999;319(7212):780–2.
5. Fiks AG, Jimenez ME. The promise of shared decision-making in paediatrics. Acta Paediatr 2010;99:1464–6.

6. Arras JD, Dubler NN. Bringing the hospital home: ethical and social implications of high-tech home care. Hastings Cent Rep 1994;24:S19.

7. Toly V, Musil C, Carl J. Families with children who are technology dependent: normalization and family functioning. West J Nurs Res 2012;34:52–71.

8. O'Brien M, Wegner C. Rearing the child who is technology dependent: perceptions of parents and home care nurses. J Spec Pediatr Nurs 2002;7:7–15.

9. Johnston SC, Pfeifer MP, McNutt R. The discussion about advance directives. Patient and physician opinions regarding when and how it should be conducted. End of Life Study Group. Arch Intern Med 1995;155:1025–30.

10. Nijs E, Cahill A. Pediatric enteric feeding techniques: insertion, maintenance, and management of problems. Cardiovasc Intervent Radiol 2010;33:1101–10.

11. Soscia J, Mahant S. Nutrition support in children with neurologic disabilities. Curr Pediatr Rev 2012;8:103–13.

12. Friedman JN, Ahmed S, Connolly B, et al. Complications associated with image-guided gastrostomy and gastrojejunostomy tubes in children. Pediatrics 2004; 114:458–61.

13. Albanese CT, Towbin RB, Ulman I, et al. Percutaneous gastrojejunostomy versus Nissen fundoplication for enteral feeding of the neurologically impaired child with gastroesophageal reflux. J Pediatr 1993;123:371–5.

14. Soscia J, Friedman JN. A guide to the management of common gastrostomy and gastrojejunostomy tube problems. Paediatr Child Health 2011; 16:281–7.

15. Sullivan P, Juszczak E, Bachlet A, et al. Gastrostomy tube feeding in children with cerebral palsy: a prospective, longitudinal study. Dev Med Child Neurol 2005;47:77–85.

16. Craig GM, Carr LJ, Cass H, et al. Medical, surgical, and health outcomes of gastrostomy feeding. Dev Med Child Neurol 2006;48:353–60.

17. Mahant S, Friedman JN, Connolly B, et al. Tube feeding and quality of life in children with severe neurological impairment. Arch Dis Child 2009;94:668–73.

18. Canadian Paediatric Society. Nutrition in neurologically impaired children. Paediatr Child Health 2009;14:395–401.

19. Marchand V, Motil KJ, NASPGHAN Committee on Nutrition. Nutrition support for neurologically impaired children: a clinical report of the North American Society for Pediatric Gastroenterology, Hepatology, and Nutrition. J Pediatr Gastroenterol Nutr 2006;43:123–35.

20. Heine RG, Reddihough DS, Catto Smith AG. Gastro-oesophageal reflux and feeding problems after gastrostomy in children with severe neurological impairment. Dev Med Child Neurol 1995;37:320–9.

21. Sullivan P, Juszczak E, Bachlet A, et al. Impact of gastrostomy tube feeding on the quality of life of carers of children with cerebral palsy. Dev Med Child Neurol 2004;46:796–800.

22. Smith S, Camfield C, Camfield P. Living with cerebral palsy and tube feeding: a population-based follow-up study. J Pediatr 1999;135:307–10.

23. Morton RE, Wheatley R, Minford J. Respiratory tract infections due to direct and reflux aspiration in children with severe neurodisability. Dev Med Child Neurol 1999;41:329–34.

24. Srivastava R, Jackson WD, Barnhart DC. Dysphagia and gastroesophageal reflux disease: dilemmas in diagnosis and management in children with neurological impairment. Pediatr Ann 2010;39:225–31.

25. Thomson M. Percutaneous endoscopic gastrostomy and gastro-oesophageal reflux in neurologically impaired children. World J Gastroenterol 2011;17:191–6.

26. Trinick R, Johnston N, Dalzell AM, et al. Reflux aspiration in children with neuro-disability—a significant problem, but can we measure it? J Pediatr Surg 2012; 47:291–8.
27. Maudsley G, Hutton JL, Pharoah PO. Cause of death in cerebral palsy: a descriptive study. Arch Dis Child 1999;81:390–4.
28. Sullivan PB, Morrice JS, Vernon-Roberts A, et al. Does gastrostomy tube feeding in children with cerebral palsy increase the risk of respiratory morbidity? Arch Dis Child 2006;91:478–82.
29. Strauss D, Kastner T, Ashwal S, et al. Tube feeding and mortality in children with severe disabilities and mental retardation. Pediatrics 1997;99:358–62.
30. Eyman RK, Grossman HJ, Chaney RH, et al. The life expectancy of pro-foundly handicapped people with mental retardation. N Engl J Med 1990; 323:584–9.
31. Ferluga ED, Sathe NA, Krishnaswami S, et al. Surgical intervention for feeding and nutrition difficulties in cerebral palsy: a systematic review. Dev Med Child Neurol 2014;56:31–43.
32. Plioplys AV, Kasnicka I, Lewis S, et al. Survival rates among children with severe neurologic disabilities. South Med J 1998;91:161–72.
33. Mahant S, Pastor AC, Deoliveira L, et al. Well-being of children with neurologic impairment after fundoplication and gastrojejunostomy tube feeding. Pediatrics 2011;128:e395–403.
34. Brotherton A, Abbott J, Aggett P. The impact of percutaneous endoscopic gas-trostomy feeding in children; the parental perspective. Child Care Health Dev 2007;33:539–46.
35. Townsend JL, Craig G, Lawson M, et al. Cost-effectiveness of gastrostomy placement for children with neurodevelopmental disability. Arch Dis Child 2008;93:873–7.
36. Craig GM. Psychosocial aspects of feeding children with neurodisability. Eur J Clin Nutr 2013;67(Suppl 2):S17–20.
37. Craig GM, Scambler G. Negotiating mothering against the odds: gastrostomy tube feeding, stigma, governmentality and disabled children. Soc Sci Med 2006;62:1115–25.
38. Petersen M, Kedia S, Davis P, et al. Eating and feeding are not the same: care-givers' perceptions of gastrostomy feeding for children with cerebral palsy. Dev Med Child Neurol 2006;48:713–7.
39. Craig G, Scambler G, Spitz L. Why parents of children with neurodevelopmental disabilities requiring gastrostomy feeding need more support. Dev Med Child Neurol 2003;45:183–8.
40. Thorne SE, Radford MJ, McCormick J. The multiple meanings of long-term gastrostomy in children with severe disability. J Pediatr Nurs 1997;12:89–99.
41. Morrow AM, Quine S, Loughlin EV, et al. Different priorities: a comparison of parents' and health professionals' perceptions of quality of life in quadriplegic cerebral palsy. Arch Dis Child 2008;93:119–25.
42. Mahadevan M, Barber C, Salkeld L, et al. Pediatric tracheotomy: 17 year review. Int J Pediatr Otorhinolaryngol 2007;71:1829–35.
43. Trachsel D, Hammer J. Indications for tracheostomy in children. Paediatr Respir Rev 2006;7:162–8.
44. Lawrason A, Kavanagh K. Pediatric tracheotomy: are the indications changing? Int J Pediatr Otorhinolaryngol 2013;77:922–5.
45. Seddon PC, Khan Y. Respiratory problems in children with neurological impair-ment. Arch Dis Child 2003;88:75–8.

46. Carr MM, Poje CP, Kingston L, et al. Complications in pediatric tracheostomies. Laryngoscope 2001;111(11 Pt 1):1925–8.
47. Carron JD, Derkay CS, Strope GL, et al. Pediatric tracheotomies: changing indications and outcomes. Laryngoscope 2000;110:1099–104.
48. Fiske E. Effective strategies to prepare infants and families for home tracheostomy care. Adv Neonatal Care 2004;4:42–53.
49. Gallagher TQ, Hartnick CJ. Pediatric tracheotomy. Adv Otorhinolaryngol 2012; 73:26–30.
50. Carnevale FA, Alexander E, Davis M, et al. Daily living with distress and enrichment: the moral experience of families with ventilator-assisted children at home. Pediatrics 2006;117:e48–60.
51. Flynn AP, Carter B, Bray L, et al. Parents' experiences and views of caring for a child with a tracheostomy: a literature review. Int J Pediatr Otorhinolaryngol 2013;77:1630–4.
52. Morrow A, Quine S, Craig J. Health professionals' perceptions of feeding-related quality of life in children with quadriplegic cerebral palsy. Child Care Health Dev 2007;33:529–38.
53. Rouse L, Herrington P, Assey J, et al. Feeding problems, gastrostomy and families: a qualitative pilot study. Br J Learn Disabil 2002;30:122–8.
54. Mahant S, Jovcevska V, Cohen E. Decision-making around gastrostomy-feeding in children with neurologic disabilities. Pediatrics 2011;127:e1471–81.
55. Deutsch ES. Tracheostomy: pediatric considerations. Respir Care 2010;55: 1082–90.
56. Özmen S, Özmen ÖA, Ünal ÖF. Pediatric tracheotomies: a 37-year experience in 282 children. Int J Pediatr Otorhinolaryngol 2009;73:959–61.
57. French LC, Wootten CT, Thomas RG, et al. Tracheotomy in the preschool population: indications and outcomes. Otolaryngol Head Neck Surg 2007;137: 280–3.

Pediatric Hospital Medicine Role in the Comanagement of the Hospitalized Surgical Patient

Joshua K. Schaffzin, MD, PhD[a],*, Tamara D. Simon, MD, MSPH[b]

KEYWORDS

- Pediatric • Hospitalist • Surgery • Comanagement • Pediatric hospital medicine
- Consultant • Service

KEY POINTS

- Surgical comanagement is one of several specialized niches emerging in pediatric hospital medicine.
- In a comanagement model, pediatric hospitalists and surgeons share responsibility and accountability for patient management and outcomes.
- Particular considerations are required in the establishment of surgical comanagement programs.
- Surgical hospitalists are poised to make contributions in the areas of clinical care, practice management, quality, education, and research.

INTRODUCTION

In the past decade, pediatric hospital medicine (PHM) has grown dramatically in breadth and in numbers. Simultaneously, as pediatric care has advanced, children who would not have survived infancy are growing into young adults with complex chronic diseases and are frequently hospitalized to address exacerbation of underlying disease processes and procedures to improve their quality of life. This article focuses on issues that arise in the comanagement of medically complex patients preoperatively and postoperatively with surgical colleagues.

Funding: NIH, K23NS062900; ULI RR025014.
[a] Division of Hospital Medicine, Cincinnati Children's Hospital Medical Center, 3333 Burnet Avenue, MLC 9016, Cincinnati, OH 45229-3033, USA; [b] Division of Hospital Medicine, Department of Pediatrics, Seattle Children's Hospital, University of Washington, Room 946, MS JMB-9, 1900 Ninth Avenue, Seattle, WA 98101, USA
* Corresponding author.
E-mail address: Joshua.schaffzin@cchmc.org

Pediatr Clin N Am 61 (2014) 653–661
http://dx.doi.org/10.1016/j.pcl.2014.04.002
0031-3955/14/$ – see front matter © 2014 Elsevier Inc. All rights reserved.

In recent years, the comanagement of surgical patients has become prevalent among PHM programs, likely due to several factors. First, hospital medicine is becoming accepted as a subspecialty of pediatrics, and comanagement is one of several specialized niches in the practice of PHM. Second, hospitalized children are more complex medically.[1,2] As pediatrics has become more specialized, so too have surgical specialties, such that training does not include as in-depth pediatric patient management as it may once have. Finally, comanagement in PHM is a natural evolution of comanagement in adult hospital medicine settings, which is a widespread practice model.

This relatively new role for PHM providers is an ideal fit within existing hospitalist practice models. PHM providers are typically involved directly in hospital safety and systems integration. They provide value to institutions in patient care coordination, excelling in the management of medically complex patients. These patients typically have multiple subspecialists involved in their care, as well as a battery of hospital-based ancillary staff. PHM providers communicate well with families, nurses, and surgical and medical providers, integrating all of the input into patient management plans that focus on the needs of the patient and family. In addition, in hospitals where sentinel events have occurred among surgical patients, PHM providers and comanagement have been identified as the solution.

As a relatively recent addition to the PHM provider repertoire, surgical comanagement suffers from a paucity of literature describing its benefits and limits. In this review, a summary of both the authors' experiences and published data are provided to outline the current state of surgical comanagement and to create a framework for presenting challenges and issues within the field.

WHAT IS COMANAGEMENT AND WHY IS IT INCREASINGLY COMMON?

Traditional models of medical care for surgical patients involve consultation of medical providers if and when a need arises. Although this model may work in some situations, it is not optimal, because it can lead to missed diagnoses and poor quality care.[3] In essence, by waiting for something to happen, an opportunity may have been missed to prevent patient harm. The solution to this issue is to bring medical providers into the care team early in the process, before any harm occurs. For example, in a child with a seizure disorder, it would be better for a medical provider to manage antiepileptic medications to prevent a seizure rather than consult someone after a seizure has occurred. The model that has emerged to provide medical care for surgical patients is one of comanagement between surgical and PHM providers.

According to the Society of Hospital Medicine (SHM), surgical comanagement is the "shared responsibility, authority, and accountability for the care of a hospitalized patient...[where] the patient's surgeon manages the surgery related treatments and a hospitalist manages the patient's medical conditions."[4] In theory, comanaging pediatricians promote valuable assets to institutions. These assets may include safety, by anticipating complications and preventing poor patient outcomes, availability for families and nurses by being present on the medical units, and resource allocation by allowing surgical colleagues to spend more time operating than managing admitted patients.[5–7]

In reality, the benefit provided by pediatric hospitalist comanagement likely differs between targeted populations and routine use.[5,6] Among pediatric patients receiving comanagement before and following surgery for neuromuscular scoliosis, length of stay was decreased in one study and unchanged in another.[8,9] Among adult populations receiving comanagement before and following knee or hip replacement surgery, results also varied, with some studies showing decreased length of stay, complication rates, and mortality among comanaged patients, but others showing no such benefit.[7,10–15] One study reported a subjective benefit to hospitalist comanagement of surgical patients, where nurses and surgeons both reported preferring the comanagement model for its delivery of prompt coordinated care.[7] However, the same study failed to show a decrease in cost or mortality for co-managed patients. Finally, there is no evidence that surgeons' time in the operating room increased in the context of comanagement.[5]

CURRENT STATE OF COMANAGEMENT IN PHM

According to a recent informal survey of PHM providers conducted on the American Academy of Pediatrics Section on Hospital Medicine Listserve©, surgical comanagement represents a portion and not the whole of time spent in care of hospitalized patients (J. Schaffzin, unpublished data, 2013). Approximately one-third of respondents reported spending between 20% and 39%, and nearly half reported spending less than 20% of their clinical time in postoperative care (**Fig. 1**). PHM providers who care for surgical patients do so mostly through consultation, with 92% of respondents reporting working in a consultative model, whereas 65% reported working in a comanagement model (**Fig. 2**). In addition, PHM providers do not work alone in providing medical care to surgical patients. At free-standing hospitals and hospitals-within-hospitals, PHM providers most often collaborate with surgical residents and midlevel providers (eg, nurse practitioners) in addition to the attending surgeons, to provide care to surgical patients.

ESTABLISHING A SURGICAL COMANAGEMENT PROGRAM

Although comanagement models provide what is thought to be quality medical care to surgical patients, comanagement may not be appropriate in all clinical settings. PHM providers may think they mediate well between different providers, but it is possible that in the instance of disagreement between medical and surgical providers, the family is left in the middle. In addition, when attending physicians take over care and work directly with each other, there is a potential for education of residents, particularly surgical residents, to suffer.[5] It may be detrimental to withhold the experience of

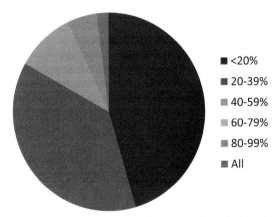

Fig. 1. Proportion of time spent in postoperative care of surgical patients by responding pediatric hospitalists. Number of respondents, 61. (*Data from* Informal SOHM survey, J. Schaffzin, unpublished data, 2013.)

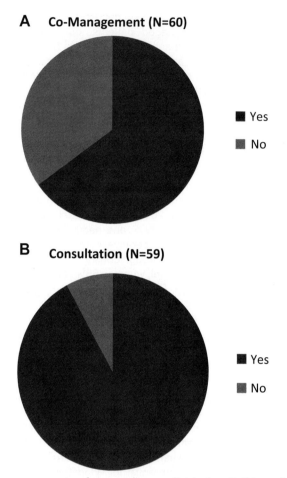

Fig. 2. Practice arrangements of responding pediatric hospitalists caring for surgical patients. (*A*) Proportion practicing in a comanagement model. (*B*) Proportion practicing in a consultative model. Number of respondents is noted for each arrangement, and responses are not mutually exclusive. (*Data from* Informal SOHM survey, J. Schaffzin, unpublished data, 2013.)

providing basic medical care to postoperative pediatric patients to future surgery attendings, because comanagement models may not be available in their future practices. On the other hand, exposure to hospitalists may enhance surgical residents' learning, given the prominent role hospitalists play in resident education.[16]

The American Medical Association, SHM, and the literature provide guidance for aspects desirable to include in comanagement models.[5,8,17,18] There are 5 aspects to consider. The first is equity, whereby all stakeholders have a similar investment in and accountability for patient outcomes, and all share the responsibility of patient management. Second, each stakeholder has clearly defined and mutually agreed-on roles, ideally in the form of a comanagement agreement (**Table 1**). Third, an equal exchange of information, education, and ideas among all providers is critical. Fourth, adequate staffing of PHM providers is necessary to ensure adequate coverage is provided for the patient volume seen. Finally, constant and open communication is required to develop and maintain the relationship between comanaging providers.

Table 1 Basic components of a comanagement agreement	
Component	**Example Questions**
Patient selection	Which patients are eligible for comanagement? How will they be selected?
Attending of record	Who will serve as attending of record? Who as consultant?
Nursing first call	Whom should bedside staff call with what concerns?
Communication with patients and families	How will a unified message be conveyed to patients and families? How will disagreements in management be addressed?
Communication between providers	How frequent should communication happen? How should one provider contact another?
Admission and discharge procedures	Who is responsible for medication reconciliation? For discharge planning? For transition of care to primary provider?
Financial and billing considerations	How will comanaged cases be billed?

Data from Society of Hospital Medicine. A white paper on a guide to hospitalist/orthopedic surgery co-management. Available at: http://www.hospitalmedicine.org/AM/Template.cfm?Section=White_Papers&Template=/CM/ContentDisplay.cfm&ContentID=25864. Accessed May 12, 2014.

To establish a viable comanagement program, an initial investment is required.[8] The number of full-time equivalent positions and a schedule framework (eg, shifts, day vs night in-house coverage) must be determined. Consideration must be given to the skill set and level of experience needed for physician providers. Many pediatric hospitalists have engaged in surgical comanagement, but new residency graduates are unlikely to have been exposed to care of surgical patients outside of an intensive care unit. Midlevel providers are becoming a more permanent fixture of PHM programs as well as surgical programs. An advantage to including midlevel providers in comanagement models is the ability to have engaged, present providers who coordinate care and give continuity to care. However, midlevels may provide most benefit when the patient populations and postoperative course are mostly homogeneous, with a potential opportunity to target physician involvement to the more complex patients. In addition, optimizing care of surgical patients may start in the preoperative period, and some programs have explored the extension of hospitalist comanagement to the preoperative time period.[8,9]

The context of practice must also be considered. The surgical services in need of medical support should be identified, and a case made to these services of the value comanagement can bring to care of their patients. An institution must be engaged and supportive to provide overhead and infrastructure to a comanagement program. Protected time is needed for administrative activities, such as committee service and administering the comanagement arrangements. In addition, education is essential, and time must be set aside to train experienced providers as well as trainees and new graduates. There are likely to be significant knowledge gaps in the care of surgical patients at all levels of experience. If teaching is an expected part of the job, expectations of teaching activities and time to perform teaching must also be provided.

CURRENT CHALLENGES AND ISSUES FOR SURGICAL COMANAGEMENT IN PHM
Clinical Practice/Practice Management

From a clinical perspective, surgical comanagement must be recognized as within the scope of general pediatric hospital practice. A recent American Academy of Pediatrics statement recognizes "perioperative surgical and medical subspecialty care" as one of the guiding principles for a PHM program.[19] However, billing and payment for services are not yet straightforward for comanagement models and are greatly influenced by local factors. Possibilities for payment for comanagement services include having the time of comanaging PHM providers being covered by institutions.[20] Alternatively, comanaging providers may bill for their time as consultants, provided there is a specific question or issue to be addressed. Routine postoperative conditions, such as constipation and pain, for which PHM providers are often responsible, are covered by the global billing fee that the surgical services collect. Thus, billing for such services is less likely to be reimbursed. PHM providers may seek to take advantage of this situation when developing comanagement agreements by allocating a portion of the global billing fee to support of the comanagement program.

Following initial establishment of a comanagement service, sustainability of the surgical comanagement role is critical. To sustain this practice, PHM providers providing care to surgical patients must develop a professional pride in their role. It is important to avoid a situation in which PHM providers may feel as though they work for the surgeons, rather than for the patient and family. Interpersonal engagement is also crucial to sustain a surgical comanagement program. Medical providers must learn to work with surgical colleagues to avoid personality conflicts. Differences in training and experience, as well as potentially underlying personality types, exist between surgeons and pediatricians, and at times approaches and personalities can clash. Finally, comanaging partners must remain acutely aware of the value of comanagement over traditional models. Traditional models of care, where medical providers are consulted after a problem is identified, are not ideal, and both surgical and PHM providers must stay vigilant to avoid reverting to such situations.

Quality

Quality care is difficult to measure, but is essential to the sustainability of surgical comanagement. PHM and surgical providers need to work to optimize postoperative outcomes, manage available personnel resources, and reduce costs to the patient and to the hospital. Surgical care lends itself to standardization, given a frequently predictable postoperative course and the need to prevent complications. One recent example of a successful quality initiative focused on efforts to recognize compartment syndrome.[21] Other areas ripe for standardization of postoperative management are those where evidence suggests best practice but implementation is variable. These areas include but are not limited to reduction of wound infection,[22,23] antibiotic stewardship,[24] deep venous thrombosis prevention,[25] pain management,[26] and lung recruitment.[27]

In addition, PHM providers, particularly those who care for surgical patients, have an opportunity to play a significant role as the Affordable Care Act is implemented. In the new Affordable Care Act model, payment is linked to patient outcomes, and institutions will be challenged to use resources judiciously for surgical patients. PHM providers can help by standardizing the processes, shortening length of stay, decreasing costs, and preventing readmission of the most complex patients.

Education

Sustainability will also rely on educating future PHM providers capable of comanaging surgical patients. Internal medicine trainees have reported training during residency of certain perioperative conditions to be lacking.[28] Although perioperative care is an important aspect of hospitalist care,[19] it does not necessarily generalize to all areas of pediatrics. Thus, it is unclear how to train whom during residency to use time and effort maximally. Currently, hospital medicine fellowships offer an opportunity for such training. Although not yet accredited by the Accreditation Council for Graduate Medical Education (ACGME), fellowships are becoming more common and stronger in the training in research and clinical management they provide.[29] The new model of specialty tracking during residency also provides an opportunity for trainees interested in hospital medicine to obtain subspecialized training, including perioperative care.[29] Finally, with the increased prevalence of children with complex chronic conditions,[1,2] there is greater need for specific training to care for these children. Perioperative management is an essential component of care of the complex child, because these children tend to have more technology than noncomplex children.[1] Training of surgical colleagues in the care of pediatric patients is also important in this new paradigm. PHM providers are potentially a source for surgical trainees to learn such care, as well to advocate for formalized training in surgical programs.

Research

Finally, perhaps the greatest challenge facing PHM providers who comanage surgical patients is the creation and execution of a research agenda. Once a clinical service is established, and providers trained, there arises a need to generate generalizable knowledge that goes beyond that individualized for a particular practice. As a result, there is also a need to share knowledge about specific practices and systems. To standardize practice, models of care and their outcomes need to be better understood.[30] This way, national benchmarks can be developed to guide optimal care for all patients.

Although some literature exists linking comanagement to outcomes, few studies were conducted in pediatrics and results have been variable. Carefully designed and analyzed studies of resource utilization (eg, length of stay and costs), safety (eg, serious safety events avoided), and patient and family-centered outcomes (eg, satisfaction, quality of life)[31] are needed. Furthermore, PHM providers are natural partners for the study of surgical procedures in children, to evaluate short-term and long-term outcomes, such as the epidemiology of neurosurgical shunt infections[32,33] and the use of fibrinolytics in spinal surgery.[34] Particularly important questions to ask are about the true long-term benefit of major surgeries, such as spinal fusion, for medically complex children, and identifying time points at which benefits outweigh the short-term risks.

SUMMARY

Surgical comanagement is one of several specialized niches emerging in PHM. This model of care seems superior to the more traditional consult model because in comanagement PHM and surgical providers share responsibility and accountability for patient management and outcomes. The establishment of such programs requires both financial and personnel investment. Once established, pediatric hospitalist programs providing care to surgical patients are poised to make contributions in the areas of quality, education, and research.

REFERENCES

1. Simon TD, Berry J, Feudtner C, et al. Children with complex chronic conditions in inpatient hospital settings in the United States. Pediatrics 2010;126(4):647–55.
2. Burns KH, Casey PH, Lyle RE, et al. Increasing prevalence of medically complex children in US hospitals. Pediatrics 2010;126(4):638–46.

3. Robie PW. The service and educational contributions of a general medicine consultation service. J Gen Intern Med 1986;1(4):225–7.

4. Society of Hospital Medicine. Hospitalist co-management with surgeons and specialists. Available at: http://www.hospitalmedicine.org/AM/Template.cfm?Section=Home&Template=/CM/HTMLDisplay.cfm&ContentID=25894. Accessed May 12, 2014.

5. Siegal EM. Just because you can, doesn't mean that you should: a call for the rational application of hospitalist comanagement. J Hosp Med 2008;3(5):398–402.

6. Whinney C, Michota F. Surgical comanagement: a natural evolution of hospitalist practice. J Hosp Med 2008;3(5):394–7.

7. Huddleston JM, Long KH, Naessens JM, et al. Medical and surgical comanagement after elective hip and knee arthroplasty: a randomized, controlled trial. Ann Intern Med 2004;141(1):28–38.

8. Rappaport DI, Adelizzi-Delany J, Rogers KJ, et al. Outcomes and costs associated with hospitalist comanagement of medically complex children undergoing spinal fusion surgery. Hosp Pediatr 2013;3(4):233–41.

9. Simon TD, Eilert R, Dickinson LM, et al. Pediatric hospitalist comanagement of spinal fusion surgery patients. J Hosp Med 2007;2(1):23–30.

10. Fisher AA, Davis MW, Rubenach SE, et al. Outcomes for older patients with hip fractures: the impact of orthopedic and geriatric medicine cocare. J Orthop Trauma 2006;20(3):172–8 [discussion: 179–80].

11. Macpherson DS, Parenti C, Nee J, et al. An internist joins the surgery service: does comanagement make a difference? J Gen Intern Med 1994;9(8):440–4.

12. Phy MP, Vanness DJ, Melton LJ 3rd, et al. Effects of a hospitalist model on elderly patients with hip fracture. Arch Intern Med 2005;165(7):796–801.

13. Zuckerman JD, Sakales SR, Fabian DR, et al. Hip fractures in geriatric patients. Results of an interdisciplinary hospital care program. Clin Orthop Relat Res 1992;(274):213–25.

14. Marcantonio ER, Flacker JM, Wright RJ, et al. Reducing delirium after hip fracture: a randomized trial. J Am Geriatr Soc 2001;49(5):516–22.

15. Southern WN, Berger MA, Bellin EY, et al. Hospitalist care and length of stay in patients requiring complex discharge planning and close clinical monitoring. Arch Intern Med 2007;167(17):1869–74.

16. Heydarian C, Maniscalco J. Pediatric hospitalists in medical education: current roles and future directions. Curr Probl Pediatr Adolesc Health Care 2012;42(5):120–6.

17. Society of Hospital Medicine. A white paper on a guide to hospitalist/orthopedic surgery co-management. Available at: http://www.hospitalmedicine.org/AM/Template.cfm?Section=Home&TEMPLATE=/CM/ContentDisplay.cfm&CONTENTID=25864. Accessed May 12, 2014.

18. American Medical Association. Ethical implications of surgical co-management. 1999. Report 5-I-99. Available at: http://www.ama-assn.org/ama/pub/physician-resources/medical-ethics/code-medical-ethics/opinion8043.page. Accessed May 12, 2014.

19. Section on Hospital Medicine. Guiding principles for pediatric hospital medicine programs. Pediatrics 2013;132(4):782–6.

20. Freed GL, Dunham KM, Switalski KE, Research Advisory Committee of the American Board of Pediatrics. Assessing the value of pediatric hospitalist programs: the perspective of hospital leaders. Acad Pediatr 2009;9(3):192–6.

21. Schaffzin JK, Prichard H, Bisig J, et al. A collaborative system to improve compartment syndrome recognition. Pediatrics 2013;132(6):e1672–9.

22. Glotzbecker MP, Riedel MD, Vitale MG, et al. What's the evidence? Systematic literature review of risk factors and preventive strategies for surgical site infection following pediatric spine surgery. J Pediatr Orthop 2013;33(5):479–87.

23. Vitale MG, Riedel MD, Glotzbecker MP, et al. Building consensus: development of a Best Practice Guideline (BPG) for surgical site infection (SSI) prevention in high-risk pediatric spine surgery. J Pediatr Orthop 2013;33(5):471–8.

24. McLeod LM, Keren R, Gerber J, et al. Perioperative antibiotic use for spinal surgery procedures in US children's hospitals. Spine 2013;38(7):609–16.

25. Raffini L, Trimarchi T, Beliveau J, et al. Thromboprophylaxis in a pediatric hospital: a patient-safety and quality-improvement initiative. Pediatrics 2011;127(5): e1326–32.

26. Greco C, Berde C. Pain management for the hospitalized pediatric patient. Pediatr Clin North Am 2005;52(4):995–1027, vii–viii.

27. Cassidy MR, Rosenkranz P, McCabe K, et al. I COUGH: reducing postoperative pulmonary complications with a multidisciplinary patient care program. JAMA Surg 2013;148(8):740–5.

28. Plauth WH 3rd, Pantilat SZ, Wachter RM, et al. Hospitalists' perceptions of their residency training needs: results of a national survey. Am J Med 2001;111(3): 247–54.

29. Maloney CG, Mendez SS, Quinonez RA, et al. The Strategic Planning Committee report: the first step in a journey to recognize pediatric hospital medicine as a distinct discipline. Hosp Pediatr 2012;2(4):187–90.

30. Wiese J, Jaffer AK. A new home awaits the hospitalist. J Hosp Med 2007;2(1):3–4.

31. Cohen E, Kuo DZ, Agrawal R, et al. Children with medical complexity: an emerging population for clinical and research initiatives. Pediatrics 2011; 127(3):529–38.

32. Tuan TJ, Thorell EA, Hamblett NM, et al. Treatment and microbiology of repeated cerebrospinal fluid shunt infections in children. Pediatr Infect Dis J 2011;30(9): 731–5.

33. Simon TD, Whitlock KB, Riva-Cambrin J, et al. Revision surgeries are associated with significant increased risk of subsequent cerebrospinal fluid shunt infection. Pediatr Infect Dis J 2012;31(6):551–6.

34. McLeod LM, French B, Flynn JM, et al. Antifibrinolytic use and blood transfusions in pediatric scoliosis surgeries performed at US Children's Hospitals. J Spinal Disord Tech 2013. [Epub ahead of print].

Family-Centered Rounds

Vineeta Mittal, MD

KEYWORDS

- Family-centered rounds • Patient satisfaction • Communication • Team-based care
- Resident education

KEY POINTS

- Family-centered rounds (FCRs) are multidisciplinary rounds that involve complete case discussion and presentation in front of the patient and family so as to involve them in the decision-making.
- FCR benefits include improved perception of parental satisfaction, communication, coordination of care, discharge planning, teamwork, quality improvement and improved trainee education.
- Key FCR barriers include lack of attending and trainees training on FCR, variability in conducting FCRs, duration, patient confidentiality, and physical constraints of large team and small room.
- As FCRs are adopted, research in needed to objectively measure outcomes such as parental satisfaction, safety, and quality improvement, and communication. These can then further improve FCR implementation.

In the last decade, in an effort to improve family-centered care, pediatric hospitalists have incorporated family-centered bedside rounds in the inpatient setting. By involving patients and families in decision making during rounds, hospitalists have given a new twist to the old concept of bedside rounds, and have called it family-centered rounds (FCRs).[1]

BEDSIDE ROUNDS AND FCRs

Forty years ago, bedside rounds were conducted in many academic centers. Physicians rounded in teams with residents and students, and 75% of teaching occurred during rounds. Teaching during ward rounds was focused on acquiring mastery in history taking and acquiring clinical skills. Sir William Osler, father of modern medicine, liked to say, "He who studies medicine without books sails an uncharted sea, but he who studies medicine without patients does not go to sea at all." His best-known saying was "Listen to your patient; he is telling you the diagnosis," which emphasizes the importance of taking a good history.[2] Bedside rounds were the norm for physician-led teaching rounds. Over the years, the proportion of teaching

Disclosure: None.

Division of General Pediatrics, Department of Pediatrics, UT Southwestern Medical Center and Children's Medical Center, 5323 Harry Hines Lane, Dallas, TX 75239, USA

E-mail address: Vineeta.Mittal@Childrens.com

Pediatr Clin N Am 61 (2014) 663–670

http://dx.doi.org/10.1016/j.pcl.2014.04.003

pediatric.theclinics.com

0031-3955/14/$ – see front matter Published by Elsevier Inc.

that occurs at the bedside decreased to 16% in 1978, and to even lower estimates in the 1990s as rounds moved away from the bedside.[3]

The 2001, the Institute of Medicine report, *Crossing the Quality Chasm: A New Health System for the 21st Century*, emphasized the need to ensure the involvement of patients and families in their own health care decisions, to better inform patients of treatment options, and to improve patients' and families' access to information.[4] As a result, the focus of practice shifted from physician-centered care toward providing patient-and family-centered care. Family-centered care in pediatrics is based on the understanding that family is the primary source of strength and support and that the child's and family's perspectives and information are important in clinical decision making. The American Academy of Pediatrics (AAP) recommended that in the inpatient setting, complete case discussion and presentation should occur in the presence of patients and family to involve them in the decision making.[5] As a result, FCRs have gained substantial momentum, and bedside rounds have returned to the inpatient setting, this time with focus on family-centered care. In a recent Pediatric Research in the Inpatient Network (PRIS) survey, over half the pediatric hospitalists reported conducting FCRs, and academic centers were more likely to conduct them.[6]

FCRs, SIT DOWN ROUNDS, HALLWAY ROUNDS, AND CONFERENCE ROOM ROUNDS

FCRs are defined as a multidisciplinary rounding model that involves planned, purposeful interaction that requires the permission of patients and families and the cooperation of physicians, nurses, and ancillary staff.[1] FCRs are multidisciplinary rounds and involve nurses, care coordinators, social workers, pharmacists, attending physicians, students, and residents. Many different types of rounds are described and practiced in the hospital setting; therefore it is important to understand how they differ from FCRs. "Sit down rounds" and "conference room" style rounds occur away from patients and families and are traditionally physician-centered rounds that involve the attending physician and students and residents rounding in a conference room to discuss a patient's plan of care. These may or may not be attended by other staff. "Hallway rounds" involve rounds in the corridors or hallway outside patient rooms. The medical team (the attending physician and students and residents) discusses a patient's case in the hallway without patient or family involvement. Traditionally, a team member (often a resident or attending physician) then updates or discusses the patient's plan of care with his or her family. FCRs, unlike the other rounds, are multidisciplinary rounds and involve complete case presentation and discussion in front of family members and their involvement in the medical decision making.

BENEFITS OF FCRs

Benefits of involving families during FCRs have been studied in the last decade. The value of FCRs in improving parental satisfaction, discharge timeliness, nursing satisfaction, communication, and resident and student education has been reported.[7–17]

Muething and colleagues[7] developed the first FCR model for improvement and described the role of FCRs in improving family-centered care, trainee education, and reducing time to discharge. They found FCRs to be efficient, and efficiency was further improved by the presence of nurses and other key ancillary staff who contributed valuable information regarding the patient's condition and progress made toward meeting discharge goals.[7] Family involvement and engagement were high in decision making. Rosen and colleagues,[9] in their quasi-experimental design, studied the impact of FCRs on parental and team satisfaction when compared with conventional rounds. They did not find any difference in parental satisfaction; however, they noted that staff satisfaction was higher on FCRs. They concluded that FCRs foster team work and empower hospital staff; additionally, the family members are engaged and are the focus point of FCRs. Rappaport and colleagues identified benefits of and barriers to FCRs for individuals who attend FCRs, including trainees, nurses, patients, and families. They reported that both patients and families were satisfied with FCRs, and FCRs were beneficial for trainee education.[9]

Parents and families are central to a child's environment, and involving them in care plan is crucial. FCRs bring everyone involved in a patient's care together in the same room at the same time, creating an environment of direct communication and providing a venue for immediate clarification of any miscommunication. Effective communication is crucial for parental understanding of a medical condition, plan of care, and discharge planning; therefore it is not surprising that FCRs are perceived to improve parental satisfaction and communication.[6,7,10,12,17–19] Both English-speaking and limited English proficient families perceive FCRs to improve communication and parental satisfaction.[13,14]

In teaching institutions with trainees (residents and students), several FCR-related benefits have been identified (**Box 1**). FCRs provide a venue for trainees to see patients in real time. They get to directly observe the attending physicians communicate

---

Box 1
Benefits of FCRs

Patient and family satisfaction

- Improved satisfaction with care
- Better understanding of plan of care
- Better understanding of discharge plan
- Feeling of involvement in care/partners in care
- Improved communication and understanding
- Better understanding of hospital workflow
- Better understanding of roles of different providers

Communication

- Improved doctor-family/patient communication
- Improved team communication
- Better understanding of the disease process

Coordination of care and discharge planning

Patient safety and quality improvement

Resident and student education

- Direct observation of patient
- Attending physician role modeling
- Improved physical examination skills
- Improved knowledge and communication skills
- Improved compassion
- Direct observation by attending physician and feedback

Improved staff satisfaction

with patients and families and with members of the multidisciplinary team. FCRs also allow attending physicians to directly observe trainees and provide real-time feedback.[17] A recent study from Johns Hopkins Medical Center reported that interns lack training on bedside etiquettes such as compassion and communication.[16] Many crucial elements of patient care and the Accreditation Council of Graduate Medical Education (ACGME) requirements such as compassion, respect, professionalism, dignity and cultural competencies, and communication with patients and families cannot be taught in a lecture room format, and FCRs might be an excellent venue to teach and directly observe trainees. In a recent study on pediatric resident perspectives about FCRs, residents reported improved nondidactic teaching and patient satisfaction, and reduced need for clarification on patient care plans.[11] In a focus group study at 2 large children's hospitals, residents perceived FCRs to improve their communication skills, especially the use of lay language. Residents noted that discharge planning during rounds helped them understand reasons for admissions, criteria for discharge, and systems-based practice required to coordinate discharge. Role modeling by the attending physician was also reported to be beneficial for resident education concerning skills such as communication, compassion, and respect and dignity when communicating with patients and family.[11,17,19]

HOW DO PATIENTS AND FAMILIES PERCEIVE ROUNDS?

Conducting daily multidisciplinary rounds with family members present can appear to be a complex task in a busy inpatient unit. Therefore, understanding how patients and families perceive FCRs is important for providers to partner with patients and family and implement FCRs into their daily practice. Contrary to popular belief, patients and families like to be included in daily rounds.[10,20] According to Osler, there should be "no teaching without a patient for a text, and the best teaching is that taught by the patient himself."[21] Parents report better doctor–patient relationships and feelings of mutual trust and respect, when involved directly during FCRs.[12–14,17] Although health care providers have expressed concerns about teaching and the impact of rounds on family members present, 93% of parents reported that they like to participate in morning rounds.[20,22] Parents reported comfort with attending rounds.[10,20,23,24] Being able to communicate, understand the plan of care, and participate with the team in decision making about their children were cited as very important to parents.[10] Often providers take their medical jargon to the bedside. As a student reported, "I realize that doctors talk to doctors in a way that doctors should not talk to patients. We need to leave the medical vocabulary out when talking to patients and families."[17] Use of lay terminology and inclusion of nurses in rounds were preferred.[6,10] Nurses share a special rapport with their patients. From admission to discharge they know about patient and family dynamics and the plan of care including timings of tests and treatment. Therefore, the bedside nurse can be a crucial partner during FCRs.[6] Parents found that careful explanation of the plan of care was most helpful when it was descriptive and directed to the parents' level of understanding.[10] Parents reported understanding that medical students and residents are in training and felt reassured to see experienced attending physicians teaching and training them during rounds.[17] Overall, parents reported being comfortable with attending and participating during FCRs.

As FCRs benefits are recognized, it is important to understand the perceptions of families with limited English proficiency (LEP). One of the core principles of family-centered care is honoring race, ethnicity, and cultural diversity.[5] Families with LEP generally reported positive experiences with FCRs and appreciated the transparency during rounds and that many providers were involved in caring for their child.[13] LEP families did not feel empowered to ask medical teams to request an interpreter for better communication and understanding.[14] Language barriers have been reported by pediatric hospitalists, and parents have reported satisfaction with FCRs when language barriers were addressed.[13,14] Addressing language and cultural competency through training improves health care professionals' knowledge, attitudes, and skills and patients' experience and ratings of health care.[13,14] Therefore, those conducting FCRs involving LEP families should pay attention to availability of trained interpreters to ensure that families understand the care plan in their primary language.

BARRIERS TO FCRs

In a busy inpatient environment, conducting multidisciplinary FCRs in a timely and efficient manner can be challenging. FCRs involve many aspects of care, including patient care; communication between patients and family and providers; team communication; decision making; teaching of trainees; discharge planning; coordination of care; answering patients, family, trainee and nursing questions; and ensuring efficiency. Therefore, if FCRs are not well organized and planned, they may not be effective. Barriers to FCRs remain. Key barriers include large team sizes, small room size, duration of FCRs, trainees' perceptions of not appearing knowledgeable in front of the families, language and cultural barriers, specific and sensitive patient conditions, efficiency, lack of training on FCRs, and variability in attending physicians' teaching and FCR styles.[6–14,17] However, because of the many recognized FCR benefits, it is not surprising that FCRs have been adopted by many physicians. Many pediatric intensive care units, neonatal intensive care units, and subspecialty services have adopted FCRs. In adult medicine, patient-centered multidisciplinary rounds are gaining momentum. Successful FCR implementation might require addressing FCR barriers (**Box 2**).

Many national workshops at Pediatric Academic Society meetings and annual Pediatric Hospitalists Medicine Conferences have discussed best practices in conducting FCRs and addressed key barriers. FCRs are planned and purposeful rounds and require organization and planning within an institution.[1] Whether FCRs will be conducted at in institution depends on medical teams' perceptions toward FCRs.[6] Defining the daily FCR process and identifying FCR personnel may help limit team size. Participation of a bedside nurse and case manager was reported as crucial in a PRIS network study.[6]

A common misconception is that FCRs will prolong the overall work day. At Cincinnati Children's Hospital FCRs were determined to take about 20% more time than traditional rounds. All participants believed that this time was utilized more efficiently as time saved later in the day.[7]

Trainees express fear of not appearing knowledgeable in front of families and patients. The attending physician can optimize their self-efficacy by creating a better and more transparent teaching and learning environment that improves trainees' comfort.[17] Workflow-related FCR barriers can be limited by developing a structured FCR process that includes educating patients, families and FCR teams about conducting FCRs, performing preround preparation, assigning roles during FCRs to facilitate work during rounds, and ensuring that trainees' fears are addressed during FCRs.[6] Attending physician variability and lack of FCR rules can make FCRs inefficient. Although this is an area for future research, having faculty development programs to streamline attending physician FCR practice might be helpful to reduce attending physician variability in conducting FCRs.[17,25]

Box 2
Barriers to conducting FCRs

Physical constraints

- Large teams
- Small rooms
- Patients on different floors

Duration of rounds

- FCRs prolong duration of rounds
- Too many parental questions

Trainees' fears of not appearing knowledgeable in front of families

Lack of formal training on conducting FCRs

- Variability in attending physicians' teaching style
- Variability in attending physicians conducting FCRs
- Lack of FCR training for trainees

Sensitive and specific patient conditions

- Child abuse
- Sexually transmitted diseases
- Patients on isolation

Confidentiality problems

Family-related barriers

- Lack of empowerment with team
- Cultural and language barriers
- Lack of interest in participation
- Absence of families

Some additional barriers are regarding the discussion of sensitive patient information in front of families, especially with adolescent patients. The need to gown and glove because of infection control precautions can be a barrier to the team entering the room. Attending physician discretion and preplanning are required to determine how FCRs should be conducted in these circumstances (see **Box 2**).

NEXT STEPS WITH FCRs

As FCRs are better operationalized, and best practices are established by programs, future research will be needed to objectively identify FCR outcomes such as impact on patient satisfaction, patient safety, quality of care, discharge planning, resident and medical student education, and clinical outcomes. Past FCR research on the educational impact of FCRs was mainly focused on perceptions of trainees using qualitative methodologies and is encouraging.[6–14,17] Future objective educational outcome measures are needed as stronger FCR models evolve. Developing and evaluating trainees' competencies in bedside communication are challenges, but very achievable ones. Future quality improvement projects should focus on innovative models to better operationalize FCRs and make them more efficient. These efforts might include developing models for faculty development programs to streamline daily FCRs, partnering with language and interpreter services to address language barriers, developing FCR rules or best practices for individual programs, and identifying strategies to improve FCR efficiency. These can then set the stage for outcomes research in FCRs.

REFERENCES

1. Bergert L, Patel S. Family-centered rounds: a new twist on an old concept. Hawaii Med J 2007;66(7):188–9.
2. Tuteur A. Listen to your patient. The skeptical OB. 2012.
3. Reichsman F, Browning FE, Hinshaw JR. Observations of undergraduate clinical teaching in action. J Med Educ 1964;39:147–63.
4. Institute of Medicine, Committee on Quality Health Care in America. Crossing the quality chasm: a new health system for the 21st century. Washington, DC: The National Academies Press; 2001.
5. Committee on Hospital Care. Family centered care and the pediatrician's role. Pediatrics 2003;112:691–6.
6. Mittal V, Sigrest T, Ottolini M, et al. Family-centered rounds on pediatric wards: a PRIS network survey of US and Canadian hospitalists. Pediatrics 2010;126:37–43.
7. Muething SE, Kotagal UR, Schoettker PJ, et al. Family-centered bedside rounds: a new approach to patient care and teaching. Pediatrics 2007;119(4):829–32.
8. Sisterhen LL, Blaszak RT, Woods MB, et al. Defining family-centered rounds. Teach Learn Med 2007;19(3):319–22.
9. Rosen P, Stenger E, Bochkoris M, et al. Family-centered multidisciplinary rounds enhance the team approach in pediatrics. Pediatrics 2009;123(4):e603–8.
10. Latta LC, Dick R, Parry C, et al. Parental responses to involvement in rounds on a pediatric inpatient unit at a teaching hospital: a qualitative study. Acad Med 2008;83(3):292–7.
11. Rappaport DI, Ketterer TA, Nilforoshan V, et al. Family-centered rounds: views of families, nurses, trainees, and attending physicians. Clin Pediatr (Phila) 2012;51(3):260–6.
12. Kuo DZ, Sisterhen LL, Sigrest TE, et al. Family experiences and pediatric health services use associated with family-centered rounds. Pediatrics 2012;130(2):299–305.
13. Lion KC, Mangione-Smith R, Martyn M, et al. Comprehension on family-centered rounds for limited English proficient families. Acad Pediatr 2013;13(3):236–42.
14. Seltz LB, Zimmer L, Ochoa-Nunez L, et al. Latino families' experiences with family-centered rounds at an academic children's hospital. Acad Pediatr 2011;11(5):432–8.
15. Young HN, Schumacher JB, Moreno MA, et al. Medical student self-efficacy with family-centered care during bedside rounds. Acad Med 2012;87(6):767–75.
16. Block L, Hutzler L, Habicht R, et al. Do internal medicine interns practice etiquette-based communication? A critical look at the inpatient encounter. J Hosp Med 2013;8:631–4. http://dx.doi.org/10.1002/jhm.2092.
17. Mittal V, Krieger E, Lee B, et al. Pediatric residents' perspectives on family-centered rounds—a qualitative study at 2 children's hospitals. J Grad Med Educ 2013;5:81–7.
18. Accreditation Council for Graduate Medical Education program requirements for residency education in pediatrics. Available at: http://www.acgme.org/acWebsite/downloads/RRC_progReq/339_child_abuse_peds_02062010.pdf. Accessed October 26, 2013.

19. LaCombe MA. On bedside teaching. Ann Intern Med 1997;126(3):217.
20. Stickney C, Ziniel S, Brett M, et al. Family participation during intensive care unit rounds: attitudes and experiences of parents and healthcare providers in tertiary pediatric intensive care unit. J Pediatr 2014;164(2):402–6.e1–4.
21. Osler W. On the need of a radical reform in our methods of teaching senior students. Med News 1903;82:49–53.
22. Lehmann LS, Brancati FL, Chen MC, et al. The effects of bedside case presentations on patients perceptions of their medical care. N Engl J Med 1997;336:1150–5.
23. Bramwell R, Weindling M. Families' views on ward rounds in neonatal units. Arch Dis Child Fetal Neonatal Ed 2005;90:F429–31.
24. Frogge MH, Vance RB, Meyer M, et al. Multidisciplinary rounds: patient-family-staff dyanamics: when the patient/family are colleagues. Cancer Pract 1998;6:258–61.
25. Ottolini M, Wohlberg R, Lewis K, et al. Using observed structured teaching exercises (OSTE) to enhance hospitalist teaching during family centered rounds. J Hosp Med 2011;6(7):423–7.

Effective Communication with Primary Care Providers

Karen Smith, MD, MEd

KEYWORDS

- Hospitalist • Primary care provider • Discharge • Communication

KEY POINTS

- Effective communication requires direct interaction between the hospitalist and the primary care provider using a standardized method of information exchange with the opportunity to ask questions and assign accountability for follow-up roles.
- The discharge summary is a part of the process, but does not provide the important aspects of handoff, such as closed loop communication and assignment of roles.
- Hospital discharge is a significant safety risk for patients, with more than half of the discharged patients experiencing at least one error.
- Effective communication with the primary care provider can eliminate errors or mitigate the effect of an error.
- Current technologies provide increased options to improve communication with limited time investment.
- Hospitalists and primary care providers need to develop measurable goals for communication and share outcomes to optimize patient care.

Hospital medicine is a relatively new designation of medical care. First described in 1996 by R. Watcher in the *New England Journal of Medicine*,[1] hospital medicine has rapidly grown among adult providers and then pediatricians. As a result, there has been a shift in the attending for hospitalized patients from the primary care physician to the hospitalist.[2] Research has demonstrated several benefits of hospital medicine, including decreased cost and length of stay; however, one unexpected consequence is the increased number of handoffs between providers.[3] The most significant handoff is the one between the hospitalist and the primary care provider.

Disclosure: The author has nothing to disclose.
Division of Hospitalist Medicine, Children's National Medical Center, 111 Michigan Avenue, Northwest, Washington, DC 20010, USA
E-mail address: ksmith@childrensnational.org

Pediatr Clin N Am 61 (2014) 671–679
http://dx.doi.org/10.1016/j.pcl.2014.04.004   **pediatric.theclinics.com**
0031-3955/14/$ – see front matter © 2014 Elsevier Inc. All rights reserved.

Before the growth of hospital medicine, the primary communication challenge for the primary care provider was with families, residents, and consultants. At its inception, hospital medicine added a new layer of care and communication challenge without a fully defined process for integration into the patient care continuum. Compounding this problem is the increased pressure to limit hospitalizations and shorten lengths of stay, resulting in the need to discharge patients "quicker and sicker."[4] The many demands of effective and efficient care highlight the need for ongoing clear communication between the hospitalist and the primary care provider, but too often the only communication is at the time of discharge in the form of the discharge summary.

Current US regulatory standards require a discharge summary to be completed within 30 days of discharge. In contrast, the discharge follow-up visit occurs much earlier, usually within 1 to 2 weeks after discharge. This disconnect demonstrates that the current use of the discharge summary does not reflect the new paradigm of care. The discharge summary simply provides documentation of the hospital stay rather than effective communication between providers. In 2006, the Joint Commission established a National Patient Safety Goal which required the adoption of a standardized approach to patient handoffs. Although this resulted in close scrutiny of handoffs within the hospital, the handoff to the primary care provider has not received the same attention. Recent literature on safe and effective handoffs recommends that a formal handoff plan be instituted at any change in service.[5] Effective handoffs include a verbal exchange of information that affords an opportunity for questions, a handoff procedure that is standardized and simplified, and uses closed looped communication with a readback/hearback technique.[5,6] Arora and colleagues[7] developed handoff recommendations for hospitalists that were peer-reviewed at the 2007 Hospital Medicine Annual Meeting (**Box 1**). However, very few of these components are used in the handoff to the primary care provider or included in the usual discharge summary.

CURRENT STATE OF COMMUNICATION

It is no surprise that half of primary care providers report communication with hospitalists as fair to poor.[8] In a large multicenter study of adult providers, Bell and colleagues[9] found that 23% of primary care providers did not know their patient was admitted to

---

Box 1
Handoff recommendations for hospitalists

- Time dedicated for a verbal exchange of information
  - ○ Interactive process
  - ○ Ill patients given priority in time
  - ○ The focus is to inform the receiving provider on what to expect and what to do after the patient is discharged
- Ability to access and record patient information during the handoff (standardized discharge summary template and access to electronic record)
- Train new users on handoff expectations
- System to identify the correct *provider* caring for a specific patient *during the discharge transition*

Data from Aora VM, Manjarrez E, Dressler DD, et al. Hospitalist handoffs: a systemic review and tack force recommendations. J Hosp Med 2009;4(7):433–40.

the hospital; less than half received a discharge summary by 2 weeks after discharge, and only 18% had direct communication with the inpatient provider. The lack of timely communication has been echoed in other studies, which found that 58% to 75% of all discharge summaries fail to arrive in a timely manner. Delay in receiving a timely hand-off of information limits the ability of the primary care provider to provide adequate care in 24% of hospital follow-up visits.[10,11] Furthermore, even when the discharge summary arrived in a timely manner, it did not provide sufficient information for appropriate transfer of care, specifically, discharge medications, pending laboratory results, and suggested follow-up testing.[12–14]

Providers describe transitions in care as "chaotic, unsystematic, and unstandardized." They ask for a system whereby all providers acknowledge and understand their role. Presently, the roles of the sender and receiver of discharge information are not clear.[15] Role confusion is most notable in the expected provider to follow-up laboratory tests pending at the time of discharge. Most hospitalists (65%) think the responsibility is the primary care provider, while most primary care providers (51%) think the responsibility lies with the ordering hospitalist.[16]

COMMUNICATION AND PATIENT SAFETY

Effective communication is crucial to patient safety. Multiple studies have shown that patients are at risk for medical errors on discharge from the hospital.[4,10–12,17,18] Almost half (49%) of the adult patients experience a medical error after discharge.[4,10] Medication errors, unviewed laboratory results or tests resulting after discharge, and missed follow-up testing are the most common adverse events. However, many of these adverse events are preventable or at least ameliorable if caught in time.[10]

Medications are the most prevalent source of error in patient transitions. Kripalani and colleagues[10] reported that 54% of patients experienced at least one unintended medication discrepancy on admission to the hospital and close to half of these errors were a potential threat to the patient. The most common error is omission of a medication taken at home. Hospitalization itself provides opportunity for error because of the various changes to a patient's medication profile during the hospital stay. Often the change is due to the hospital formulary restrictions requiring substitution of one medication for another. By the time of discharge, 49% of patients have an unexplained discrepancy between admission and discharge medications.[10,18] After discharge, patients are still at risk for error due to prescription-related problems. Patients on more than 5 medications were most likely to have a medication discrepancy. Inhaled medications are the most common group of medications for a prescription-related problem.[17] However, a recent study found that patients were 70% less likely to have a medication discrepancy at the time of follow-up when their inpatient provider communicated with their primary care provider before discharge and the primary care provider called the patient within 24 hours of discharge.[18]

Pending laboratory or microbiology tests at the time of discharge are a frequent occurrence. Although many pending test results may not impact or change treatment, nearly 10% to 15% of pending tests have potentially actionable results.[10] Likewise, microbiology results finalized after discharge were noted to be clinically important and required a change in treatment in 2% to 4% of discharges.[12] The current handoff process between the hospitalist and primary care provider still lacks the assignment of responsibility for the follow-up of pending tests.[16]

Many patients require continued outpatient workup after discharge for either their primary condition or new findings discovered during their hospital stay. Moore and colleagues[19] found that 54% of all discharge summaries did not document the recommended outpatient workup identified in the patient's inpatient medical record. Furthermore, the authors found that patients who did not receive the suggested outpatient workup were 6 times more likely to be rehospitalized within 3 months.

A coordinated and comprehensive handoff to the primary care provider can help mitigate or eliminate many of these errors.[10,18] Discharge follow-up with a provider that knows the patient well and follow-up phone calls have also been shown to improve outcomes and decrease errors (**Box 2**). Although reduction in errors should lead to better long-term outcomes, recent research on discharge communication has failed to demonstrate consistent improvement in several key indicators: emergency room visits, readmission rates, and mortality.[9,20,21] Some studies have been limited by the inclusion of all readmissions both planned and unplanned, although other observational studies have found that communication with primary care providers only occurred with the more complex patients who are at a higher risk readmission after discharge. The lack of clear and consistent improvement in the prevention of 30-day readmission rates has led many to consider whether a focused intervention with high-risk populations may demonstrate effectiveness compared with broad implementation with multiple patient populations.[22] Pediatric populations at high risk for readmission include patients between 15 and 18 years of age with public insurance, increased number of secondary diagnoses, and increased length of stay.[20,23]

WHAT DO OUR PRIMARY CARE PROVIDERS WANT?

Primary care providers desire to work together with the hospitalist for the care of their patient. As with all critical handoffs, verbal communication provides the opportunity for clarifying questions and closed loop communication. Pantilat and colleagues[24] found that primary care providers "very much prefer" to communicate with the hospitalist by telephone (77%) or e-mail at admission and discharge.[25] Although there are a few differences in how hospitalists and primary care providers wish to communicate, there are many areas in common (**Table 1**). Hospitalists are committed to the electronic medical record and desire that all providers have access to the electronic record for both inpatient and outpatient information. However, many primary care providers

---

Box 2
Interventions that improve outcomes after discharge

Continuity: follow-up with a provider that knows the patient well:

- Follow-up appointments with the same inpatient provider can result in a lower combined readmission and 30-day mortality[11]
- Patients followed up with same provider of inpatient care—5% decrease in relative risk of death or readmission[13]
- Follow-up with the primary care provider that knew the patient before hospitalization decreased risk of urgent readmissions[27]

Follow-up phone calls:

- Patients who received a phone call from their primary care provider within 24 hours of discharge were 70% less likely to have a medication discrepancy[18]
- Telephone follow-up increased patient satisfaction and medication adherence, decreased preventable adverse drug events, and decreased emergency department visits and readmissions[10]
- Telephone follow-up by the insurance provider reduced readmissions for select conditions[28]

Table 1		
What do hospitalists and primary care providers want for effective communication?		
	Hospitalist View	**Primary Care Provider View**
Method of contact	Electronic medical record	Phone calls, faxes, or e-mails
Contact information required	Primary care provider directory with phone, fax, and e-mail	Name and contact information of the treating hospitalist
Access to patient records	Electronic medical record viewable by both parties with inpatient and outpatient information	
Critical information	Diagnoses, medications, follow-up plans	
Timing	Discharge, admission, and major clinical changes	

Data from Harlan G, Srivastava R, Harrison L, et al. Pediatric hospitalists and primary care providers: a communication needs assessment. J Hosp Med 2009;4:187–93.

have not yet been able to transition to an electronic record and have difficulty accessing the hospital's electronic record. Primary care providers still prefer a phone call to discuss their patient, although other communication methods are acceptable, such as fax and e-mail. Asynchronous communication through fax or e-mail should include a contact number for the hospitalist in case of questions or if more information is needed. Hospitalists and primary care providers do agree on the type of information that should be shared and the timing of communication.[8]

A limitation in communicating by e-mail or fax is the inability to assign responsibility for future tasks, such as who will contact the patient immediately after discharge, which provider will follow-up on pending laboratory results and tests, and who will schedule follow-up procedures and tests.[4,26] A 2-way conversation is required to ensure both the sending and the receiving providers understand their role in the transition of care. The discharge summary should contain standard elements (**Box 3**) and be available to the primary care provider immediately after discharge. The use of headers for key categories will aid in quick reference to critical information.[18]

A CALL TO ACTION

Communication with the primary care provider must move from being considered a courtesy to a key component of a safe and effective handoff. Multiple studies have

Box 3
Primary care provider preference for discharge information

- Primary and secondary diagnoses
- Pertinent physical findings
- Results of procedures and laboratory tests
- Test results pending on discharge
- Discharge medications AND reasons for changes from home medications
- Details of follow-up arrangements
- Specific follow-up needs
- Information given to family

Data from Kripalani S, LeFevere F, Phillips CO, et al. Deficits in communication and information transfer between hospital-based and primary care physicians. JAMA 2007;297(8):831–41.

documented that patients are at high risk for medical error at the time of discharge. This rate of error would be unacceptable to the hospitalist during the inpatient stay. Similarly, no hospitalist would tolerate an incomplete paper handoff delivered by the exiting hospitalist several hours after the start of their shift. Why should the primary care provider be expected to tolerate a handoff of an incomplete discharge summary 2 weeks after the patient was discharged? As it is endeavored to continually improve patient care and decrease errors, communication with the primary care provider and the discharge handoff must be addressed.

STRATEGIES TO IMPROVE HOSPITALIST AND PRIMARY CARE PROVIDER COMMUNICATION AND PARTNERSHIP

All hospital medicine programs should develop a standardized handoff process for communication with the primary care provider similar to the handoff process from one hospitalist to another. The handoff process should address key periods in the hospitalization: admission, major clinical change, and discharge. One strategy is the use of template letters in the electronic medical record that can be quickly modified for each patient and faxed directly to the provider. The template can be prepopulated with an introduction, contact numbers, and the best time to contact the hospitalist. The busy hospitalist just needs to add 1 to 2 lines describing the admission diagnosis or updates and plan of care. To make this process successful, the electronic record needs to have an updated referring provider directory with accurate fax numbers and/or e-mail addresses. It is essential that this list be constantly updated with any changes and additions of new referring providers. Hospitalists should partner with their community providers to encourage them to update their office contact information at regular intervals and identify handoff times such as 7 to 8 AM, 12 noon to 1 PM, or 5 to 6 PM for verbal handoffs via the phone to avoid disrupting clinic schedule and rounding. Primary care practices should also provide "back line" numbers to bypass the main office recorded message. Another novel way to collaborate on care is to include the primary care provider in family meetings or during family centered rounds. The use of video communication via "Face time" or "Skype" allows for complete integration of the health care team with minimal interruption in the daily schedule.

Clear metrics are vital to ensure that all providers understand the expectation for communication. Such metrics include communication with the primary care provider within 24 hours of admission, every week that the patient is admitted, at transfer to the intensive care unit, and before discharge. As with any metric, performance needs to be measured and reported to the members (**Fig. 1**). The author's division places a short note in the chart for every provider communication. The electronic medical record is able to generate a report that documents every communication note in relation the time of admission, allowing the division to track the provider's ability to contact all providers within 24 hours of admission.

Accountability extends beyond whether contact was made. Handoffs must include assigning roles for follow-up care verbally or by e-mail. Simply sending a discharge report or note with a list of the pending tests that need follow-up is destined for failure. Either no one will follow-up or both the hospitalist and primary care provider will expend the time to follow-up on the pending test resulting in duplication of effort. Both are unsafe and inefficient uses of time. One-way communication does not allow for closed loop communication to ensure that the primary care provider understands and accepts responsibility for follow-up. Technology provides some options for the future. Many electronic records can forward a laboratory or test result to a specific provider. The provider can document in the record when the result was reviewed

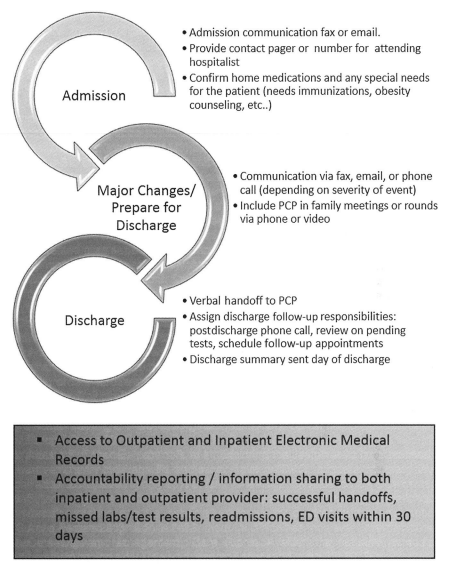

Admission

- Admission communication fax or email.
- Provide contact pager or number for attending hospitalist
- Confirm home medications and any special needs for the patient (needs immunizations, obesity counseling, etc..)

Major Changes/ Prepare for Discharge

- Communication via fax, email, or phone call (depending on severity of event)
- Include PCP in family meetings or rounds via phone or video

Discharge

- Verbal handoff to PCP
- Assign discharge follow-up responsibilities: postdischarge phone call, review on pending tests, schedule follow-up appointments
- Discharge summary sent day of discharge

- Access to Outpatient and Inpatient Electronic Medical Records
- Accountability reporting / information sharing to both inpatient and outpatient provider: successful handoffs, missed labs/test results, readmissions, ED visits within 30 days

Fig. 1. Recommended communication plan for hospitalists and primary care providers. ED, emergency department; PCP, primary care provider.

and acted on, if needed. If the result is not reviewed in a certain amount of time, the electronic record can send the result to the next provider until appropriate action is taken. However, electronic solutions require a sophisticated system and appropriate information technology support to create. As these safety concerns are raised, more information technology providers are building these programs into their electronic record platform.

Collaboration is necessary to continually improve the care provided to patients. As payers focus on readmissions, emergency department visits, and preventable morbidity; hospitalist and primary care providers need to share this data with each other. Many community providers may be unaware of which patients are readmitted or frequently use the emergency room. Likewise, a hospitalist may not be aware of a readmission or morbidity that occurs after discharge. By sharing this data between providers, hospitalists can continue to improve the transition process to optimize patient outcomes. Last of all, because the ultimate goal is to improve patient health, hospitalization provides an opportunity to address any gaps in care and improve access to resources available in a large health care system. The hospitalist has the opportunity to address many chronic health concerns, such as immunizations, patient nutrition, either limited resources in terms of food insecurity or excess, as in obesity, and exposures, including smoking, environmental, and violence. Health care reform demands that we move from silos to full partnership with all health care providers. Communication is the mode to creating these partnerships and improving child health.

REFERENCES

1. Watcher RM. The hospitalist field turns 15: new opportunities and challenges. J Hosp Med 2011;6(4):E1–4.
2. Fletcher K, Sharma G, Dong Z, et al. Trends in inpatient continuity of care for a cohort of Medicare patients, 1996-2006. J Hosp Med 2011;6:438–44.
3. Landrigan CP, Conway PH, Edwards S, et al. Pediatric hospitalists: a systematic review of the literature. Pediatrics 2006;117(5):1736–44.
4. McLeod L. Patient transitions from inpatient to outpatient: where are the risks? Can we address them? J Healthc Resour Manag 2013;32(3):14–9.
5. Joint Commission Center for Transforming Healthcare. Improving transitions of care: hand-off communications. Available at: http://www.centerfortransforminghealthcare.org/assets/4/6/CTH_Hand-off_commun_set_final_2010.pdf. Accessed February 17, 2014.
6. Steitenberger K, Breen-Reed K, Harris C. Handoffs in care – can we make them safer? Pediatr Clin North Am 2006;53(6):1185–95.
7. Arora VM, Manjarrez E, Dressler DD, et al. Hospitalist handoffs: a systemic review and task force recommendations. J Hosp Med 2009;4(7):433–40.
8. Harlan G, Srivastava R, Harrison L, et al. Pediatric hospitalists and primary care providers: a communication needs assessment. J Hosp Med 2009;4:187–93.
9. Bell CM, Schnipper JL, Auerbach AD, et al. Association of communication between hospital-based physicians and primary care providers with patient outcomes. J Gen Intern Med 2009;24(3):381–6.
10. Kripalani S, Jackson A, Schnipper J, et al. Promoting effective transitions of care at hospital discharge: a review of the key issues for hospitalists. J Hosp Med 2007;2(5):314–23.
11. Kripalani S, LeFevere F, Phillips CO, et al. Deficits in communication and information transfer between hospital-based and primary care physicians. JAMA 2007;297(8):831–41.
12. El-Kareh R, Roy C, Brodsky G, et al. Incidence and predictors of microbiology results returning postdischarge and requiring follow-up. J Hosp Med 2011;6(5):291–6.
13. Roy CL, Poon EG, Karson AS, et al. Patient safety concerns arising from test results that return after hospital discharge. Ann Intern Med 2005;143(2):121–8.
14. Walz SE, Smith M, Cox E, et al. Pending laboratory tests and the hospital discharge summary in patients discharged to sub-acute care. J Gen Intern Med 2011;26(4):393–8.

15. Davis MM, Devoe M, Kansagara D, et al. "Did i do as best as the system would let me?" Healthcare professional views on hospital to home care transitions. J Gen Intern Med 2012;27(12):1649–56.
16. Ruth JL, Geskey JM, Shaffer ML, et al. Evaluating communication between pediatric primary care physicians and hospitalists. Clin Pediatr 2011;50(10):923–8.
17. Kripalani S, Price M, Vigil V, et al. Frequency and predictors of prescription-related issues after hospital discharge. J Hosp Med 2008;3:12–9.
18. Lindquist LA, Yamahiro A, Garrett A, et al. Primary care physician communication at hospital discharge reduces medication discrepancies. J Hosp Med 2013;8: 672–7.
19. Moore C, Wisnivesky J, Williams S, et al. Medical errors related to discontinuity of care from an inpatient to an outpatient setting. J Gen Intern Med 2003;18:646–51.
20. Coller RJ, Klitzner TS, Lerner CF, et al. Predictors of 30-day readmission and association with primary care follow up plans. J Pediatr 2013;163:1027–33.
21. Oduyebo I, Lehmann CU, Pollack CE, et al. Association of self-reported hospital discharge handoffs with 30-day readmissions. JAMA Intern Med 2013;173(8): 624–9.
22. Auger KA, Kenyon CC, Feudtner C, et al. Pediatric hospital discharge interventions to reduce subsequent utilization: a systemic review. J Hosp Med 2014;9: 251–60.
23. Spehar AM, Campbell RR, Cherrie C, et al. Seamless care: safe patient transitions from hospital to home. Available at: http://www.ahrq.gov/qual/advances. Accessed February 8, 2014.
24. Pantilat SZ, Lindenauer PK, Katz PP, et al. Primary care physician attitudes regarding communication with hospitalists. Am J Med 2001;111(9B):15S–20S.
25. Walsh C, Siegler EL, Cheston E, et al. Provider-to-provider electronic communication in the era of meaningful use: a review of the evidence. J Hosp Med 2013;8: 589–97.
26. Lye PS, American Academy of Pediatrics. Committee on Hospital Care and Section on Hospital Medicine. Clinical report-physician's roles in coordinating care of hospitalized children. Pediatrics 2010;126(4):829–32.
27. Van Walraven C, Taljaard M, Etchells E, et al. The independent association of provider and information continuity on outcomes after hospital discharge: implications for hospitalists. J Hosp Med 2010;5:398–405.
28. Tang N. A primary care physician's ideal transitions of care – where's the evidence? J Hosp Med 2013;8:472–7.

Pediatric Hospitalists Working in Community Hospitals

 CrossMark

Jack M. Percelay, MD, MPH, MHM

KEYWORDS

- Advocacy • Community hospital • Hospitalist • Intermediate care • Training

KEY POINTS

- Pediatric hospital medicine (PHM) programs are now commonplace in community hospitals with medium-sized to large pediatric inpatient services and vary significantly based on local needs and resources.
- Clinical capabilities of Community Hospital Pediatric Hospital Medicine (CHPHM) programs depend on the hospitalists' skill sets, nursing expertise, subspecialist and surgeon availability, and proximity to neonatal and pediatric critical care services.
- CHPHM programs create value by increasing quality, satisfaction, and efficiency while reducing costs, but are not financially self-supporting based on professional fee revenues.
- Training needs for community hospitalists reflect the diversity of clinical practice with an emphasis on procedural competency.
- CHPHM programs have a responsibility to advocate for children's interests throughout the hospital through participation on key committees and nurturing of key liaison relationships.

BACKGROUND
Terminology and Overview

This article uses the term pediatric hospitalists in community hospitals or the shorter term community hospitalists to identify pediatricians who practice the discipline of PHM in general, nonuniversity, nonchildren's hospitals. Community Hospital Pediatric Hospital Medicine programs are referred to as CHPHM programs. Although other entities, most notably the Medical Group Management Association, may use the terms community and academic to distinguish between different management models for

---

Financial Disclosure: The author has no financial relationships relevant to this article to disclose.
Funding: No external funding.
Potential Conflict of Interest: The author has no potential conflicts of interest to disclose.
Department of Physician Assistant Studies, Pace University College of Health Professions, 163 William Street, Room 517, New York, NY 10038, USA
E-mail address: JPercelayMD@gmail.com

Pediatr Clin N Am 61 (2014) 681–691
http://dx.doi.org/10.1016/j.pcl.2014.04.005
0031-3955/14/$ – see front matter © 2014 Elsevier Inc. All rights reserved.

pediatric.theclinics.com

compensation and productivity surveys, this article explicitly avoids the term academic hospitalists in favor of pediatric hospitalists in university or children's hospitals. This language has been carefully chosen to avoid the implication that PHM programs in community hospitals are necessarily nonacademic.[1] In addition, this article focuses on community hospitals with limited pediatric resources and the challenges community hospitalists face caring for children without the infrastructure and support of a tertiary care referral center or a complete pediatric department, regardless of whether that department is housed in a larger community hospital, a children's hospital within a hospital, or a free-standing children's hospital.

Growth of CHPHM Programs

Tracking the number of pediatric hospitalists currently practicing in community hospitals is problematic. The Kid's Inpatient Database uses descriptors of children's versus nonchildren's hospitals, and separately classifies hospitals by size (small, medium, or large). There is no comprehensive national database of community hospitals with pediatric services. Similarly, pediatric hospitalists lack a unique subspecialty identifier (such as subboard certification or eligibility), and all hospitalist data are self-reported. Estimates of the growth of pediatric hospitalists in community hospitals are largely extrapolated from growth of the PHM community in general and by anecdotal observations of leaders in the field. Overall, the author believes that CHPHM programs have grown in frequency similar to the growth of adult hospital medicine programs in general and PHM programs at children's and university hospitals, but firm data are lacking. The key distinguishing feature between adult and pediatric hospital medicine programs in community hospitals is that every adult hospital is large enough to support a hospitalist; this is not the case in pediatrics. In rural community hospitals with small inpatient pediatric services, office-based general pediatricians still cover the hospital on-call, attend deliveries, consult in the emergency department (ED), and manage their own inpatients without benefit of hospitalists.

The most recent American Academy of Pediatrics (AAP) Section on Hospital Medicine (SOHM) survey indicates that 31% of respondents work in community hospitals (17% in hospitals with limited or no pediatric subspecialty and surgical services, 8% in community hospitals with significant services, and 6% in hospitals with nearly complete pediatric services).[2] The increasing importance of pediatric hospitalists in community hospitals is recognized by the creation of (1) a community hospitalist subcommittee within the AAP SOHM beginning in about 2010, (2) a specific community hospitalist track at the annual PHM 20XX meeting beginning 2013, and (3) dedicated community hospitalist seats on both the AAP SOHM Executive Committee and the Joint Council of Pediatric Hospital Medicine also in 2013.

Variability of CHPHM Programs

CHPHM programs vary widely in terms of size, scope of practice, available resources, coverage models, and nonclinical duties, including teaching of house staff and medical students, as well as other learners. All programs share a common focus of care of the hospitalized child on the general pediatric ward, but from there it varies greatly. **Table 1** lists different potential responsibilities for pediatric hospitalists in community hospitals. The ability of the community hospitalists to multitask across settings and services adds value to the local pediatric services. CHPHM programs are often established to enable smaller hospitals to continue to provide local pediatric inpatient care in the face of trends to hospitalize children at children's hospitals and larger community hospitals.[3] CHPHM programs are not profitable in and of themselves. They are mission driven, not margin driven. The individuals working in these settings need to

Table 1	
Range of potential responsibilities for community hospitalists	
Area	**Comments**
General pediatric ward	Core activity
Well-baby nursery	Frequent activity, particularly for unassigned newborns
Labor and delivery	Newborn resuscitation skills are key
Step-down unit/intermediate care	Often intermediate level of care within a general pediatric unit
Neonatal intensive care unit	Typically for after-hours coverage only
Pediatric intensive care unit	Only in larger community hospitals, after-hours coverage only
Emergency department	As consultant or potentially as primary provider
Other	Sedation, consultant for diagnostic dilemmas, occasional outpatient follow-up

be comfortable functioning independently, triaging simultaneous clinical demands, and working in different parts of the hospital. It is a source of both frustration and satisfaction, and makes practice in smaller community hospitals unique compared with the narrower range (but admittedly higher acuity) of practice in larger community hospitals, university hospitals, and children's hospitals.

CLINICAL ISSUES
Unique Aspects of Small Community Hospital Programs

CHPHM programs demonstrate significant more variability than the traditional resident teaching service at children's and university hospitals. Larger community hospitals with larger volumes may have multiple hospitalists assigned to the inpatient unit at a time or may have one hospitalist assigned to the inpatient unit and another to the ED/urgent care or well-baby nursery (WBN). In smaller community hospitals, a single hospitalist may be simultaneously responsible for the general pediatric ward, the WBN, and ED consultations. Maryland hospital regulations permit shared ED and inpatient pediatric units. These units are designed to accommodate both short- and long-term ED visits/ observation stays, as well as short inpatient stays.[4] Nurses and physicians working in these units must be skilled and comfortable managing both patient populations. The flexible staffing and common physical space create efficiencies and economic savings more than what separate inpatient and outpatient (ie, ED) units would offer and allow these community programs to continue to provide low-acuity inpatient pediatric services instead of automatically transferring out any child who requires hospitalization.

For CHPHM programs in which a single pediatrician covers the entire hospital, flexibility is required to manage simultaneous demands. This situation requires the aptitude and ability to triage requests effectively and the flexibility for other team members to expand their practice beyond their usual role. For example, when a hospitalist is attending a delivery for fetal distress, most other responsibilities have to wait. But if there is a child acutely decompensating in the ED while the hospitalist is attending an elective C-section, perhaps the ED physician can manage the child in the ED until the pediatrician arrives or an appropriately trained nurse can recover the newborn and the hospitalist can leave the delivery room (DR). On-call backup from home in the form of another hospitalist, a neonatologist, or a community pediatrician may also be part of contingency planning.

Subspecialty and Surgical Resources

Hospitalist staffing considerations have less impact on patient selection for community hospitals than does the availability of pediatric subspecialty and/or surgical resources. Community hospitals should develop admission, discharge, and transfer (ADT) criteria collaboratively and proactively with PHM program leadership, surgical and subspecialty representatives, and nursing leadership to address likely scenarios. For example, should the community hospital perform a barium enema to attempt to diagnose and reduce on intussusception, or should such patients be referred to a tertiary care center where an air contrast enema could be performed? Without a pediatric surgeon, what is the lower age limit for appendectomies by a general adult surgeon? Similar questions can be asked of medical subspecialists. When pediatric subspecialty and surgical expertise is readily available at a nearby hospital, local standards of care typically direct most subspecialty care to tertiary care centers. In more rural settings where pediatric expertise is several hours away, adult trained physicians may of necessity be more comfortable and experienced caring for younger children. The availability of pediatric hospitalists to comanage the general medical care of pediatric patients contributes additional comfort for adult providers. Telemedicine can further augment the ability of rural community hospitals to deliver more expert pediatric inpatient care.

Patient Acuity and Intermediate Care

Acuity is the other main concern driving patient selection. For hospitals without a pediatric intensive care unit (PICU), patient admission to a community hospital may depend on the ability of the hospital to provide intermediate level care. Intermediate level care is most appropriate for patients in whom there is potential for deterioration, but the likelihood is low. It includes cardiorespiratory monitoring and intermediate nursing staffing ratios. The definition refers to a level of care and not a geographically defined unit such as a step-down unit. Intermediate level care may be provided on a general pediatric ward or in a PICU.[5] Criteria for intermediate care should be determined in advance of admission by program leadership including nursing and not on the fly, after-hours, by junior personnel.

Intermediate level care is certainly appropriate for hospitalists to initiate in the ED. These patients may be quickly transferred to a tertiary care hospital with a PICU if their status does not rapidly improve and the referral hospital is nearby. Alternatively, in more rural settings where transfer to referral centers involves greater distances, hospitalists may choose to provide intermediate level care on the ward for a longer period before transferring patients, as long as the child's initial status meets predefined physiologic parameters, the patient's status does not worsen, and the duration of intermediate care therapy does not exceed predefined limits. Sample criteria frameworks are highlighted in **Table 2**.

Relationships with Tertiary Care Centers

Preexisting relationships between the community hospital and tertiary care referral centers facilitate transfers when needed and consultation when not. Certainly, telemedicine facilities need to be arranged in advance to assure compatibility of receiving and sending equipment, as well as to address credentialing issues for consultation services for patients who are not transferred out. As part of the relationship, the tertiary care facility can offer external feedback and validation on decisions of whether or not to transfer patients. Collaborative Quality Improvement (QI) meetings that review all transfers between community hospitals and tertiary care facilities can help identify

Table 2 Intermediate care considerations			
Disease and Therapy	**Physiologic Parameters**	**Treatment Parameters**	**Miscellaneous**
Asthma Continuous albuterol	Mental status Respiratory rate, respiratory distress score Oxygen saturation P_{CO_2}	Oxygen requirement Continuous albuterol dose Improvement within x hours	No pneumothorax No prior history of intubation
Diabetic ketoacidosis Insulin	pH Initial glucose HCO_3 Mental status	Continuous insulin Duration of therapy Response to therapy	New-onset diabetes vs established patient Patient age

transfers that may have been initiated later than desirable, as well as transfers that might have been avoided with minimal additional training or support for the community hospital. Accountable Care Organizations (ACOs) and consolidation of care may further drive affiliations between community hospitals and tertiary care referral centers.

LOGISTICAL ISSUES
Staffing

Staffing a CHPHM program varies depending primarily on the range of responsibilities of the program, predicted volumes, and coverage model (24/7 in-house vs on-call from home). For an inpatient-only service, the author believes 15 patient contacts (ignoring normal newborns) per weekday shift is a sustainable workload for community hospitalists. Acuity is lower than that in children's or university hospitals, but typically the hospitalist does not have any residents to help with paperwork, phone calls, and procedures. The number of patient contacts is a much more appropriate metric than daily census. Community PHM programs tend to have short lengths of stay. If the average length of stay is 1 day and the average midnight census is 15, there are 30 patient contacts per day.

The calculations become more challenging when the CHPHM program covers multiple areas of the hospital. Coverage models are best based on historical norms and adjusted based on experience. Predictable periods of increased clinical demands may lead smaller programs to incrementally increase staff at selected times of the day—mornings to cover the WBN and evenings to cover the ED and admissions. Seasonal variations further complicate staffing. On-call backup systems and/or short shifts offer creative, cost-effective staffing solutions. Nighttime coverage is inherently inefficient but is often used to meet requirements for neonatal intensive care unit (NICU) and DR coverage while providing increased quality, safety, and patient, registered nurse, and referring physician satisfaction.

A sample staffing calculation for a typical 24/7 program with 1 person in house is provided in **Table 3**.

When comparing workloads among programs, it is helpful to consider the expected number of hours one is in the hospital performing clinical duties in a year, taking continuing medical education and paid time off into account. (Monthly calculations do not reflect seasonal variability and frequently fail to account for variable numbers of days and weekends per month.) Weekend and weeknight obligations should be clarified along with holiday expectations, sick leave, and jeopardy call. The total number of nights worked per year, as well as the amount of sleep one can expect on

Table 3
Sample staffing calculation for a typical 24/7 program

Metric	Sample Calculation	Comments
Total physician hours per year	365 d × 25 h/d = 9125 h	Assumes no double coverage except for sign-out period, could double staff for predictable high volume hours/seasons
Expected average number of in-house hours per week	40 h/wk	Varies by local market, workload, range 36–48
Total number of weeks physician works per year	47 wk	(Assumes 4-wk vacation, 1-wk continuing medical education, add more for holidays and sick leave)
Total hours per full-time equivalent (FTE) per year	40 × 47 =1880 h	Crucial to calculate per year
Total number of FTEs required clinically	9125/1880 = 4.85 FTEs	
Administrative FTE requirement	0.05 × 4.85 = 0.25 admin FTE	0.05 admin FTE per clinical FTE is a useful starting point, adjust up or down based on individual program experience/needs
Total staffing needs	4.85 + 0.25 = 5.2 FTEs total	Flexibility is greater if instead of 5 individuals working full time, there are some part-timers willing to pick up extra work and a pool of moonlighters

average are other crucial considerations, as are the expected numbers of phone calls and trips to the hospital (after midnight) if one takes call from home.

Productivity

Productivity data for PHM programs in general and small CHPHM programs in particular are woefully inadequate. The most common metric used is work relative value units (wRVUs). The numbers are especially meaningful for programs that operate at a full census, and are certainly followed closely by program administrators. These figures are most useful to examine intragroup and year-to-year comparisons for a given practice. Pediatric hospitalists have little chance of hitting adult productivity norms, but annual growth of 5% to 10% may be a reasonable target. (Given the inherently low productivity of nights, programs should consider separately reporting night vs daytime wRVU productivity. Nighttime coverage is usually a service requested by the hospital, not one the hospitalists choose to provide to increase revenue.)

Determining Added Value

Work RVUs are often a misleading measure of the community hospitalist's contribution to patient care and to the health care system. It is not uncommon for a community hospitalist to spend an hour trying to place an intravenous (IV) tube and be credited with no wRVUs for the service. On the cost side, hospitalists can promote their value by avoiding unnecessary testing and therapies such as those identified in the Choosing Wisely campaign,[6] shortening lengths of stay and preventing unnecessary admissions altogether. In an ACO model of care, the hospital is a cost center, not a revenue generator, and these cost savings are significant. In addition, from a system standpoint, hospitalists contribute to the overall efficiency and productivity of the system by allowing pediatricians to remain in their offices where they are maximally productive. Hospitalists facilitate management and retention of appropriately selected pediatric subspecialty and surgical patients through comanagement and consultation. Overall, the goodwill that is generated by preserving local pediatric services and caring for the children of the community is probably the most important yet most difficult to quantify value of CHPHM programs.

TRAINING OF COMMUNITY HOSPITALISTS
Residency and Fellowship Training

Training needs for community hospitalists vary based on the clinical services provided. Compared with hospitalists in university and children's hospitals who practice exclusively on the pediatric ward, less expertise is required in the management of children with medical complexity and the coordination of multiple subspecialists. Community hospitalists practicing in the DR, ED, NICU, or PICU require more procedural competency and the ability to stabilize higher acuity patients for transport. Recent residency program requirements and work hours restrictions have reduced residents' inpatient experiences. Many CHPHM program leaders believe current pediatric residency graduates are less prepared to care for patients in community hospital settings than their predecessors.

As a result of these concerns and others, there is active discussion in the PHM community at large to petition the American Board of Pediatrics (ABP) for a formal subspecialty designation for PHM. The proposal involves a 2-year fellowship as opposed to the traditional 3-year fellowship model. In addition to additional clinical and procedural training and a scholarly project, fellowships would also include instruction in systems of care, QI science, and program management.[7] From a community hospital perspective, there is a strong desire to include experience in community hospitals as part of the clinical training of these fellowships. Such training would not only prepare future hospitalists for work in community settings but also inform future researchers and children's hospital faculty of the reality of practice in community settings. It is expected that not all community hospitalists will be fellowship trained in the future. Many will be general pediatricians practicing as community hospitalists. This situation is similar to the ED, where generally trained pediatricians often work clinically but rarely head pediatric emergency medicine programs.

Procedural Skills and Simulation

Community hospitalists regularly identify vascular access, airway management, and newborn resuscitation as key procedural skills they require for their practice. Simulation is one way to practice these skills, but no one has found a high-fidelity model for intubation of newborns. This is a particularly problematic area. Most senior hospitalists mastered this technique in bygone eras when meconium-stained babies, even the vigorous ones, were routinely intubated. At present, graduating residents have less opportunity to acquire newborn intubation skills in the first place, and practicing hospitalists have fewer opportunities to exercise and maintain it. One option is established programs such as Neonatal Resuscitation Program, Pediatric Advanced Life Support, Pediatric Fundamentals of Critical Care Support, and Advanced Pediatric Life Support. National meetings such as PHM 20XX offer training workshops, simulation experiences, and the all-important opportunity to network with colleagues about how their program addresses these same training needs. Locally, community hospitalists should practice mock codes within their own program alongside their own nursing staff. Most community hospitalists maintain proficiency at IVs, arterial punctures, and lumbar punctures through regular clinical practice. Other procedures may be simulated or proctored under the guidance of affiliated subspecialists and tertiary care partner institutions to help hospitalists develop those skills they do not regularly exercise in clinical practice.

ADVOCACY
The Hospitalist as Advocate for Pediatrics in General

In children's hospitals, hospitalists advocate for the care of children cared for on the general pediatric ward. They may focus on other populations such as children with medical complexity or processes such as patient and family-centered care (see the article by Mittal elsewhere in this issue), but they need not advocate for children in general. The entire hospital focuses on children. In contrast, in community hospitals with a small pediatric department and few if any subspecialists, pediatric hospitalists are often the ones best suited to advocate for the care of children throughout the hospital. If present, pediatric emergency medicine physicians concentrate on care in the ED and neonatologists on care provided in the NICU; in other areas of the hospital, the hospitalists are likely more knowledgeable, available, and capable as serving as physician advocates for Pediatrics in collaboration with office-based primary care providers (PCPs) who are members of the pediatric department.

Department Chair and Committee Roles

Pediatric hospitalists advocate clinically for children by proactively developing ADT criteria for patients based on patient acuity and availability of pediatric and adult subspecialty and surgical expertise. But just as the Pediatric Hospital Medicine Core Competencies emphasize clinical competencies, so too do they emphasize systems-based competencies and administrative skills.[8] Before the advent of hospitalists, department chair duties were most frequently rotated among volunteer office-based PCPs who served a 1- to 2-year term, perhaps longer, with minimal support. Committee assignments were similarly rotated among physicians who (were) volunteered for the position. This model continues in many small community hospital pediatric departments. In others, the head of the CHPHM group serves as the department chair. Regardless of the particular arrangement, community hospitalists should expect to be asked to represent pediatrics on various committees and working groups. In particular, the committees listed in **Table 4** represent opportunities for hospitalists to improve their professional workflow and environment and, more importantly, to improve the care of children and families cared for in the hospital.

Liaison Relationships

Outside of the committee structure and relationships, the CHPHM group benefits from established liaison relationships with Case Management/Social Work, Volunteer Services, Child Life services (if present), and Occupational, Physical, and Respiratory Therapy. In smaller community hospitals, these are most often informal personal relationships. CHPHM group leaders may decide to designate different staff hospitalists to be the designated liaisons for their group to involve every hospitalist in at least one systems issue. In other groups, the CHPHM group leader is automatically the contact person for all external departments.

Nursing

The most important relationship hospitalists have with other departments is the relationship with the pediatric nursing staff. This relationship merits special attention.

Table 4
Important committees for CHPHM program participation

Committee	Comments
Pharmacy and Therapeutics	Crucial for medication selection, including pediatric preparations, medication safety
Code Blue	Assures appropriate personnel, equipment, and regular simulation training for pediatric codes
Quality Improvement	Assures attention and resources are devoted to pediatric QI efforts on the general pediatric unit (and not just NICU or WBN). Pediatric QI should have established process to either jointly review or refer issues detected in pediatric review to other departments, most importantly Surgery, Emergency Medicine, Obstetrics, and Radiology
Safety	Assures attention to unique pediatric safety concerns in all areas of the hospital
Credentials	Provides advance notice of new (adult) physician resources/ skills in hospital; facilitates proactively addressing issues of appropriate patient selection
Disaster Preparedness	Assures attention to unique pediatric concerns in Disaster Preparedness training
Informatics/Medical Records	Facilitates pediatric friendly modifications in computerized physician order entry, electronic charting
Patient Satisfaction	Provides opportunity to lobby for pediatric resources based on complaints, highlight accomplishments based on successes (eg, patient and family-centered rounds)
Accreditation Preparation/ Joint Commission	Assures resources and attention are devoted to unique pediatric accreditation and regulatory concerns. Facilitates early clarification of policies not relevant to pediatrics
Medical Executive	Generally reserved for Pediatric Department Chair. If not a hospitalist, PHM group leader needs close working relationship with Department Chair with regular and timely updates
Laboratory (and Imaging)	Assures availability of appropriate laboratory and radiology services. Useful venue to address overuse

Hospitalists cannot assume that they are knowledgeable about nursing protocols, policies, and standards and should be careful not to cross professional boundaries. Systems issues, competency issues, unresolved interpersonal conflicts, and other sensitive issues typically are best handled by having the CHPHM group leader discuss the issue privately with the parallel nursing leader. Physicians can provide basic lectures on pediatric illnesses, patient presentation, and expected therapies and interventions, but hospitalists should not underestimate the value of advanced pediatric nursing support and specialized nurse educators. Pediatric hospitalists may be most effective by advocating for the local hospital to recruit external part-time or consultant pediatric-specific nurse educators to help the nursing staff expand its skill sets and capabilities, rather than assuming that the hospital's adult nurse educators can provide this expertise.

CHPHM groups should consider creating an Advisory Committee consisting of referring physicians, nurses, and other members of the pediatric health care team, including interested parents when appropriate. This Advisory Committee can provide feedback on where and how the CHPHM group can perform as a group. Committee members can serve as allies to advocate for the CHPHM group to get the resources the group needs to achieve these goals.

Advocacy Outside of the Hospital

Community hospitalists can also play important roles in advocacy and education beyond the boundaries of the hospital walls. Outreach to referring PCPs (family medicine physicians and pediatricians) may address issues such as office preparedness for emergencies. Alternatively, community hospitalists may lead educational sessions in the community on topics such as obesity, asthma, and concussions. Health promotion may take the form of reach out and read activities in the hospital or promoting vaccinations during ED visits. Community hospitalists may collaborate with local school systems or county health departments. Hospitalists will have direct experiences with children whose care is profoundly impacted by Medicaid availability and access to health care. These vignettes can be used locally and at the state and federal levels with the support (and advocacy and media training) of the AAP to advocate for specific programs that promote child welfare in and outside of the hospital.

SUMMARY

The practice of PHM in community hospitals offers career satisfaction from providing direct patient care in a wide variety of settings to a wide variety of patients outside the hierarchy of residents and fellows. The variety of roles pediatric hospitalists are asked to perform and the range of support they have from adult and pediatric subspecialists and surgeons vary significantly, which create challenges in both appropriate patient selection and the staffing and economics of programs, especially for small community hospitals with limited pediatric subspecialty support. Advance planning and careful monitoring of patient outcomes supported by collaborative, structured relationships with tertiary care referral centers is crucial to balance the benefits of care in one's local community hospital versus referral to a more distant tertiary care facility. Pediatric hospitalists in community hospitals require additional procedural training compared with pediatric hospitalists in children's or university hospitals. Residency, fellowship, and on-the-job training must recognize these unique considerations. In addition to advocating for the care of their individual patients, pediatric hospitalists in community hospitals often serve as advocates for all children cared for in the hospital, even those outside of the pediatric ward.

REFERENCES

1. Roberts K, Brown J, Quinonez R, et al. Institutions and individuals: What makes a hospitalist "academic"? Pediatr Hosp Med, in press.
2. Fisher ES, Percelay JM, Quinonez RA, et al. Growing strong: findings from the American Academy of Pediatrics hospital medicine workforce survey 2013-2014. Abstract #1760, presented at Pediatric Academic Societies Meeting. Vancouver, May 3, 2014.
3. Aragona E, Rauch DA. Changing demographics of pediatric hospitalizations. Abstract # 4345.5, presented at Pediatric Academic Societies Meeting. Boston, May 1, 2012.
4. Krugman S, Sugs A, Photowala HY, et al. Redefining the community pediatric hospitalist: the combined pediatric ED/inpatient unit. Pediatr Emerg Care 2007; 23(1):33–7.

5. Jaimovich DG, Committee on Hospital Care, and Section on Critical Care. Admission and discharge guidelines for the pediatric patient requiring intermediate care. Pediatrics 2004;113(5):1430–3.
6. Quinonez RA, Garber MD, Schroeder AR, et al. Choosing wisely in pediatric hospital medicine: five opportunities for improved healthcare value. J Hosp Med 2013;8(9):479–85.
7. Carney S, Hill V. Should pediatric hospitalists seek formal subspecialty status? Hosp Pediatr 2011;1(1):4–6.
8. Stucky ER, Maniscalco J, Ottolini MC, et al. The pediatric hospital medicine core competencies supplement: a framework for curriculum development. J Hosp Med 2010;5(Suppl 2):i–xv, 1–114.

Quality Improvement and Comparative Effectiveness
A Review for the Pediatric Hospitalist

 CrossMark

Paul E. Manicone, MD*, Jimmy Beck, MD

KEYWORDS

- Pediatric hospitalist • Quality improvement • Comparative effectiveness research

KEY POINTS

- Engaging in meaningful quality improvement (QI) activities begins with education.
- By being informed and engaged, pediatric hospital medicine (PHM) physicians will have a key role in shaping the health care transformation expected over the next decade and beyond.
- The magnitude of the role that the community of PHM physicians plays in future health care transformation is predicated on a commitment to gaining mastery of QI and comparative effectiveness research (CER) through various educational mechanisms and other related activities.

INTRODUCTION TO QUALITY IMPROVEMENT

In the past 10 to 15 years, there has been an enormous focus on the quality of health care in the United States. Several major reports placed a spotlight on quality improvement (QI) and threw the gauntlet down for change. Among these were the Institute of Medicine (IOM) National Roundtable on Health Care Quality Report, "The Urgent Need to Improve Health Care Quality,"[1] To Err is Human,[2] and IOM's Crossing the Quality Chasm.[3] There have been many definitions of quality and operational frameworks. The most highly referenced of these come from the IOM report, Crossing the Quality Chasm, whereby quality is defined as "the degree to which healthcare services increase the likelihood of desired health outcomes and are consistent with current professional knowledge." The framework to measure quality included 6 dimensions: effectiveness, equity, efficiency, patient-centered, safety, and access.[3]

The US health care system is the most costly in the world, accounting for 17% of the gross domestic product with estimates that percentage will grow to nearly 20% by

Hospitalist Division, Children's National Health System - Sheikh Zayed Campus for Advanced Children's Medicine, 111 Michigan Avenue, Northwest, Washington, DC 20010, USA
* Corresponding author.
E-mail address: pmanicon@cnmc.org

Pediatr Clin N Am 61 (2014) 693–702
http://dx.doi.org/10.1016/j.pcl.2014.04.006
0031-3955/14/$ – see front matter © 2014 Elsevier Inc. All rights reserved.

2020 (National Healthcare Expenditure Projections, 2010–2020).[4] A recent report from the Robert Wood Johnson Foundation Commission to Build a Healthier America warns that the health in America is worse than other developed nations on more than 100 measures. Furthermore, they report 30 countries having lower infant mortality rates, and people in 26 countries can expect to live longer than Americans. The trend of this latter statistic was of even more concern because life expectancy in the United States ranked 15th among affluent countries in 1980, and by 2009 had slipped to 27th place.[5]

In 2007, the Institute for Healthcare Improvement (IHI) launched the Triple Aim Initiative, which is composed of 3 key goals: improving the patient experience of care, improving the health of populations, and reducing the per capita cost of health care. This broad concept brings the attention to individuals, populations, and cost, along with the necessary integration of systems (health care, social services, public health, community organizations, and school systems). In the US environment, many areas of health reform can be furthered and strengthened by Triple Aim thinking, including accountable care organizations, bundled payments, and other innovative financing approaches; new models of primary care, such as patient-centered medical homes; sanctions for avoidable events, such as hospital readmissions or infections; and the integration of information technology.[6] The following hyperlink to the IHI Web site provides a short video on "design of a triple aim enterprise": www.IHI.org/ TripleAim.

As the emphasis on QI grows in the hospital arena, so does the emphasis in other arenas as well. In government, as policy makers work to increase the incentives for quality in government programs, in the insurance arena, as health plans evaluate providers based on quality indicators, in the provider arena, as hospitals and practices are investing in information technology to improve efficiency and effectiveness of care, and in the consumer arena, patients are seeking transparent information from health care organizations before choosing a physician or hospital for their care.[7] Pediatric hospital medicine (PHM) physicians can play an important role in linking QI activities to these other arenas by way of national QI collaboratives, partnerships and networks, professional organizations, and the federal government via funding sources, such as the Agency for Healthcare Research and Quality (AHRQ), the National Institutes of Health, and the Centers for Medicare and Medicaid Services (CMS).

QI EDUCATION FOR THE PEDIATRIC HOSPITALIST

Engaging in meaningful QI activities begins with education. Many practicing PHM physicians received little or no formal education in QI as a medical student or pediatric resident. More QI educational and mentorship opportunities exist for physicians engaged in PHM fellowships; however, they are a minority of the workforce. Much of the education comes on the job, which is meaningful, applicable, and relevant to the PHM physician. There are a number of well-established conferences that focus on QI, such as the Academic Pediatrics Association (APA) conference on QI research conducted in conjunction with the Pediatric Academic Societies meeting. The Children's Hospital Association Implementing Quality Improvements in Children's Health Conference offers the opportunity to participate in an educational series with a wider range of pediatric health care professionals. The American Board of Pediatrics Maintenance of Certification Program involves completing a Web-based performance improvement module that provides a basic understanding of QI methods, including key steps, such as assessing baseline performance, collecting data, identifying gaps in quality, implementing change, reassessing performance through repeated cycles, and reporting gains. The American Board of Pediatrics (ABP) also has approved externally developed Web-based QI modules, such as the American Academy of Pediatrics' (AAP's) Education in Quality Improvement for Pediatric Practice modules.[8] Last, a rigorous form of QI education now exists as graduate course work, including online distance education formats, such as the Masters of Science in Health Sciences in Health Care Quality at the George Washington University.[9] Programs such as these are time-consuming and costly; however, they provide a comprehensive curriculum to gain mastery of QI research, leadership, implementation science, and organizational change.

QI COLLABORATIVES IN PHM

The role of QI collaboratives is critical to the translation of research to practice and the dissemination of newly established best practices. Adoption delay is endemic in health care research, and QI breakthroughs are no exception. QI collaboratives are organized with 5 features:

1. A specific topic, typically one with large variations between current and best practice
2. Clinical and QI experts to provide ideas and support for improvement
3. A critical mass of multiprofessional teams from multiple sites willing to share ideas
4. A collaborative process involving a series of structured activities (eg, webinars, conference calls, in-person meetings, and online discussion boards)
5. A model for improvement focusing on setting clear and measurable targets, collecting data and testing changes[10]

The translation of research into practice demands the involvement of practicing clinicians in the research design and by active participation. This can lead to the incorporation of results into the culture of a practice and then to spread throughout an organization.[11] One notable example of this is the QI research collaborative, Pediatric Research in the Inpatient Setting (PRIS), which is jointly supported by the APA, AAP, and Society of Hospital Medicine (SHM). PRIS has been active in QI research for more than a decade, and has moved forward important work such as the Prioritization Project, which identified the inpatient conditions with high prevalence, high cost, and wide variations in resource utilization.[12] This work provided 43 CHA (Children's Hospital Association) hospitals with scientifically rigorous data to prioritize their QI resources, and engaged the clinical leadership to improve care within their hospital.[13] Another exciting PRIS collaborative includes the Pediatric Health Information System Plus (PHIS+), which links not only administrative data, but clinical data from 6 participating children's hospitals affording the opportunity for comparative effectiveness research (CER), as well as QI research. Last, the most recent success of the PRIS network was evident in the work published by Starmer and colleagues[14] in the *Journal of the American Medical Association* regarding the I-PASS project whereby 11 academic institutions implemented a handoff communication bundle (standardized communication, handoff training, a verbal mnemonic, and a new team handoff structure), which resulted in a decrease in medical errors from 33.8 per 100 admissions to 18.3 per 100 admissions, and preventable adverse events decreased from 3.3 to 1.5 per 100 admissions. In the spirit of dissemination, the PRIS Study Group has made these handoff bundle materials downloadable, for free, by any individual or institution at www.ipasshandoffstudy.com. This type of open source content will benefit the greater PHM community to implement, evaluate, and, if needed, tailor these practices to meet to their local needs.

PUBLICATION OF QI WORK

Publishing QI work offers the possibility of accelerating the translation of research into practice. Additionally, it provides pediatric hospitalists the opportunity for academic promotion through a different body of scholarly work other than traditional scientific research or educational research. The clinical demands of most pediatric hospitalists, combined with a lack of education in QI methodology and/or manuscript writing, present challenges for QI publication and recognition for these efforts. Guidelines do exist for QI publication. The Standards for Quality Improvement Reporting Excellence (SQUIRE) Guidelines for Quality Improvement Reporting were initially drafted in 2005 and revised in 2007. These guidelines have been accepted by editors of some journals relevant to PHM, which include *Pediatrics* and *Hospital Pediatrics*, and the *Journal of Hospital Medicine*. More recently, the SQUIRE guidelines were supplemented with an Explanation and Elaboration document, which is a companion to the SQUIRE guidelines that provides 1 or 2 examples from the published improvement literature, followed by an analysis of the example with respect to the specific guidelines intent. Further details are available at www.squire-statement.org.

INTRODUCTION TO COMPARATIVE EFFECTIVENESS

Comparative effectiveness studies have been conducted for the past several decades. However, the term "comparative effectiveness research" did not garner much attention until the passage of the American Reinvestment and Recovery Act of 2009, which allotted $1.1 billion to support this type of research. In 2009, the IOM Committee on Comparative Effectiveness Research Prioritization[15] and the Federal Coordinating Council for Comparative Effectiveness Research[16] submitted complementary reports with recommendations on how to prioritize topics for allocation of the new CER funds. The council has been superseded by the Patient-Centered Outcomes Research Institute, which was created under the Patient Protection and Affordable Care Act to foster comparative effectiveness and to formulate a "research project agenda."

The IOM Committee on Comparative Effectiveness has defined CER as the "generation and synthesis of evidence that compares the benefits and harms of alternative methods to prevent, diagnose, treat, and monitor a clinical condition or to improve the delivery of care." The purpose of CER is "to assist consumers, clinicians, purchasers, and policy makers to make informed decisions that will improve health care at both the individual and population level."[15] Other definitions of CER are available from the Federal Coordinating Council for Comparative Effectiveness Research (The US Department of Health and Human Services) and the AHRQ, which all share common themes.

The principal methods of CER are grounded in the traditions of clinical research (ie, randomized trials and observational research), outcomes research, decision analysis, and health services research.[17] The types of evidence that are considered CER include both the review of existing studies and data, in addition to the completion of new trials.[18] The following are the distinguishing elements of CER[17]:

1. Direct comparisons of active treatments
2. Studying patients and interventions that are representative of those who would receive the intervention in usual practice, thereby making the results more generalizable
3. Seeking patient-specific characteristics that account for variability in response to treatment
4. Patient/family-centered focus: Measuring all outcomes that are important to patients and their caregivers, including adverse ones

General questions that CER may answer include which drug is best for a given condition, which laboratory or radiologic studies are necessary to diagnose a certain condition, and which diagnostic tests are needed to monitor a chronic condition to improve delivery of care. Specific questions that are unique to the field of pediatric hospital medicine include the following:

1. What is the most effective treatment option for recurrent aspiration pneumonia: Gastrojejunostomy tube placement versus gastrostomy tube placement with Nissen fundoplication versus medical management and what are the specific patient characteristics that can guide our recommendations to families?
2. What is the best way to follow the response to treatment in patients with acute osteomyelitis?
3. What is the best approach for discharging our growing population of medically complex patients with special health care needs, which should include soliciting family reported outcomes of this process?

The quest that drives CER is to discover which interventions will lead to improved health for individual patients, as well as the population as a whole, with the fewest adverse effects.

COST-EFFECTIVENESS AND COMPARATIVE EFFECTIVENESS

It should be noted that none of the aforementioned definitions of CER explicitly make mention of cost or cost-effectiveness, although initial descriptions of CER did include discussion of cost.[19] This omission may have been out of fear that health care reform was the first step toward rationing.[20] By determining necessary tests and formulating cost-effective treatments, CER will identify wasteful practices that do not benefit patients. Potentially, there will be significant monetary savings, as 20% of routine practices are "rooted in outmoded habits" that add no value to patient outcomes.[21] This makes CER more in line with the term "parsimonious care," which "utilizes the most efficient means to effectively diagnose a condition and treat a patient."[22] It also is consistent with the Choosing Wisely initiative of the American Board of Internal Medicine, which has sparked specialty societies, including the SHM to identify specific ways in which physicians can reduce the overuse of tests and procedures to reduce costs.[23]

Including cost and cost-effectiveness analysis alongside CER seems both logical and necessary to significantly improve the value of health for patients. The American College of Physicians recently highlighted the need to provide cost-effectiveness data as part of the CER.[24] Their opinions are consistent with the recent push for a "value-based" national health care system, which may be one of the cornerstones of reimbursement in the future.[25] This concept of maximizing "value" was first proposed by Porter,[26] who defined value as the outcomes and services that matter to patients achieved relative to the costs incurred.

$$\text{Value} = \frac{\text{Quality}}{\text{Cost}}$$

Using that definition, improving quality is necessary but not sufficient. Most people would argue that it makes sense to substitute more costly diagnostic regimens and treatment for cheaper ones, as long as the quality of care is not adversely affected. However, the challenge of determining thresholds for what constitutes "cheaper" clinical strategies and determining thresholds for what constitutes "similar" levels of quality of care is one of the reasons why the debate over whether or not to include cost-effective analysis in CER remains.

EXAMPLES OF CER IN PEDIATRIC HOSPITAL MEDICINE

In recent years, pediatric researchers have used administrative databases to perform comparativeness effectiveness studies to investigate commonly encountered inpatient diagnoses, such as skin and soft tissue infections,[27] and urinary tract infections.[28] In addition, Zaoutis and colleagues[29] compared prolonged intravenous therapy versus early transition to oral antibiotic therapy for children with osteomyelitis and found that early transition was not associated with a higher risk of treatment failures. Treatment of children hospitalized with pneumonia has been extensively examined using comparative effective studies.[30–32] One example compared narrow versus broad-spectrum antimicrobial therapy for community-acquired pneumonia.[33] This study showed that narrow therapy was just as effective as broad-spectrum therapy.

Databases are attractive alternatives to clinical trials because they contain large numbers of patients, are readily accessible, and are relatively inexpensive.[34] Although they can provide crude knowledge about regional variations in utilization rates, they have significant limitations. For instance, they lack patient-reported validated measures of outcomes and are vulnerable to different types of confounding. Clinicians and policy makers will therefore need to be cautious about interpreting the results of observational studies and will need to incorporate and balance findings from other types of CER studies.

Studies have shown that the current evidence base is inadequate for half of all clinical decisions that a physician makes.[15] The need for CER is particularly urgent in the field of pediatric hospital medicine. First, we know there are significant and unwarranted variations in the resource utilization for the same conditions at different centers across the country.[12] Second, it remains unclear "what quality care actually represents"[13] for some of the most common inpatient diagnoses. For many years we have used "process measures" as proxies for quality measures. This is understandable because these are the easiest metrics to measure. Hospitalists need to come to together through collaboratives, such as the Value in Inpatient network, to decide what to compare, what to measure, and what "quality" actually means. Although the IOM committee identified 100 specific CER topics, very few were relevant to the pediatric inpatient setting.[35] As introduced earlier, a recent study by Keren and colleagues[12] used the Pediatric Health Information System (PHIS) administrative database to identify inpatient conditions that met the following 3 criteria: high prevalence, high total standardized cost, and a significant amount of variation in standardized cost per encounter. In this analysis of nearly 3.5 million admissions to 38 children's hospitals, there were 3 conditions that met all 3 criteria: surgical procedures for hypertrophy of tonsil and adenoids, tympanostomy tube place for otitis media, and acute appendicitis without peritonitis. The investigators highlighted 2 implications from the significant variation in the use of resources. Despite evidence that exists to support best practices, physicians are not following clinical practice guidelines, as has been shown in other studies.[36–38] More importantly, they concluded that the variation was a "symptom of major evidence gaps regarding best practices and highlight the need for more CER." Although the conditions they identified previously were surgical procedures, they also discovered numerous other conditions that are more relevant to pediatric hospitalists. Identification of these specific conditions is a tremendous first step. It allows for future targets of research to promote CER. The challenge will be in determining ways to prioritize these topics.

THE ROLE OF PEDIATRIC HOSPITALISTS IN CER

In preparing this article, the authors asked the following question to Dr Patrick Conway, Deputy Administrator for Innovation and Quality and CMS Chief medical officer: In 5 to 10 years, do you think value-based reimbursement will impact PHM and, if so, what can hospitalists do to be both informed and involved in this process? He said, "*I think that value-based reimbursement will start to impact pediatric hospitalists in 5 years or less. Specifically, hospitals will increasingly be paid based on quality performance and cost efficiency and hospital contracts will move toward more accountable care models. Pediatric hospitalists should consider learning about pediatric quality measures, reimbursement, and skills to improve quality across their system.*"

Currently there is a lack of education and training opportunities for those interested in becoming more informed and involved in CER.[39] There are 27 pediatric hospital medicine fellowships in 2014, some of which offer opportunities to obtain advanced degrees in research and/or training in CER methodology.[40] For hospitalists who work in university settings, there are also a number of university-affiliated federal training programs in CER.[41] Pursing a pediatric hospital medicine fellowship or an advanced degree in research methods is not a practical option for many. Although there is a lack of experienced faculty in QI methods, this gap is even more pronounced in the field of CER. The SHM executive committee recently established a mentorship program that matches mentors/mentees based on mutual interests.[42] To date, there have been 34 matched dyads. QI has been the most commonly listed area of interest/expertise by mentors, whereas CER thus far has not been listed as an area of expertise by any of the mentors who have submitted applications. The PHM and SHM annual meetings now include specific QI tracks in their programs. Future planning committees should consider complementing curricula with CER content to develop a more robust CER workforce. Finally, a recent study of pediatric hospitalists and residents demonstrated the lack of knowledge of physicians of the cost of a variety of medications and laboratory and radiologic tests.[43] Because cost is such an integral part of a value-based health care system and CER, hospitalists need to become more aware of health care costs to improve this value proposition.[44]

THE FUTURE OF QI AND CER IN PEDIATRIC HOSPITAL MEDICINE

The magnitude of the role in which the community of PHM physicians plays in the coming health care transformation is predicated on the following activities:

1. A commitment to
   a. Gaining mastery of QI and CER through a variety of educational mechanisms.
   b. Active participation in local projects and implementation of other's successes.
   c. The engagement of hospital leadership to provide support, mentorship, and the necessary infrastructure for continuous QI.
2. Participation in national collaboratives, networks, and partnerships to advance the rigor of QI and CER products that are generalizable and focused on patient outcomes.
3. Determining organizational-level metrics, consistent with accountable care organizations, that can be used as benchmarks for continuous QI and evidence of high-quality care.
4. Soliciting the support of professional societies, state and federal funding sources, and finding common threads with the private sector with vested interests in high-quality care and cost reduction.
5. The production of a rigorous body of scholarly work that will prioritize change, motivate the PHM community to examine local practices, adopt best practices, and ultimately stimulate further inquiries and produce future QI leaders.

REFERENCES

1. Chassin MR, Galvin RW. The urgent need to improve health care quality. Institute of Medicine national roundtable on health care quality. JAMA 1998;280(11): 1000–5.
2. Kohn LT, Corrigan JM, Donaldson MS. To err is human: building a safer health system. Washington, DC: National Academies Press; 2000.
3. Institute of Medicine. Crossing the quality chasm: a new health system for the 21st century. Washington, DC: National Academies Press; 2001.
4. Centers for Medicare and Medicaid Services. Available at: www.cms.gov/Research-Statistics-Data-and-Systems/Statistics-Trends-and-Reports/NationalHealthExpend Data/NationalHealthAccountsHistorical.html. Accessed January 30, 2014.
5. Robert Wood Johnson Foundation. Time to act: investing in the health of our children and communities. 2014. Available at: http://www.rwjf.org/en/research-publications/find-rwjf-research/2014/01/recommendations-from-the-rwjf-commission-to-build-a-healthier-am.html. Accessed January 30, 2014.
6. Institute of HealthCare Improvement. The IHI triple aim. Available at: https://ihi.org. Accessed January 30, 2014.
7. Ranso E, Joshi M, Nash D, et al, editors. The healthcare quality book. 2nd edition. Chicago: Health Administration Press; 2008.
8. Miles PV, Moyer VA. Quality improvement and maintenance of certification. Acad Pediatr 2013;13(Suppl 6):S14–5. http://dx.doi.org/10.1016/j.acap.2013.08.001.
9. The George Washington University. School of medicine and health sciences. Available at: http://smhs.gwu.edu. Accessed January 30, 2014.
10. Devers KJ, Foster L, Brach C. Nine states' use of collaboratives to improve children's health care quality in Medicaid and CHIP. Acad Pediatr 2013;13(Suppl 6): S95–102. http://dx.doi.org/10.1016/j.acap.2013.04.008.
11. Kairys S, Wasserman R, Pace W. Practice-based quality improvement/research networks: full speed forward. Acad Pediatr 2013;13(Suppl 6):S12–3. http://dx.doi.org/10.1016/j.acap.2013.02.001.
12. Keren R, Luan X, Localio R, et al. Prioritization of comparative effectiveness research topics in hospital pediatrics. Arch Pediatr Adolesc Med 2012;166(12): 1155–64. http://dx.doi.org/10.1001/archpediatrics.2012.1266.
13. Simon TD, Starmer AJ, Conway PH, et al. Quality improvement research in pediatric hospital medicine and the role of the Pediatric Research in Inpatient Settings (PRIS) network. Acad Pediatr 2013;13(Suppl 6):S54–60. http://dx.doi.org/10.1016/j.acap.2013.04.006.
14. Starmer AJ, Sectish TC, Simon DW, et al. Rates of medical errors and preventable adverse events among hospitalized children following implementation of a resident handoff bundle. JAMA 2013;310(21):2262–70. http://dx.doi.org/10.1001/jama.2013.281961.
15. Institute of Medicine. Initial national priorities for comparative effectiveness research. Washington, DC: National Academies Press; 2009.
16. US Department of Health and Human Services. Federal coordinating council for comparative effectiveness research report to the president and the congress. Washington, DC: US Department of Health and Human Services; 2009.
17. Garber AM, Sox HC. The role of costs in comparative effectiveness research. Health Aff (Millwood) 2010;29(10):1805–11. http://dx.doi.org/10.1377/hlthaff.2010.0647.
18. Prosser LA. Comparative effectiveness and child health. Pharmacoeconomics 2012;30(8):637–45. http://dx.doi.org/10.2165/11633830-000000000-00000.

19. Wilensky GR. Developing a center for comparative effectiveness information. Health Aff (Millwood) 2006;25(6):w572–85. http://dx.doi.org/10.1377/hlthaff.25. w572.

20. Weinstein MC. Comparative effectiveness and health care spending—implications for reform. N Engl J Med 2010;362(5):460–5.

21. Berwick DM, Hackbarth AD. Eliminating waste in US health care. JAMA 2012; 307(14):1513–6. http://dx.doi.org/10.1001/jama.2012.362.

22. Snyder L, American College of Physicians Ethics, Professionalism, and Human Rights Committee. American College of Physicians ethics manual: sixth edition. Ann Intern Med 2012;156(1 Pt 2):73–104. http://dx.doi.org/10.7326/0003-4819-156-1-201201031-00001.

23. Cassel CK, Guest JA. Choosing wisely: helping physicians and patients make smart decisions about their care. JAMA 2012;307(17):1801–2. http://dx.doi.org/10.1001/jama.2012.476.

24. American College of Physicians. Information on cost-effectiveness: an essential product of a national comparative effectiveness program. Ann Intern Med 2008;148(12):956–61.

25. United States Department of Health & Human Services. Value-driven health care home. Available at: http://www.hhs.gov/valuedriven/index.html. Accessed January 18, 2014.

26. Porter ME. What is value in health care? N Engl J Med 2010;363(26):2477–81. http://dx.doi.org/10.1056/NEJMp1011024.

27. Williams DJ, Cooper WO, Kaltenbach LA, et al. Comparative effectiveness of antibiotic treatment strategies for pediatric skin and soft-tissue infections. Pediatrics 2011;128(3):e479–87. http://dx.doi.org/10.1542/peds.2010-3681.

28. Conway PH, Keren R. Factors associated with variability in outcomes for children hospitalized with urinary tract infection. J Pediatr 2009;15(6):789–96.

29. Zaoutis T, Localio AR, Leckerman K, et al. Prolonged intravenous therapy versus early transition to oral antimicrobial therapy for acute osteomyelitis in children. Pediatrics 2009;123(2):636–42. http://dx.doi.org/10.1542/peds.2008-0596.

30. Leyenaar JK, Shieh MS, Lagu T, et al. Comparative effectiveness of ceftriaxone in combination with a macrolide compared with ceftriaxone alone for pediatric patients hospitalized with community acquired pneumonia. Pediatr Infect Dis J 2014;33(4):387–92. http://dx.doi.org/10.1097/INF.0000000000000119.

31. Shah SS, Hall M, Newland JG, et al. Comparative effectiveness of pleural drainage procedures for the treatment of complicated pneumonia in childhood. J Hosp Med 2011;6(5):256–63. http://dx.doi.org/10.1002/jhm.872.

32. Queen MA, Myers AL, Hall M, et al. Comparative effectiveness of empiric antibiotics for community-acquired pneumonia. Pediatrics 2014;133(1):e23–9. http://dx.doi.org/10.1542/peds.2013-1773.

33. Williams DJ, Hall M, Shah SS, et al. Narrow vs broad-spectrum antimicrobial therapy for children hospitalized with pneumonia. Pediatrics 2013;132(5):e1141–8. http://dx.doi.org/10.1542/peds.2013-1614.

34. Billings J. Using administrative data to monitor access, identify disparities, and assess performance of the safety net. Agency for Healthcare Research and Quality. Available at: http://archive.ahrq.gov/data/safetynet/billings.htm. Accessed January 15, 2014.

35. Institute of Medicine. Initial national priorities for comparative effectiveness research. Available at: http://www.iom.edu/~/media/Files/Report%20Files/2009/ComparativeEffectivenessResearchPriorities/CER%20report%20brief%2008-13-09.pdf. Accessed January 15, 2014.

36. Pronovost PJ. Enhancing physicians' use of clinical guidelines. JAMA 2013; 310(23):2501–2. http://dx.doi.org/10.1001/jama.2013.281334.

37. Cabana MD, Rand CS, Powe NR, et al. Why don't physicians follow clinical practice guidelines? A framework for improvement. JAMA 1999;282(15): 1458–65.

38. Kalu SU, Hall MC. A study of clinician adherence to treatment guidelines for otitis media with effusion. WMJ 2010;109(1):15–20.

39. Simpson LA, Peterson L, Lannon CM, et al. Special challenges in comparative effectiveness research on children's and adolescents' health. Health Aff (Millwood) 2010;29(10):1849–56. http://dx.doi.org/10.1377/hlthaff.2010.0594.

40. American Academy of Pediatrics. Section of hospital medicine—pediatric hospital medicine fellowship programs. Available at: http://www.aap.org/en-us/about-the-aap/Committees-Councils-Sections/Section-on-Hospital-Medicine/Pages/Hospitalist-Fellowship-Programs.aspx. Accessed January 15, 2014.

41. Agency for Health Care Research and Quality. Federal training programs in comparative effectiveness research. Available at: http://www.ahrq.gov/research/findings/final-reports/learningcollab/learningapb.html. Accessed January 14, 2014.

42. American Academy of Pediatrics. Section on hospital medicine—mentorship. Available at: http://www.aap.org/en-us/about-the-aap/Committees-Councils-Sections/Section-on-Hospital-Medicine/Pages/Mentorship.aspx. Accessed January 16, 2014.

43. Rock TA, Xiao R, Fieldston E. General pediatric attending physicians' and residents' knowledge of inpatient hospital finances. Pediatrics 2013;131(6): 1072–80. http://dx.doi.org/10.1542/peds.2012-1753.

44. Sachdeva R. The need for physician education in health care costs to enhance efficiencies in care delivery. Pediatrics 2013;131(6):1184–5. http://dx.doi.org/10.1542/peds.2013-0823.

Pediatric Sedation

Yasmeen N. Daud, MD, Douglas W. Carlson, MD*

KEYWORDS

- Sedation • Pediatric • Pre-sedation assessment • Patient selection
- Risk assessment • Monitoring • Credentialing • Pediatric hospitalist

KEY POINTS

- The roles, responsibilities, and skills of providers administering pediatric sedation continue to advance globally.
- Pediatric sedation providers should be trained in the principles and practice of sedation, which include patient selection, performing pre-sedation assessments to determine risks during sedation, selection of optimal of sedation medication, monitoring requirements, and post-sedation care.
- Collaboration with other sedation providers to partner in the training, certification, and ongoing maintenance of sedation skills are important in creating safe systems for pediatric sedation to be performed by pediatric hospitalists.

INTRODUCTION

The roles, responsibilities, and skills of providers administering pediatric sedation continue to advance globally. Pediatric sedation is a growing field involving not only new pharmacologic innovation but also the emerging roles of the sedation provider. Across the world, several different practitioners are currently providing pediatric sedation. This extensive list includes anesthesiologists, emergency medicine physicians, dentists, intensivists, pediatric hospitalists, pediatric subspecialists, radiologists, surgeons, nurse anesthetists, advanced nurse practitioners, and nurses.[1–3] Each of these specialties carries their own skill set for providing mild, moderate, and deep pediatric sedation. Providers of pediatric sedation must adhere to the principles and practices of pediatric sedation and maintain the skills necessary to provide safe sedation and recovery. In the United States several groups have published guidelines regarding the practice of pediatric sedation, including the American Academy of Pediatrics,[4] the American Academy of Pediatric Dentistry,[5] the American College of Emergency Physicians,[6] and the American Society of Anesthesiologists (ASA).[7] Accordingly, the

Disclosures: None.
Division of Pediatric Hospital Medicine, St. Louis Children's Hospital, Washington University School of Medicine, 660 South Euclid Avenue, NWT9, St Louis, MO 63049, USA
* Corresponding author.
E-mail address: carlson@wustl.edu

Pediatr Clin N Am 61 (2014) 703–717
http://dx.doi.org/10.1016/j.pcl.2014.05.003   **pediatric.theclinics.com**

Joint Commission of Healthcare Organization has incorporated these sedation guidelines into their Comprehensive Accreditation Manual for Hospitals.[8] Sedation services should be governed by institutional standards that incorporate national guidelines for pediatric sedation. Quality improvement measures must be used to monitor and review sedation practices. Credentialing and training programs should be available to non-Anesthesia providers to assure safe sedation practices.

PATIENT SELECTION AND PRE-SEDATION ASSESSMENT

Appropriate patient selection is a critical element in providing safe sedation. A thorough pre-sedation assessment must be completed for every pediatric patient before sedation. This evaluation should be focused on identifying potential risks for sedation and difficulty with airway management, and should include the reason for the sedation, active medical problems, and past medical problems (**Box 1**).

Certain patients have medical conditions that put them at high risk for complications during sedation. In general, patients with significant craniofacial abnormalities or history of upper airway abnormalities may have anatomic alterations to upper airway structures that would put them at risk for respiratory complications and difficult intubation.[9] Recognition of the increased risks of sedation in young infants must be appreciated. Infants younger than 6 months are at risk for respiratory depression and apnea.[9] Infants younger than 3 months should be sedated by anesthesiologists or intensivists. Given the same concerns with infants 3 to 6 months old, careful assessment and monitoring should be performed in this age group. Caution should be exercised with obese patients whose body mass index is greater than 95% on standard pediatric growth curves.[9] These children can be subject to reduction in lung volumes and compliance, are at risk for upper airway obstruction, can be difficult to ventilate using a bag-valve mask (BVM) technique, and can be difficult to intubate. Obese children also may have cardiac complications including hypertension and increased left ventricular mass/hypertrophy. Obese children who have significant symptoms or a diagnosis of obstructive sleep apnea should be sedated by an anesthesiologist or intensivist.

The patients' family history in relation to anesthesia/sedation complications or psychiatric history should also be obtained. It is important to document any allergies or sensitivities to medications and to list all current medications the patient is taking. Postmenarchal females and any girl 12 years and older should have a documented negative human chorionic gonadotropin before sedation.

Elective and urgent sedation cases should adhere to individual institution guidelines, which vary among pediatric facilities. Most institutions adopt standard ASA nil-by-mouth (NPO) guidelines for elective cases of 2 hours for liquids, 4 hours for breast milk, and 6 hours for formula/nonhuman milk in infants 6 months and younger, and 6 hours for solids for infants older than 6 months.[7] NPO status is controversial in the urgent setting. The risks and benefits must be considered before attempting to sedate patients in urgent situations.[10] Consideration must be made for available resources should complications arise during sedations performed for relatively urgent procedures. Anesthesia consultation should be sought if the procedure must happen emergently, NPO guidelines are not met, and there is a high risk for aspiration.

ASA classification should be determined for each patient to determine his or her current disease state (**Table 1**). It is important to identify which patients require further Anesthesia consultation or are more appropriate to be sedated by an anesthesiologist or intensivist. In general, patients with an ASA classification of I or II are appropriate for sedation by a trained sedation provider.[1–3,11–13] ASA class III patients should require a minimum of an anesthesiologist/intensivist consultation, and are best served by

---

Box 1
Potential risks for sedation

Active Medical Problems

Fever

Head/facial trauma

Depressed level of consciousness

Obesity

Reduced intravascular volume

Symptoms of sleep apnea

Snoring

Upper/lower airway issues

Upper respiratory infection (URI) symptoms

Uncontrolled seizures

Unfasted

Unstable psychiatric disorder

Past Medical Problems

Apnea

Craniofacial abnormalities

Genetic syndromes (eg, Down syndrome)

Hematologic/oncologic disease

History of postoperative nausea/vomiting

History of prior sedation complications

Liver dysfunction

Metabolic disorders

Myopathy or neurologic condition

Prematurity

Renal disease

Risk of aspiration

Significant cardiac disease

Significant dental problems/devices

Significant gastrointestinal condition

Tracheal abnormalities

Upper/lower airway issues

---

sedation providers with advanced training in sedation. Patients with ASA classification of IV or more should be sedated by an anesthesiologist or intensivist.

A detailed physical examination should be performed before any sedation, focusing on key elements that could pose potential risks or complications to the patient while under sedation. It is equally important to obtain baseline vital signs including temperature, heart rate, respiratory rate, blood pressure, oxygen saturation, weight, and pain score. The physical examination should include a thorough examination of the

Table 1	
Physical status classification of the American Society of Anesthesiologists	
Status	**Disease State**
I	A normal healthy patient
II	A patient with mild systemic disease
III	A patient with severe systemic disease
IV	A patient with severe systemic disease that is a constant threat to life
V	A moribund patient who has little chance of survival but is submitted to surgery as a last resort
VI	A declared brain-dead patient whose organs are being removed for donor purposes

From American Society of Anesthesiologists. Physical status classification system. Available at: http://www.asahq.org/For-Members/Clinical-Information/ASA-Physical-Status-Classification-System.aspx. Accessed April 1, 2014.

head and neck. Specific attention should be paid to craniofacial characteristics such as a short neck, small mandible, dysmorphic features, small mouth opening, large tongue, and enlarged tonsils. This evaluation will help to determine which patients are at more risk for difficult intubation or airway complications arising from sedation.

The Mallampati classification relates tongue size to pharyngeal size, and should be performed on every patient who is able to cooperate. This test is performed with the patient in the sitting position, the head held in a neutral position, the mouth wide open, and the tongue protruding to the maximum, with no vocalization. The subsequent classification is assigned based on the pharyngeal structures that are visible (**Box 2, Fig. 1**). Infants and children who are uncooperative should undergo a visual inspection of the oropharynx with a tongue depressor for any abnormalities. Referral to an anesthesiologist for sedation should be considered for patients with a Mallampati classification of IV.

A focused clinical examination including the cardiovascular and pulmonary systems is crucial. Any significant or unexpected findings such as a pathologic murmur, significant wheezing, or respiratory distress should be evaluated and treated before providing sedation. After performing a thorough sedation history and physical examination, the sedation provider must assess the proposed procedure or study for guidance in the selection of appropriate sedation agents.

INDICATIONS FOR SEDATION

It is important to consider the need for sedation, and which properties of sedation or combination thereof will be required to perform a procedure or study. These properties include mild/moderate/deep sedation, analgesia, amnesia, anxiolysis, and degree of immobility. It is equally important to ascertain the anticipated length of the procedure, as this plays an important role in determining optimal medications, redosing, or combinations of sedation agents. The pre-sedation assessment and physical

Box 2	
Mallampati classification	
Class	**Structures Visualized**
I	Soft palate, fauces, uvula, anterior and posterior pillars
II	Soft palate, fauces, uvula
III	Soft palate and base of the uvula
IV	Soft palate is not visible at all

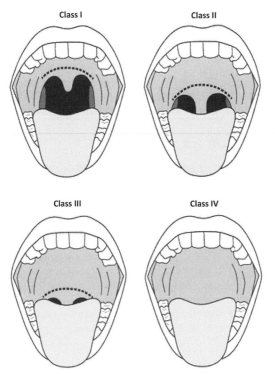

Fig. 1. Visual image of Mallampati classification. (*From* Vargo JJ, DeLegge MH, Feld AD, et al. Multisociety sedation curriculum for gastrointestinal endoscopy. Gastrointest Endosc 2012;76(1):e1–25; with permission.)

examination should alert the sedation provider as to which medications may pose greater sedation risks and complications, or which medications are contraindicated for specific patients. Providers who are relatively inexperienced should ask for assistance or Anesthesia consultation should they be asked to perform a sedation they think exceeds their abilities. The request for evening and overnight urgent sedations at risk for complications may be best delayed until appropriate personnel are available. Sedation providers must also be aware of institutional policies regarding which children are considered appropriate candidates for sedation, which targeted depth of sedation is acceptable, monitoring requirements, recovery and discharge criteria, and necessary documentation.

CHOOSING THE OPTIMAL SEDATION AGENT

Common medications used for pediatric sedation include midazolam, nitrous oxide, ketamine, pentobarbital, dexmedetomidine, and propofol. Of importance is that some of these medications used alone may not achieve the level of sedation required to complete a procedure or study. Several of these medications are used in combination to achieve optimal sedation; it is imperative that experienced, advanced sedation providers provide this type of sedation. It has been shown that the use of multiple sedation medications significantly increases the rates of adverse events.[14] Sedation providers must be aware of personal limitations in addition to those institutional policies and procedures that govern sedation. Sedation providers should have the ability to manage and rescue patients who progress to a deeper sedation level than was planned.[8] Appreciation of these issues is an important element in providing consistently safe sedation. For sedation providers with less experience or training, a one-drug sedation plan should be adopted. Sedation is much more predictable using one medication only to complete a study or procedure. It is imperative that the sedation provider be in control of all sedation medications, and supervises or personally discards the unused medication. **Boxes 3–8** summarize the general guidelines for medication selection for uncomplicated pediatric sedation.

LOCATION AND EQUIPMENT FOR SEDATION

Sedations should be performed in a location with which the sedation provider is familiar, thus aiding the ability of the sedation practitioner to manage unexpected complications with confidence in regard of the location of necessary rescue equipment.[32] The area should have monitoring and nearby oxygen available. There should be immediate access to rescue equipment, including crash cart, airway equipment, and rescue medications. It is important to assemble all of the equipment that may be needed for the sedation before administering medications. A common pneumonic (SOAPME) can be used to remind the sedation practitioner of all of the appropriate equipment that should be gathered before the sedation (**Table 2**).[4] Before undertaking a sedation, the sedation practitioner must understand which resources (anesthesia, critical care, respiratory therapy, immediately available nursing staff) are available should they be required, and how to access these resources rapidly.

THE SEDATION TEAM

Before performing sedation, it is best to assemble the team who will be providing direct care to the patient. The team leader should be the practitioner performing the sedation. A nurse or medical technician with sedation skills and/or pediatric advanced life support (PALS) training should also be with the patient at all times during both the sedation and recovery phases. The nurse should not have any other duties than monitoring the patient and assisting the physician when sedation complications arise. The team may also involve other physicians or staff when performing the procedure, such as a surgeon for abscess drainage or a radiology technician. Child life services and distraction

---

Box 3
Midazolam

Sedation properties	Anxiolysis, mild sedation	
Indications	Radiology examinations	**Examples**
	Brief studies/procedures (local anesthetic medications should be used for analgesia during procedures)	Bladder catheterization, computed tomography (CT), intravenous (IV) placement, lumbar puncture, minor laceration repair
Contraindications	Relative	
	Patients at high risk for respiratory depression	
	Previous prolonged agitation with midazolam	
Dosing	Inhaled IV	By mouth (PO)
	0.4 mg/kg 0.05 to 0.2 mg/kg	0.5 mg/kg
Adverse effects	Agitation, respiratory depression	

Box 4		
Nitrous oxide		
Sedation properties	Anxiolysis, amnesia, mild analgesia, mild/moderate sedation, relative immobility	
Indications	Short painful procedures Painful/difficult examinations	**Examples** Abscess incision and drainage (I&D), burn/wound debridement, bladder catheterization, Botox injection, Foreign body removal, joint aspiration/ injection, IV placement, laceration repair, lumbar puncture, examination for sexual assault, voiding cystourethrogram, wound care
Contraindications	**Relative** Current/previous bleomycin treatment Elevated intracranial pressure Methylene tetrahydrofolate reductase deficiency Vitamin B_{12} deficiency	**Absolute** Bowel obstruction Pneumothorax Recent intraocular surgery Recent tympanoplasty
Dosing	Inhaled 30% to 70% (higher concentrations provide enhanced analgesia and sedation)[12,15,16] PO oxycodone 0.2 to 0.3 mg/kg (maximum 10 mg) given 60 minutes prior can augment analgesia and sedation[12]	
Adverse effects	Nausea, vomiting, hallucinations, agitation	

techniques can greatly improve the comfort of the patient and sedation. There should be a discussion before sedation with the team that should include the intended procedure to be performed, the anticipated duration of procedure, the sedation plan including medications and dosages, anticipated difficulties, and reversal medications.

MONITORING, DOCUMENTATION, AND RECOVERY

Depending on the level of sedation, different monitoring devices may be used to observe the sedated patient. National guidelines should be followed and incorporated into individual institutional guidelines with regard to monitoring and documentation criteria.[4–8] The use of approved standard sedation documents provides assistance to the sedation provider in regard of monitoring guidelines and documentation. Sedation providers should be familiar with definitions regarding the depth of sedation. The University of Michigan Sedation Scale is a commonly used and reliable scoring system for the assessment of sedation level (**Table 3**).[33,34] Patients must be observed carefully with mild sedation, and will need regular assessment of the depth of sedation until they are fully awake.

Moderate sedation requires continuous monitoring of heart rate, and pulse oximetry to be recorded at regular intervals. Respiratory rate, blood pressure, and depth of sedation should be recorded at regular intervals on a sedation document. The same

Box 5 Ketamine			
Sedation properties	Amnesia, analgesia, dissociative (deep) sedation, relative immobility		
Indications	Brief painful procedures	**Examples**	
	Painful/difficult examinations		
	Short radiology procedures	Abscess I&D, burn/wound debridement, bone marrow biopsy, central line placement, chest tube placement, CT scan, foreign body removal, fracture reduction, joint aspiration/injection, laceration repair, lumbar puncture, medication implants, postoperative wound care, renal biopsy, examination for sexual assault	
Contraindications[17]	**Relative**	**Absolute**	
	Cardiac disease	Infants younger than 3 months	
	Current URI	Schizophrenia	
	Current pulmonary infection/ disease		
	Glaucoma, open globe injury		
	Hydrocephalus		
	Known/suspected intracranial tumor/disease		
	Procedures with manipulation in posterior pharynx		
	Porphyria		
	Thyroid disease		
Dosing[12,17–21]	IV	Intramuscular (IM)	
	Induction dose 1 to 2 mg/kg	Dose 3 to 4 mg/kg	
	Bolus dosing 0.5 to 1 mg/kg		
Adverse effects	Brief apnea, emesis; emergency reactions: agitation, hallucinations, laryngospasm, respiratory depression		

monitoring requirements should be used for deep sedation, recorded at 5-minute intervals. The use of end-tidal CO_2 monitoring should be considered during deep sedation and should be mandatory during prolonged radiology examinations when continuous medication infusions are used.[4] Changes in the numeric display or waveform can indicate hypoventilation, airway obstruction, and impeding apnea. Decreasing oxygen saturations occur late in hypoventilation and apnea, so it is important to use capnography to intervene before a significant respiratory event occurs. When administering nitrous oxide, nitrous gas monitoring should be used.

The recovery of sedated patients is as important as monitoring the patient during sedation. Patients who have undergone painful procedures and are still deeply sedated no longer have stimulus during the recovery phase. Hypoventilation and apnea are common events that may occur. The sedation provider should observe

Box 6
Pentobarbital

Sedation properties	Amnesia, deep sedation, immobility	
Indications	Radiology examinations	**Examples**
		CT, magnetic resonance imaging (MRI)
Contraindications	**Relative**	**Absolute**
	Patients with high risk for respiratory depression	Porphyria
Dosing	IV[22,23]	
	Induction dose 2 to 3 mg/kg	
	Bolus dose for induction 1 to 3 mg/kg, titrate maximum 6 mg/kg	
	May be augmented with IV midazolam 0.05 to 0.1 mg/kg	
Adverse effects	Agitation, prolonged recovery, respiratory depression	

sedated patients until they reach a level of sedation that may be transferred to the care of nursing staff, or are fully awake and ready for discharge. A commonly used tool is the Modified Aldrete Recovery Score, which assesses the level of recovery following sedation (**Table 4**).[35]

Specific criteria for discharge, transfer, or admission of a patient to another location should be strictly adhered to. Patients who are discharged home should be back to the pre-sedation state and Aldrete score. If the patient is returning to a hospital bed and the pre-sedation state and Aldrete score have not been reached, the patient should be closely monitored with continued observation and oxygen saturation until the

Box 7
Dexmedetomidine

Sedation properties	Deep sedation, Immobility	
Indications	Radiology examinations	**Examples**
	Brief studies	CT, MRI, electroencephalogram
Contraindications	**Relative**	**Absolute**
	Patients with reduced intravascular volume, URI	Active cardiac disease, arteriovenous malformations, hypotension, Moyamoya disease, patients receiving digoxin or α-blockers, recent stroke, symptoms of stroke
Dosing	Short Procedures[23–29]	Prolonged sedation IV[22,28]
	IV induction dose 2 μg/kg over 10 min	Induction dose 2 to 3 μg/kg over 10 min
	IV bolus dose for induction 1 to 2 μg/kg, titrate	Bolus dosing for induction 2 to 3 μg/kg, titrate × 2 doses
	IV maintenance infusion rate 1 μg/kg/h	Maintenance infusion rate 1 to 2 μg/kg/h, titrate to desired effect
	IM 1.0 to 4.5 μg/kg	
Adverse effects	Bradycardia, hypotension, transient hypertension, sinus arrest	

Box 8		
Propofol		
Sedation properties	Amnesia, deep sedation, immobility	
Indications	Prolonged radiology examinations	**Examples**
	Short procedures	Abscess I&D, burn/wound debridement, bone marrow biopsy, chest tube placement, central line placement, CT scan, foreign body removal, fracture reduction, joint aspiration/injection, laceration repair, lumbar puncture with intrathecal chemotherapy administration, medication implants, MRI, renal biopsy
Contraindications	**Relative**	**Absolute**[24]
	Patients with reduced intravascular volume, URI	Hypersensitivity to eggs, egg products, soybeans, or soy products; hypotension
Dosing	Short procedures IV[22,30] Induction dose 1 mg/kg Bolus dosing 0.5 to 1 mg/kg, titrate to desired effect	Prolonged sedation IV[22,31] Induction dose 2 mg/kg Bolus dosing for induction 1 to 2 mg/kg, titrate to desired effect Maintenance infusion rate 100 to 200 μg/kg/min, titrate to desired effect
Adverse effects	Apnea, bradycardia, hypotension, metabolic acidosis, respiratory depression, rhabdomyolysis	

Table 2		
SOAPME checklist for pediatric sedation		
S	Suction	Suction should be functioning and turned on before medications are administered with the appropriate suction catheter sizes
O	Oxygen	O_2 should be turned on and connected to a CPAP bag or BVM with the appropriate mask size
A	Airway	Airway equipment should be available with appropriate sizes, including nasal cannula, simple face masks, masks for CPAP/BVM, oral airways, nasopharyngeal airways, endotracheal tubes, laryngeal mask airways, and laryngeal blades
P	Pharmacy	Quick access to pharmacologic agents including reversal agents
M	Monitors	Electrocardiogram, respiratory rate, blood pressure, O_2 saturation, $\pm$ inspired N_2O/end-tidal N_2O and $\pm$ end-tidal CO_2 capnography should be placed on the patient before administration of sedation medication
E	Equipment	Nearby crash cart and defibrillator should be available

Abbreviations: BVM, bag-valve mask; CPAP, continuous positive airway pressure.

Data from American Academy of Pediatrics, American Academy of Pediatric Dentistry, Coté CJ, et al. Guidelines for monitoring and management of pediatric patients during and after sedation for diagnostic and therapeutic procedures: an update. Pediatrics 2006;118(6):2587–602.

Table 3 University of Michigan Sedation Scale	
Sedation Score	Description of Sedation Level
0	Awake and alert
1	Minimally sedated; tired/sleepy, appropriate response to verbal conversation and/or sound
2	Moderately sedated; somnolent/sleeping, easily aroused with light tactile stimulation or a simple verbal command
3	Deeply sedated; deep sleep, arousable with purposeful response to significant physical stimulation
4	Unarousable or nonpurposeful response to significant physical stimulation

Data from Malviya S, Voepel-Lewis T, Tait AR, et al. Depth of sedation in children undergoing computed tomography: validity and reliability of the University of Michigan Sedation Scale (UMSS). Br J Anaesth 2002;88:241–5; and Malviya S, Voepel-Lewis T, Ludomirsky A, et al. Can we improve the assessment of discharge readiness? A comparative study of observational and objective measures of depth of sedation in children. Anesthesiology 2004;100:218–24.

pre-sedation state is achieved. When transferring a patient, direct communication with the accepting physician and nursing staff regarding the procedure, sedation, complications, and current status of the patient should be initiated. Pain scores should also be assessed. When discharging patients, parents should be informed to monitor their children carefully while driving home if they are in car seats, as they may develop airway obstruction should they fall asleep en route.[4]

Table 4 Modified Aldrete Recovery Score	
Activity	Score
Able to move 4 extremities voluntarily or on command	2
Able to move 2 extremities voluntarily or on command	1
Able to move 0 extremities voluntarily or on command	0
Respiration	
Able to deep breathe and cough freely	2
Dyspnea or limited breathing	1
Apneic	0
Circulation	
BP $\pm$ 20% of preanesthetic level	2
BP $\pm$ 20%–50% of preanesthetic level	1
BP $\pm$ 50% or more of preanesthetic level	0
Consciousness	
Fully awake	2
Arousable with verbal stimulation	1
Not responding	0
Oxygen saturation	
O_2 saturation >92% on room air	2
Supplemental oxygen to maintain O_2 saturation >90%	1
O_2 saturation <90% with supplemental oxygen	0

Abbreviation: BP, blood pressure.
Data from Aldrete JA. The post-anesthesia recovery score revisited. J Clin Anesth 1995;7:89–91.

TRAINING, CREDENTIALING, AND CONTINUING EDUCATION

Perhaps the best way to ensure safe sedation practices among providers within an institution is to create a sedation service governed by a body that outlines clear guidelines of sedation practices within the scope of specialty.[36–38] Training, credentialing, and ongoing education of dedicated practitioners performing sedation is paramount to providing excellent clinical care.

A training program should be implemented for sedation providers, which may include didactic teaching sessions and simulation,[39] shadowing of sedations or exposure to various procedures such as intubation, laryngeal mask airway, and BVM maneuvers, in addition to documentation of adequate completion of the program.[37] Documentation via sedation and procedure logs can help to verify that practitioners have met the guidelines of the training program. A training program may be an adjunct to specific institutional policies regarding credentialing, or will align with the hospital credentialing process.

A sedation credentialing program should be used by pediatric institutions to provide the skills necessary for providers to perform safe sedation. The overall goals should be to train the provider to perform safe sedation while being able to manage airway complications, rescue patients who become more deeply sedated than planned, and deal with possible cardiovascular compromise. All sedation practitioners must be PALS certified. The principles of sedation should be reviewed. Training should include didactic teaching sessions regarding commonly used sedation medications, adverse reactions, contraindications, and rescue medications. A thorough understanding of the commonly used sedation medications is critical to performing safe sedation. There should also be a discussion of pre-sedation assessment of patients to determine which patients are appropriate for sedation and when Anesthesia should be consulted. Specific medical comorbidities that could pose a risk to the sedated patient should be reviewed. Before attempting independent sedations, practitioners should learn and practice advanced airway skills with anesthesiologists in the operating room, and perform supervised sedations with an experienced sedation provider.

Some form of annual continuing education will also need to take place to assess the knowledge and skills of current sedation providers and thereby ensure that safe practices are being met. This course could include scheduled simulation modules, a written test,[40] attendance at a pediatric sedation conference, online teaching tools, or scheduled lectures within an institution. The program should also include regular ongoing continuing sedation education for the provider. There should be a system in place to track each sedation and provider, such as quality improvement reports.

Pediatric hospitalists across the United States are providing safe sedation for pediatric patients in dedicated sedation units, emergency units, inpatient units, outpatient locations, radiology suites, and urgent care facilities.[1–3,13,22,31,36,37] As this practice continues to expand and the demand for sedation services continues to grow, pediatric hospitalists must be educated with the skills necessary to perform safe sedation.[1,13,22,31,36,37] Collaboration with other sedation providers to partner in the training, certification, and ongoing maintenance of sedation skills are important in creating safe systems for pediatric sedation to be performed by pediatric hospitalists.

REFERENCES

1. Monroe KK, Beach M, Reindel R, et al. Analysis of procedural sedation provided by pediatricians. Pediatr Int 2013;55(1):17–23.

2. Couloures KG, Beach M, Cravero JP, et al. Impact of provider specialty on pediatric procedural sedation complication rates. Pediatrics 2011;127(5): e1154–60.
3. Cravero JP, Beach ML, Blike GT, et al. The incidence and nature of adverse events during pediatric sedation/anesthesia with propofol for procedures outside the operating room: a report from the Pediatric Sedation Research Consortium. Anesth Analg 2009;108(3):795–804.
4. American Academy of Pediatrics, American Academy of Pediatric Dentistry, Coté CJ, et al. Guidelines for monitoring and management of pediatric patients during and after sedation for diagnostic and therapeutic procedures: an update. Pediatrics 2006;118(6):2587–602.
5. American Academy of Pediatric Dentistry. Guideline for monitoring and management of pediatric patients during and after sedation for diagnostic and therapeutic procedures. Pediatr Dent 2008-2009;30(Suppl 7):143–59. Available at: http://www.aapd.org/policies.
6. Mace SE, Brown LA, Francis L, et al. Clinical policy: critical issues in the sedation of pediatric patients in the emergency department. Ann Emerg Med 2008; 51(4):378–99, 399.e1–57.
7. American Society of Anesthesiologists Task Force on Sedation and Analgesia by Non-Anesthesiologists. Practice guidelines for sedation and analgesia by non-anesthesiologists. Anesthesiology 2002;96(4):1004–17.
8. Joint Commission on Accreditation of Healthcare Organizations. Sedation and anesthesia care standards. Oakbrook Terrace (IL): Joint Commission on Accreditation of Healthcare Organizations; 2003.
9. Ferrari LR. The pediatric airway: anatomy, challenges, and solutions. In: Mason KP, editor. Pediatric sedation outside of the operating room: a multispecialty international collaboration. New York: Springer Science + Business Media, LLC; 2012. p. 61–76.
10. Green SM, Roback MG, Miner JR, et al. Fasting and emergency department procedural sedation and analgesia: a consensus-based clinical practice advisory. Ann Emerg Med 2007;49(4):454–61.
11. Caperell K, Pitetti R. Is higher ASA class associated with an increased incidence of adverse events during procedural sedation in a pediatric emergency department? Pediatr Emerg Care 2009;25(10):661–4.
12. Mallory MD, Baxter AL, Yanosky DJ, et al. Emergency physician-administered propofol sedation: a report on 25,433 sedations from the Pediatric Sedation Research Consortium. Ann Emerg Med 2011;57(5):462–8.e1.
13. Srinivasan M, Carlson DW. Procedural sedation by pediatric hospitalists: analysis of the nature and incidence of complications during ketamine and nitrous oxide sedation. Hosp Pediatr 2013;3(4):342–7.
14. Coté CJ, Karl HW, Notterman DA, et al. Adverse sedation events in pediatrics: analysis of medications used for sedation. Pediatrics 2000;106(4):633–44.
15. Zier JL, Liu M. Safety of high-concentration nitrous oxide by nasal mask for pediatric procedural sedation: experience with 7802 cases. Pediatr Emerg Care 2011; 27(12):1107–12.
16. Babl FE, Oakley E, Seaman C, et al. High-concentration nitrous oxide for procedural sedation in children: adverse events and depth of sedation. Pediatrics 2008;121(3):e528–32.
17. Green SM, Roback MG, Kennedy RM, et al. Clinical practice guideline for emergency department ketamine dissociative sedation: 2011 update. Ann Emerg Med 2011;57(5):449–61.

18. Green SM, Roback MG, Krauss B, et al. Predictors of airway and respiratory adverse events with ketamine sedation in the emergency department: an individual-patient data meta-analysis of 8,282 children. Ann Emerg Med 2009; 54(2):158–68.e1–4.

19. Green SM, Roback MG, Krauss B, et al. Predictors of emesis and recovery agitation with emergency department ketamine sedation: an individual-patient data meta-analysis of 8,282 children. Ann Emerg Med 2009;54(2):171–80.e1–4.

20. Roback MG, Wathen JE, MacKenzie T, et al. A randomized, controlled trial of IV versus IM ketamine for sedation of pediatric patients receiving emergency department orthopedic procedures. Ann Emerg Med 2006;48(5):605–12.

21. Green SM, Krauss B. Clinical practice guideline for emergency department ketamine dissociative sedation in children. Ann Emerg Med 2004;44(5):460–71.

22. Carlson DW. The Pediatric Hospital Medicine Sedation Service; models, protocols, and challenges. In: Mason KP, editor. Pediatric sedation outside of the operating room: a multispecialty international collaboration. New York: Springer Science + Business Media, LLC; 2012. p. 61–76.

23. Mason KP, Prescilla R, Fontaine PJ, et al. Pediatric CT sedation: comparison of dexmedetomidine and pentobarbital. AJR Am J Roentgenol 2011;196(2): W194–8.

24. Mason KP, Lubisch N, Robinson F, et al. Intramuscular dexmedetomidine: an effective route of sedation preserves background activity for pediatric electroencephalograms. J Pediatr 2012;161(5):927–32.

25. McMorrow SP, Abramo TJ. Dexmedetomidine sedation: uses in pediatric procedural sedation outside the operating room. Pediatr Emerg Care 2012;28(3): 292–6.

26. Mason KP, Lerman J. Review article: Dexmedetomidine in children: current knowledge and future applications. Anesth Analg 2011;113(5):1129–42.

27. Mason KP, Lubisch NB, Robinson F, et al. Intramuscular dexmedetomidine sedation for pediatric MRI and CT. AJR Am J Roentgenol 2011;197(3):720–5.

28. Mason JP, Zurakowski D, Zgleszewski SE, et al. High dose dexmedetomidine as the sole sedative for pediatric MRI. Paediatr Anaesth 2008;18:403–11.

29. Mason KP, Zgleszewski SE, Dearden JL, et al. Dexmedetomidine for pediatric sedation for computed tomography imaging studies. Anesth Analg 2006; 103(1):57–62.

30. Miner JR, Burton JH. Clinical practice advisory: emergency department procedural sedation with propofol. Ann Emerg Med 2007;50:182–7, 187.e1.

31. Srinivasan M, Turmelle M, DePalma LM, et al. Procedural sedation for diagnostic imaging in children by pediatric hospitalists using propofol: analysis of the nature, frequency, and predictors of adverse events and interventions. J Pediatr 2012;160(5):801–6.e1.

32. Metzner J, Posner KL, Domino KB. The risk and safety of anesthesia at remote locations: the US closed claims analysis. Curr Opin Anaesthesiol 2009;22(4): 502–8.

33. Malviya S, Voepel-Lewis T, Tait AR, et al. Depth of sedation in children undergoing computed tomography: validity and reliability of the University of Michigan Sedation Scale (UMSS). Br J Anaesth 2002;88:241–5.

34. Malviya S, Voepel-Lewis T, Ludomirsky A, et al. Can we improve the assessment of discharge readiness? A comparative study of observational and objective measures of depth of sedation in children. Anesthesiology 2004;100:218–24.

35. Aldrete JA. The post-anesthesia recovery score revisited. J Clin Anesth 1995;7: 89–91.

36. Doctor K, Roback MG, Teach SJ. An update on pediatric hospital-based sedation. Curr Opin Pediatr 2013;25(3):310–6.
37. Turmelle M, Moscoso LM, Hamlin KP, et al. Development of a pediatric hospitalist sedation service: training and implementation. J Hosp Med 2012;7(4):335–9.
38. Yamamoto LG. Initiating a hospital-wide pediatric sedation service provided by emergency physicians. Clin Pediatr (Phila) 2008;47(1):37–48.
39. Shavit I, et al. Enhancing patient safety during pediatric sedation: the impact of simulation-based training of nonanesthesiologists. Arch Pediatr Adolesc Med 2007;161(8):740–3.
40. Srinivasan M, Carlson DW. A proposed mechanism to assess knowledge of pediatric hospitalists to identify and manage rare events during procedural sedation. Hosp Pediatr 2013;3(4):381–5.

Pediatric Palliative Care

Preface

Caring for Children Living with Life-Threatening Illness: A Growing Relationship Between Pediatric Hospital Medicine and Pediatric Palliative Care

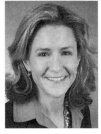
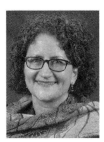

Christina K. Ullrich, MD, MPH   Joanne Wolfe, MD, MPH
Editors

HOSPITAL CARE FOR CHILDREN LIVING WITH LIFE-THREATENING ILLNESS

Recent decades have produced a host of medical and technological innovations for children with life-threatening illness (LTI). These advances, while potentially life-prolonging, only sometimes offer the possibility of cure. As a result, many conditions once acute and fatal have been transformed into chronic LTI with which children may live for years.

While some treatment advances have resulted in unquestionable benefits for children, they often have collateral effects on the child and family. One significant effect, increased hospital-based care, is the focus of this issue. Frequent or prolonged hospitalizations may afford children opportunities to benefit from tremendous treatments and technologies. They often simultaneously result in child distress and family disruption. And while hospitals are equipped to provide highly technical treatments and afford meticulous physical care, they are not necessarily geared to comprehensively meet the emotional, social, and spiritual needs of children and families.

Furthermore, the landscape of hospital care that families must navigate today is progressively more fragmented and complex. Transitions to and from the acute care hospital setting for children with complex conditions are increasingly common.[1] Adolescents/young adults with LTI, living longer, also face transitions to adult care settings. As they make these transitions, patients and families need models of care emphasizing clear communication, attention to complexities of care, and a focus on their values and goals.

Pediatr Clin N Am 61 (2014) xxi–xxiii
http://dx.doi.org/10.1016/j.pcl.2014.05.004
0031-3955/14/$ – see front matter © 2014 Elsevier Inc. All rights reserved.

pediatric.theclinics.com

THE CHALLENGE: ENSURING MORE CARE IS BETTER CARE

The rising tide of treatment options for families to consider has also outpaced the development of strategies to assist them as they consider the full range of benefits and burdens of treatments before their adoption. Treatments are often presented by subspecialists focused on a single organ system or pathophysiologic process, in a cure-oriented and intervention-oriented setting. For clinicians with a hospital-based vantage point, the lived experience of the "whole person" beyond the walls of acute care hospital is often obscured.[2]

Hospital clinicians, as experts in the care of acutely ill children, play a key role in the care of children with LTI, including communicating with families about prognosis and exploring treatment options and implications for the child and family. However, hospital clinicians often function in a fragmented and uncoordinated health care system with frequently rotating staff and mounting time and fiscal pressures. They are often challenged to find the time and availability to delve sufficiently into the beliefs, values, hopes, fears, and lived experience of the hospitalized child and family to provide optimal care centered around the overall well-being of the child and family.

HOSPITAL MEDICINE AND PEDIATRIC PALLIATIVE CARE TOGETHER: OPTIMIZING CARE FOR CHILDREN WITH LTI

Increased collaboration between hospital-based clinicians and pediatric palliative care (PPC) teams to care for children with LTI is a promising strategy to address many of the challenges described above. Through an interdisciplinary approach, PPC emphasizes honest and clear communication to support family understanding of diagnosis, prognosis, and the full range of treatment options, with their attendant benefits and burdens, with an eye toward maximizing well-being, comfort, quality of life, and meaningful experiences for both the child and the family. The number of hospital-based PPC programs has increased dramatically in recent years[3] to help meet the growing needs of hospitalized children with LTI.[4]

At the same time, palliative care need not be delivered solely by PPC specialists.[5] Hospital clinicians are positioned to provide "primary" palliative care, such as prioritizing honest, clear, and compassionate communication to discuss goals of care or medical decisions with families, or promoting comfort and quality of life. A palliative care approach, which begins with eliciting family values and hopes for the child and allows families to integrate relevant information and make the best decisions for their child, can be used by hospital-based palliative care "generalists" and palliative care specialists alike. In certain more complex or challenging situations, PPC specialists and hospital clinicians may collaborate, each lending complementary expertise and perspectives.

Regardless of who provides PPC, it must not be reserved solely for end of life. Families benefit from PPC throughout the course of illness. If the child dies, PPC may allow them to be better prepared for those difficult moments at the close of their child's life. Because this process takes time, PPC should be implemented as early as possible.

In that same vein, PPC is provided concurrently with disease-directed/life-extending treatment. PPC aims to optimize the well-being of children with LTI and their families, with an eye toward goal-consistent care. Families often hope that their child may live as long as possible and as well as possible. Hopes and efforts to support these dual goals can coexist.

Given these considerations, it is evident that the topics of PPC and hospital medicine are fitting counterparts for an issue of *Pediatric Clinics of North America*. We have assembled a series of articles focused on optimizing the care and well-being of hospitalized children with LTI, which is relevant to the practice of all clinicians caring for seriously ill children in the hospital setting. Caring for children with LTI may present challenges, but it is also immensely inspiring and gratifying. It is our hope that this issue is of interest and value to those who have the honor of caring for such children and their families.

Christina K. Ullrich, MD, MPH
Division of Pediatric Palliative Care
Department of Psychosocial Oncology and Palliative Care
Department of Pediatric Hematology/Oncology
Dana-Farber Cancer Institute
450 Brookline Avenue
Dana 1102
Boston, MA, 02215, USA

Joanne Wolfe, MD, MPH
Division of Pediatric Palliative Care
Department of Psychosocial Oncology and Palliative Care
Dana-Farber Cancer Institute
450 Brookline Avenue
Dana 2012
Boston, MA 02215, USA

E-mail addresses:
Christina_Ullrich@dfci.harvard.edu (C.K. Ullrich)
Joanne_Wolfe@dfci.harvard.edu (J. Wolfe)

REFERENCES

1. Berry JG, Hall DE, Kuo DZ, et al. Hospital utilization and characteristics of patients experiencing recurrent readmissions within children's hospitals. JAMA 2011;305(7):682–90.
2. Lamas D. Chronic critical illness. N Engl J Med 2014;370(2):175–7.
3. Feudtner C, Womer J, Augustin R, et al. Pediatric palliative care programs in children's hospitals: a cross-sectional national survey. Pediatrics 2013;132(6): 1063–70.
4. Feudtner C, Kang T, Hexem K, et al. Pediatric palliative care patients: a prospective multicenter cohort study. Pediatrics 2011;127(6):1094–101.
5. Quill T, Abernethy A. Generalist plus specialist palliative care—creating a more sustainable model. N Engl J Med 2013;368(13):1173–5.

Pediatric Hospital Care for Children with Life-threatening Illness and the Role of Palliative Care

Jori F. Bogetz, MD[a],*, Christina K. Ullrich, MD, MPH[b],
Jay G. Berry, MD, MPH[c]

KEYWORDS

- Pediatric • Child • Palliative care • Chronic disease • Life-threatening illness
- Hospitalization • Hospital care • Health care reform

KEY POINTS

- Hospitals are challenged to provide high-quality care to an increasingly complex group of children with life-threatening illness (LTI) who sometimes receive suboptimal care.
- All medical providers have the potential to improve care for hospitalized children with LTI by understanding and maintaining competence in palliative care practices.
- Health care reforms led by the Patient Protection and Affordable Care Act and Medicaid and state-based initiatives are broadening access to palliative care for children with LTI and their families.

OVERVIEW

The landscape of hospital care for children is changing. Hospital providers are challenged to provide high-quality care to an increasingly complex group of children with life-threatening illness (LTI). These children often have disabling comorbid conditions that worsen over time through acute exacerbations and chronic relapses. Hospitalizations for children with LTI are prevalent, lengthy, and costly. Often children with LTI experience suboptimal care that is characterized by fragmented and

Disclosure: The authors have no disclosures or conflicts of interests to report.
[a] Division of General Pediatrics, Department of Pediatrics, Lucile Packard Children's Hospital, Stanford University School of Medicine, 770 Welch Road, Suite 100, Palo Alto, CA 94304, USA; [b] Pediatric Palliative Care and Pediatric Hematology/Oncology, Dana-Farber Cancer Institute and Boston Children's Hospital, Harvard Medical School, 450 Brookline Avenue, Boston, MA 02215, USA; [c] Division of General Pediatrics, Department of Pediatrics, Boston Children's Hospital, Harvard Medical School, Room 212.2, 21 Autumn Street, Boston, MA 02115, USA
* Corresponding author.
E-mail address: jbogetz@stanford.edu

Pediatr Clin N Am 61 (2014) 719–733
http://dx.doi.org/10.1016/j.pcl.2014.05.002
0031-3955/14/$ – see front matter © 2014 Elsevier Inc. All rights reserved.

pediatric.theclinics.com

uncoordinated decision making, poor health information management, reactive care planning, overmedicalization, and inadequate involvement of family caregivers.[1–3]

Incorporation of pediatric palliative care for children with LTI throughout the course of their lives may improve the quality of care these children receive. For hospitalized children with LTI, pediatric palliative care is ideally delivered when integrated concurrently with disease-directed therapies. However, the workforce of pediatricians who specialize in palliative care is not sufficiently large to care for all hospitalized children who have palliative care needs. Pediatric hospital providers of all kinds (eg, hospitalists, specialists, surgeons, nurses, social workers) are increasingly being required to provide basic pediatric palliative care. These hospital providers should understand and maintain competence in palliative care practices.

Hospitals may also benefit from a better understanding of how children with LTI, pediatric palliative care, and health care reform are related. Emerging evidence suggests that palliative care is associated with improved quality of care and decreased hospital use for patients with LTI.[4–6] National health care reform efforts such as the Patient Protection and Affordable Care Act (ACA) and state and Medicaid-based initiatives are enabling early palliative care for children with LTI. In time, investigations of these reform efforts and others will help determine the most effective way to deliver palliative care to children with LTI and to optimize their health and well-being.

PART 1: THE CURRENT LANDSCAPE OF PEDIATRIC HOSPITAL CARE

CASE VIGNETTE

At birth, Jonathan's parents thought he was healthy. However, within days they noticed that his muscles were floppy and that breastfeeding was a challenge for him. Jonathan's doctors were concerned about him too. Magnetic resonance imaging of his brain revealed lissencephaly, a rare congenital malformation of the brain with a poor prognosis. The doctors told Jonathan's parents that he would not develop like a normal child and he would not survive as long either. Jonathan's parents were devastated to hear this news.

Over the following 2 years, Jonathan developed disabling comorbid conditions, including oromotor dysfunction, gastroesophageal reflux, and hip dysplasia. He developed pneumonia often and was hospitalized 5 times. Each time Jonathan was hospitalized, a new team of hospital doctors and nurses cared for him and they consistently sent Jonathan and his family home with more things to do in an effort to keep him healthy, such as more suctioning, more nebulizer treatments, more oxygen, and more medications. His parents were not sure whether these treatments were helping him.

During Jonathan's sixth hospitalization, his doctors recommended a Nissen fundoplication and gastrostomy tube to help with his gastroesophageal reflux and difficulty feeding. His family agreed. His surgery was complicated by postoperative agitation, which required 2 extra weeks in the hospital. The agitation never fully went away after the surgery, but Jonathan and his family left the hospital because there was nothing else the hospital team could do to help. A week after being home, Jonathan was readmitted to the hospital with a skin infection around his gastrostomy tube. The infection worsened his agitation. Jonathan's parents noticed that he was becoming increasingly weak and less interactive. They were frustrated and worried about him.

Hospital providers are challenged to provide high-quality care to an increasingly complex group of children with LTI. Children with LTI have chronic illnesses such as cancer, cerebral palsy spastic quadriplegia, congenital heart disease, cystic fibrosis, metabolic disorders, and sickle cell anemia.[7,8] Although many chronic illnesses in children have no cure, advances in surgical, intensive, and home care have enabled many of these children to live longer through control of their underlying illness and related comorbid conditions.[9] Despite constituting less than 1% of the pediatric population, there is also a growing presence of children with LTI in hospitals (**Fig. 1**).[2,3,10,11] Over the past 2 decades, rates of hospitalizations for children with LTI have doubled.[12] As of 2006, children with LTI accounted for approximately 10% of all hospital admissions, 25% of all hospital bed days, and 40% of all hospital charges in the United States.[13] Between 2006 and 2010, children with LTI and comorbid conditions affecting multiple organ system were the fastest growing population of patients to use children's hospitals.[10] In 2010 these children accounted for about one-third of patients and one-half of inpatient costs in children's hospitals.[10]

Many hospitalizations for children with LTI are for the treatment of disabling comorbid conditions that tend to worsen over time.[14–18] For example, nearly 50% of children with severe cerebral palsy develop comorbidities that substantially impair their digestive, respiratory, musculoskeletal, and urinary systems.[14–16] In recent years, invasive procedures (eg, spinal fusion for scoliosis) and initiation of medical technology (eg, gastrostomy tube for digestive impairment) in the inpatient setting have been increasingly used to treat these comorbidities.[15,19] In most cases, these treatments do not cure children of their LTI or their related comorbidities.[17,18,20–22] In fact, nearly one-third of children with severe neurologic impairment (eg, those children living in a minimally conscious state) do not survive 3 years after gastrostomy[21] and one-half do not survive 5 years after tracheotomy.[22] Moreover, these treatments are associated with their own complications and adverse events that are also predominately treated in the inpatient setting and that lead to more hospitalizations.[11,23,24] Illness categories for various LTI are shown in **Table 1**.

Many children with LTI experience multiple recurrent hospitalizations because of their fragile health status and substandard hospital discharge and follow-up care. The presence of LTI in a hospitalized child greatly increases the likelihood that their health will worsen after discharge and that an unplanned hospital readmission will occur.[23,25–27] Children with LTI such as sickle cell disease, hydrocephalus, or tracheostomy experience 30-day readmission rates at or greater than 25%.[24,25] Nearly one-quarter of inpatient costs in children's hospitals are attributable to children with LTI who experience 5 or more recurrent readmissions in a year.[11] Hospital discharge care for a child with LTI can be challenging, especially when the hospital providers are unfamiliar with the child and family, and when the child relies on multiple medications

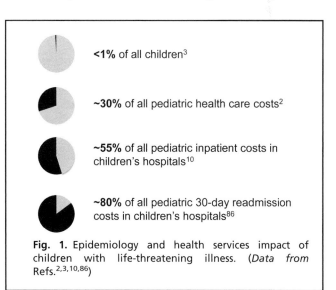

<1% of all children[3]

~30% of all pediatric health care costs[2]

~55% of all pediatric inpatient costs in children's hospitals[10]

~80% of all pediatric 30-day readmission costs in children's hospitals[86]

Fig. 1. Epidemiology and health services impact of children with life-threatening illness. (*Data from* Refs.[2,3,10,86])

Table 1	
Categories of life-threatening illness and example diagnoses of children who might benefit from palliative care	
Illness Category	Diagnoses
Conditions that can be cured but have the possibility of death	Acute leukemia Transposition of the great arteries Severe sepsis
Conditions that have no cure and premature death may be inevitable but whose symptoms can be managed	Down syndrome Sickle cell anemia Diabetes mellitus type I
Conditions requiring intensive medical therapy that are ultimately terminal	Cystic fibrosis Liver transplantation after liver failure Tracheostomy for respiratory failure
Severe neurologic impairments in which complications may lead to early death	Leukodystrophy Severe cerebral palsy Spina bifida

Adapted from Widdas D, McNamara K, Edwards F. A core care pathway for children with life-limiting and life-threatening conditions. 3rd edition. Bristol (UK): Together for Short Lives; 2013. Available at: http://www.togetherforshortlives.org.uk/assets/0000/4121/TfSL_A_Core_Care_Pathway__ONLINE_.pdf.

and medical equipment[9] without sufficient postdischarge community and home care support.[2] Children with LTI are also more likely to experience recurrent hospitalizations when their parents think that their child is not ready to leave the hospital and when their parents are uncertain about how to manage their child's health after discharge.[28] These remain important areas for research and care improvement initiatives in the future.

At the end-of-life, hospitals are still the usual site for death in children with LTI. About 60% of children with LTI die in the hospital, with one-half of those deaths occurring in an intensive care unit.[29,30] Cardiovascular, neuromuscular, and oncologic diagnoses are the most common types of LTI in children who die in the hospital. One-fourth of children with LTI who die in the hospital have LTI affecting multiple organ systems and many die after a prolonged hospitalization that includes life-sustaining treatments (eg, mechanical ventilation) or major surgery.[29] Children pursuing curative or restorative treatment such as bone marrow transplantation for cancer[31] or lung transplantation for cystic fibrosis[32] are more likely to die with fewer opportunities to plan for end-of-life care compared with other children with LTI. Hospital teams must attend to the physical, emotional, and spiritual needs of a dying child and their family. Unmet end-of-life needs may have lasting consequences for the bereaved. For example, inadequate relief from pain or psychological symptoms and a difficult moment of death are associated with increased guilt in bereaved parents.[33]

In other care settings many children with LTI experience suboptimal care that is characterized by fragmented and uncoordinated decision making, poor health information management, reactive care planning, overmedicalization, and inadequate involvement of family caregivers.[1–3] In many cases, these children do not have an outpatient or community provider who oversees their care and is knowledgeable of their overall health status and well-being. Without guidance from such a provider, attending to acute health problems in the context of the child's overall health is challenging for hospital providers. Adverse events can occur when these providers are unfamiliar with the nuances of the child's condition and there is poor communication among providers.[34] In addition, hospital staff may be hesitant to initiate discussions about the child's long-term prognosis and goals of care because they lack prognostic information and long-standing communication with these children and their families.[35] Without these discussions, uninformed decisions to pursue inpatient and postdischarge treatments and procedures that may not benefit the child are more likely to occur. Whenever possible, the child's end-of-life care should be discussed in advance of the child's death. Most hospitalists do not acknowledge the possibility of dying with seriously ill patients and focus on the biomedical issues instead.[36] The increasing prevalence of children with LTI and the complex nature of their illnesses implore inpatient health care providers to find better ways to improve care for children with LTI. Early concurrent integration of pediatric palliative care may be one strategy to achieve this goal.

PART 2: THE CONNECTION BETWEEN PALLIATIVE CARE AND HOSPITAL CARE FOR CHILDREN

CASE VIGNETTE

When Jonathan turned 3 years old, he developed pneumonia again. This pneumonia was severe and he was admitted to the intensive care unit for mechanical ventilation. After many weeks, his doctors mentioned placing a tracheostomy tube to help him breathe, clear his secretions, and treat his pneumonia. To Jonathan's parents a tracheostomy tube was a scary idea.

Over time, Jonathan's parents connected with his hospital team. Together, they talked about Jonathan's prognosis and quality of life. They shared their hopes and fears about caring for Jonathan as he got older and bigger. Hospital staff explained to his parents the connection between his lissencephaly and many of the health problems he was experiencing. They explained that, even with a tracheotomy, they could not cure Jonathan's problems. For the first time, Jonathan's parents felt like they could understand his health conditions and that their concerns were being heard.

Over the following weeks, Jonathan's pneumonia resolved and his family decided not to place the tracheostomy tube. Before leaving the hospital, Jonathan's mother expressed her concerns about what they should expect the next time he became acutely ill and about what medical decisions they might face. The palliative care team was invited to meet Jonathan and his parents to discuss this further. They decided to work together to plan, in advance, for what treatments were best for Jonathan to undergo and forgo when he got sick again.

The palliative care needs of children with LTI are increasingly recognized throughout the course of their lives.[29,30] A philosophy of care that intersects with the aims of curing and comforting (**Fig. 2**),[37] pediatric palliative care is meant to be instituted when "diagnosis, intervention, and treatment are not limited to a disease process, but rather become instrumental for improving the quality-of-life, maintaining the dignity, and ameliorating the pain and suffering of seriously ill or dying children in ways that are appropriate to their upbringing, culture, and community."[31–33] Pediatric palliative care seeks to prevent or relieve the harm and distress produced by a LTI and to enable the best life possible for patients with LTI and their families.[38] The focus of palliative care is not to provide more or less care for children with LTI, but rather the right care that is congruent with the family's goals, preferences, and priorities. Pediatric hospital providers of all kinds (eg, hospitalists, intensivists, specialists, surgeons) are well positioned to provide palliative care to children with LTI throughout the course of their lives- and not just at the end-of-life.

For hospitalized children with LTI, pediatric palliative care is ideally delivered when integrated with disease-directed care rather than delivered as an alternative to it.[38–41] In this way, treatment of a child's acute health problems can occur concurrently with practices of palliation. These practices include attention to the child's comfort, quality

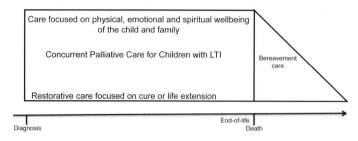

Fig. 2. Integrated model of pediatric palliative care for children with life-threatening illness. (*Adapted from* Sourkes B, Wolfe J. The child and adolescent in palliative care. In: Chochinov HM, Breitbart W, editors. Handbook of psychiatry in palliative medicine. 2nd edition. Oxford University Press; 2009: 531–43; with permission; and Feudtner C. Collaborative communication in pediatric palliative care: A foundation for problem-solving and decision-making. Pediatr Clin North Am 2007;54(5):590; with permission.)

of life, and family support. This type of care is typically delivered through comanagement of a hospitalized child with LTI by a primary team (eg, general hospitalist service) and a consulting palliative care team. Palliative care providers enhance the care offered by the primary team by discussing a family's understanding of prognosis and treatment options, holistic care plans, and recommendations for advance care planning. In general, families of children with LTI often perceive that their child's health care needs are more appropriately met with receipt of these care activities.[42] Palliative care providers are ideally positioned to assist with a child's end-of-life because most pediatric clinicians have less expertise in this area.

However, the workforce of pediatricians who specialize in palliative care is not sufficiently large to care for all hospitalized children with LTI who have palliative care needs. Consultative support from pediatric palliative care providers is not always available and nearly one-third of children's hospitals do not offer pediatric palliative care services and many programs are underresourced.[43] As a result, many children with LTI and their families are making life-altering treatment decisions in the hospital with non–palliative care providers.[42,44] Therefore, pediatric hospital staff should understand and have competency in palliative care practices.[45,46] Keeping the palliative care philosophy in mind may influence several key processes of inpatient care for children with LTI at the time of admission, during their hospital stay, and at hospital discharge. Proficiencies in palliative care for pediatric hospital providers are described below and summarized in **Box 1**.

Assess the short-term and long-term prognosis as well as the quality of life of hospitalized children with LTI. Understanding the trajectory of the child's health and quality of life in the context of their admission heavily influences the approach to the child's care during hospitalization.[47–49] Projecting prognosis accurately for children with LTI is challenging, even for clinicians trained in palliative care.[50] Without an active dialogue with the child's family and their outpatient care team, hospital providers who observe the child only in the setting of an acute illness may underestimate or overestimate the child's quality of life.[51] Higher parent ratings of physician care are associated with providers giving clear information about what to expect during the course of a child's illness.[52] Feudtner and Blinman's[44] surgical palliative care core tasks can help guide this dialogue. Although some parents may not share the same perceptions of prognosis as the inpatient care team and they may find discussions of prognosis about

---

Box 1
Pediatric palliative care tasks for hospital providers

Task 1: Assess the child's short-term and long-term prognosis and quality of life at every admission

- Recognize when a child has a chronic life-threatening illness
- Understand how primary diagnosis and comorbidities contribute to prognosis
- Assess pain or other symptoms that are not well controlled
- Converse with other providers who know the child best

Task 2: Ensure that families are fully involved when making decisions about hospital treatments

- Recognize the full range of benefits and burdens of treatment options
- Create time and space for discussing treatment options with families
- Involve the child and members of the family's support network when appropriate
- If helpful to the family, offer a medical recommendation that incorporates the family's goals, values, and preferences

Task 3: Maximize the family's understanding of their child's health and well-being

- Ask families what they understand about their child's illness and prognosis
- Ask families to elaborate on quality of life, hopes, and fears
- Consult pediatric palliative specialists if appropriate

Task 4: Address factors that could influence the child's well-being and care planning after discharge

- Assess feasibility and effectiveness of contingency plans
- Assess caregiving burden needed to keep the child safe and healthy
- Assess postdischarge providers' comfort and competency to care for the child

---

their child distressing,[46] most parents desire as much information about their child's prognosis as possible.[53]

Ensure that children and families are involved when making decisions about hospital treatments for a child with a LTI. Conversations about treatment goals, options, risks, benefits, and outcomes are absent, limited, or delayed for children with LTI and their families.[49] Such conversations take time, are challenging to initiate, are emotionally charging to sustain, and can result in distress or loss of hope.[53–56] Moreover, these conversations can reveal unrealistic parent expectations for treatment, differences in clinician and patient/family perceptions of care goals, and lack of parental readiness to discuss prognosis.[57] Many families report that hospital care for children with LTI is confusing and that hospital providers are sometimes uncaring when discussing treatment options,[58,59] which emphasizes the importance of compassionate and consistent communication with families of children with LTI throughout their hospital course.

Maximize families' understanding of their child's health and well-being. Families of children with LTI must be given ample time to reflect on, respond to, and convey their understanding of their child's illness with their care teams.[60] Parents' comprehension of their child's health may be hampered by unrealistic visions of treatment, inaccurate health information, anxiety about their child's health status, and limited health literacy.[61–64] Hospital providers should pay attention to these issues and do what they can to overcome them. Separate conversations with the family outside of morning hospital rounds and return visits to the bedside may be necessary. It may take multiple conversations before hospital providers and families can agree.[65–67] Teach-back, a question-and-answer activity during which families verbalize, their child's health issues, can serve to verify understanding and elucidate any misconceptions about care plans.[68] Hospital education methods using teach-back have been associated with increased health literacy[50,60] as well as better knowledge acquisition and retention of care plans.[61]

Prepare the child and family for life after leaving the hospital. This preparation can be accomplished by discussing the hospital course and the possibility of recurrence of a similar acute illness responsible for the child's admission with the family.[69,70] Hospital providers can also talk about the expected stability of the child's comorbid conditions and their functional abilities over time.[69,70] Because children with LTI have high readmission rates and are at risk for recurrent hospitalizations, discussions with families about the likelihood and nature of subsequent hospitalizations is important. Hospital staff can also get a sense of the child's home environment, community support, and the family burden of caregiving associated with keeping the child healthy after discharge.[71,72] Answers to questions such as "How well does the family understand management of the child's health after discharge?" and "Why might this child experience an unplanned readmission after they are discharged?" can be helpful in care planning with families before they go home.[28,69] Consideration and planning for the ongoing palliative care needs that the child and family have may circumvent future hospitalizations and decrease unmet care needs when the child leaves the hospital. Suggested questions to prompt discussions about prognosis, goals of care, and advance care planning with families of children with LTI are shown in **Table 2**.

PART 3: THE RELATIONSHIP BETWEEN HEALTH CARE REFORM AND PALLIATIVE CARE FOR CHILDREN WITH LTI

CASE VIGNETTE

Jonathan was fortunate that he lived in a state that had recently passed legislation to offer community-based palliative care for children who were not necessarily in the last 6 months of their lives. After Jonathan's hospital discharge, the community-based palliative care team met together with Jonathan, his parents, and his other outpatient health care providers to make sure that Jonathan's needs were met, that his family was supported, and that plans were in place to keep him out of the hospital, while maintaining his comfort and quality of life should he become sick again.

Hospitals are under increasing pressure to provide high quality of care while containing costs. Hospitals can benefit from considering how pediatric palliative care and health care reform can improve care for children with LTI and their families. At present, hospital care accounts for four-fifths of health care spending for children with LTI.[2,73] Policy makers nationally are striving to reduce hospital use for these children by avoiding hospitalizations and/or by reducing length of stay and cost during admission. It is possible that improvements in care delivery for children with LTI will result in a substantial reduction of hospital use. To accomplish this, more attention to the overuse of tests and treatments in the hospital setting[74] and consideration of a palliative approach are important.

Emerging evidence suggests that palliative care is associated with improved quality of care and decreased hospital use for children with LTI. In adult patients, receipt of palliative care is associated with lower hospitalization rates,[75] less use of the intensive care unit,[76,77] decreased length of hospital stay,[78] and fewer readmissions.[79] Children receiving pediatric palliative care similarly experience fewer hospitalizations, fewer

Table 2
Questions to engage families of hospitalized children with life-threatening illness in palliative care conversations

Conversation Topic	Example Questions
Prognosis	What is your understanding of your child's health problem(s)?
	How do you see your child's health over time?
	How often are you worried or concerned about your child's health?
	What are your expectations about your child's health?
	What do you think the future may hold for your child?
Quality of life	Can you tell me about your child as a person?
	What brings your child joy?
	How does your child communicate with you and with others?
	How would you describe your child's quality of life?
	What is your child's daily routine?
	Tell me about how your child's illness affects your child's and your family's lives?
	What would life be like for your child if his/her health gets worse/better?
Goals of care	What is the most challenging aspect of your child's condition?
	What care needs are not being met for your child?
	What worries you about your child's care?
	Describe the health that you want your child to achieve.
	Describe the things and activities that are important for your child to be able to do.
	What are your goals for your child?
Advance care planning	In light of your understanding of your child's illness, what is most important to you?
	Although we continue to hope for the best, how can we prepare for other possibilities?
	How could your child's health problems impact how long he/she lives?
	What do you know about treatment decisions that might arise if your child's health worsens?
	What are your hopes for your child?

days spent in the hospital, fewer interventions (eg, mechanical ventilation, surgical procedures), and less total health care spending.[4,6] At the end of life, children receiving palliative care are less likely to experience hospitalization[9] and are more likely to experience death in the home setting.[5]

National health care reform in the ACA enables concurrent pediatric palliative care for children with LTI. One initiative in this reform, the Concurrent Care for Children Requirement (CCCR), has eliminated the requirement that children with LTI forgo curative or life-prolonging medical treatment to receive hospice care in their last 6 months of life. This reform enables access to hospice care for children assisted with life-prolonging technology (eg, tracheostomy and ventilator) near their end of life. Although the provision of concurrent curative life-prolonging treatment and hospice services for hospice-eligible children is now required of Medicaid programs in every state, progress in implementing concurrent care has varied widely.

Although the CCCR may expand access to hospice care for children with LTI who have a prognosis of 6 months or less, it does not address the fact that these same hospice services may benefit children with LTI and their families well before end-of-life. In recent years, state-based initiatives have addressed this gap through efforts of pediatric palliative care coalitions, Medicaid waivers, state plan amendments, and bridging programs of home care agencies that can provide palliative care services to children who do not yet meet hospice eligibility criteria. Preliminary results of community-based palliative care in California reveal that such services are associated with less inpatient hospital care and reduced health care costs.[4] Massachusetts has a state-funded program to provide palliative care for children throughout the common-wealth with LTI who are 18 years of age or younger.[80] Outcomes of this program on health care use are still being assessed. Another state-level initiative for children with LTI financially incentivizes care management through an enhanced fee-for-service payment arrangement. Some states (eg, Michigan) are incentivizing care management specifically for children with LTI by increasing fee-for-service reimbursement (eg, up to $100 monthly per patient) for care plan oversight, multidisciplinary team meetings, telephone calls, and home visits.[81]

The Accountable Care Organization (ACO) is another initiative that may help children with LTI by provisioning groups of providers and institutions across the care contin-uum to join together to provide care for a defined group of patients.[82] ACO providers and institutions share in cost savings if targets of quality measures and reduction of costs are achieved for their patients. It is hoped that ACOs will align resources and payment with care management processes (eg, care coordination, goal setting) that typically have little or no financial reimbursement in traditional fee-for-service arrangements.[83]

Health care reform specific to hospital readmission and the meaningful use of elec-tronic health records are also particularly important for hospitalized children with LTI. Under the ACA, the Centers for Medicare and Medicaid Services (CMS) reduces Medi-care payments to hospitals with excess readmissions.[84] In part because children with LTI have an increased risk of hospital readmission, the Pediatric Quality Measurement Program, created by CMS and the Agency for Healthcare Research and Quality, is currently developing hospital readmission measures for use in children with Medicaid throughout the United States.[85] This standardized measurement allows comparison of pediatric readmission rates across hospitals and may help improve discharge care for children with LTI. Meaningful use requirements are also emerging for the develop-ment, documentation, and sharing of care plans in electronic health records. These care plans are intended for longitudinal use and will include patients' health goals and outcomes, instructions on how to stay healthy, care team members for health sys-tem navigation, and advanced directives. It is hoped that these health care reforms will improve the quality of care for children with LTI by more broadly incorporating pallia-tive care practices.

SUMMARY

Hospitals are challenged to provide high-quality care to an increasingly complex group of children with LTI. Pediatric palliative care is an essential component of optimal delivery of hospital care for children with LTI and their families. When hospital providers understand and are competent in practices of palliative care, providers of all kind can improve hospital care for children with LTI. By assessing prognosis, focusing on quality of life, involving families in treatment decisions, maximizing the family's un-derstanding of their child's health, and making plans to prepare the child and family for life after discharge- hospital providers can deliver high quality care for children with LTI that supports the child and family. Health care reforms enabled by the ACA and Medicaid are designed to improve health care value by broadening the access to pediatric palliative care. Together, these efforts can enhance health for children with LTI and their families by focusing on care that benefits their quality of life and well-being.

REFERENCES

1. Berry J, Agrawal R, Cohen E, et al. The landscape of medical care for children with medical complexity. Alexandria (VA): Children's Hospital Association; 2013. p. 1–16.
2. Cohen E, Berry J, Camacho X, et al. Patterns and costs of health care use of children with medical complexity. Pediatrics 2012;130(6):e1463–70. http://dx.doi.org/10.1542/peds.2012-0175.
3. Kuo D, Cohen E, Agrawal R, et al. A national profile of caregiver challenges among more medically complex children with special health care needs. Arch Pediatr Adolesc Med 2011;165(11):1020–6. http://dx.doi.org/10.1001/archpediatrics.2011.172.
4. Gans D, Kominski G, Roby D, et al. Better outcomes, lower costs: palliative care program reduces stress, costs of care for children with life-threatening conditions. Los Angles (CA): UCLA Center for Health Policy Research; 2012. p. 1–8.
5. Schmidt P, Otto M, Hechler T, et al. Did increased availability of pediatric palliative care lead to improved palliative care outcomes in children with cancer? J Palliat Med 2013;16(9):1034–9. http://dx.doi.org/10.1089/jpm.2013.0014.
6. Keele L, Keenan H, Sheetz J, et al. Differences in characteristics of dying children who receive and do not receive palliative care. Pediatrics 2013;132(1): 72–8. http://dx.doi.org/10.1542/peds.2013-0470.
7. Cohen E, Kuo D, Agrawal R, et al. Children with medical complexity: an emerging population for clinical and research initiatives. Pediatrics 2011; 127(3):529–38. http://dx.doi.org/10.1542/peds.2010-0910.
8. Feudtner C, Christakis D, Connell F. Pediatric deaths attributable to complex chronic conditions: a population-based study of Washington state, 1980–1997. Pediatrics 2000;106(Suppl 1):205–9. http://dx.doi.org/10.1542/peds.106.1.S1.205.
9. Fraser L, Miller M, Hain R, et al. Rising national prevalence of life-limiting conditions in children in England. Pediatrics 2012;129(4):e923–9. http://dx.doi.org/10.1542/peds.2011-2846.
10. Berry J, Hall M, Hall D, et al. Inpatient growth and resource use in 28 children's hospitals: a longitudinal, multi-institutional study. JAMA Pediatr 2013;167(2): 170–7. http://dx.doi.org/10.1001/jamapediatrics.2013.432.
11. Berry J, Hall D, Kuo D, et al. Hospital utilization and characteristics of patients experiencing recurrent readmissions within children's hospitals. JAMA 2011; 305(7):682–90. http://dx.doi.org/10.1001/jama.2011.122.
12. Burns K, Casey P, Lyle R, et al. Increasing prevalence of medically complex children in US hospitals. Pediatrics 2010;126(4):638–46. http://dx.doi.org/10.1542/peds.2009-1658.
13. Simon T, Berry J, Feudtner C, et al. Children with complex chronic conditions in inpatient hospital settings in the United States. Pediatrics 2010;126(4):647–55. http://dx.doi.org/10.1542/peds.2009-3266.
14. Venkateswaran S, Shevell M. Comorbidities and clinical determinants of outcome in children with spastic quadriplegic cerebral palsy. Dev Med Child Neurol 2008;50(3):216–22. http://dx.doi.org/10.1111/j.1469-8749.2008.02033.x.
15. Berry J, Graham R, Roberson D, et al. Patient characteristics associated with in-hospital mortality in children following tracheotomy. Arch Dis Child 2010;95(9): 703–10.
16. Srivastava R, Berry J, Hall M, et al. Reflux related hospital admissions after fundoplication in children with neurological impairment: retrospective cohort study. BMJ 2009;339:b4411. http://dx.doi.org/10.1136/bmj.b4411.

17. Strauss D, Brooks J, Rosenbloom L, et al. Life expectancy in cerebral palsy: an update. Dev Med Child Neurol 2008;50(7):487–93. http://dx.doi.org/10.1111/j. 1469-8749.2008.03000.x.

18. Strauss D, Shavelle R, Reynolds R, et al. Survival in cerebral palsy in the last 20 years: signs of improvement? Dev Med Child Neurol 2007;49(2):86–92. http:// dx.doi.org/10.1111/j.1469-8749.2007.00086.x.

19. Berry J, Poduri A, Bonkowsky J, et al. Trends in resource utilization by children with neurological impairment in the United States inpatient health care system: a repeat cross-sectional study. PLoS Med 2012;9(1):e1001158. http://dx.doi.org/ 10.1371/journal.pmed.1001158.s001.

20. Coppus A. People with intellectual disability: what do we know about adulthood and life expectancy? Dev Disabil Res Rev 2013;18(1):6–16. http://dx.doi.org/10. 1002/ddrr.1123.

21. Strauss D, Ashwal S, Day S, et al. Life expectancy of children in vegetative and minimally conscious states. Pediatr Neurol 2000;23(4):312–9.

22. Gale R, Namestnic J. Life expectancy of brain impaired, chronically ventilated children. Pediatr Neurol 2013;48(4):280–4.

23. Berry J, Graham D, Graham R, et al. Predictors of clinical outcomes and hospital resource use of children after tracheotomy. Pediatrics 2009;124(2):563–72.

24. Berry J, Toomey S, Zaslavsky A, et al. Pediatric readmission prevalence and variability across hospitals. JAMA 2013;309(4):372–80.

25. Berry J, Agrawal R, Kuo D, et al. Characteristics of hospitalizations for patients who use a structured clinical care program for children with medical complexity. J Pediatr 2011;159(2):284–90.

26. Feudtner C, Levin J, Srivastava R, et al. How well can hospital readmission be predicted in a cohort of hospitalized children? A retrospective, multicenter study. Pediatrics 2009;123(1):286–93. http://dx.doi.org/10.1542/peds.2007-3395.

27. Feudtner C, Pati S, Goodman D, et al. State-level child health system performance and the likelihood of readmission to children's hospitals. J Pediatr 2010;157(1):98–102.e1.

28. Berry J, Ziniel S, Freeman L, et al. Hospital readmission and parent perceptions of their child's hospital discharge. Int J Qual Health Care 2013;25(5):573–81. http://dx.doi.org/10.1093/intqhc/mzt051.

29. Brandon D, Docherty S, Thorpe J. Infant and child deaths in acute care settings: implications for palliative care. J Palliat Med 2007;10(4):910–8. http://dx.doi.org/ 10.1089/jpm.2006.0236.

30. Feudtner C, Kang T, Hexem K, et al. Pediatric palliative care patients: a prospective multicenter cohort study. Pediatrics 2011;127(6):1094–101. http://dx. doi.org/10.1542/peds.2010-3225.

31. Ullrich C, Dussel V, Hilden J, et al. End-of-life experience of children undergoing stem cell transplantation for malignancy: parent and provider perspectives and patterns of care. Blood 2010;115(19):3879–85. http://dx.doi.org/10.1182/blood-2009-10-250225.

32. Dellon E, Leigh M, Yankaskas J, et al. Effects of lung transplantation on inpatient end of life care in cystic fibrosis. J Cyst Fibros 2007;6(6):396–402. http://dx.doi. org/10.1016/j.jcf.2007.03.005.

33. Surkan P, Kreicbergs U, Valdimarsdóttir U, et al. Perceptions of inadequate health care and feelings of guilt in parents after the death of a child to a malignancy: a population-based long-term follow-up. J Palliat Med 2006;9(2):317–31. http://dx.doi.org/10.1089/jpm.2006.9.317.

34. Fortescue E, Kaushal R, Landrigan C, et al. Prioritizing strategies for preventing medication errors and adverse drug events in pediatric inpatients. Pediatrics 2003;111(4):722–9.
35. Davies B, Sehring S, Partridge J, et al. Barriers to palliative care for children: perceptions of pediatric health care providers. Pediatrics 2008;121(2):282–8. http://dx.doi.org/10.1542/peds.2006-3153.
36. Anderson W, Kools S, Lyndon A. Dancing around death: hospitalist-patient communication about serious illness. Qual Health Res 2012;23(1):3–13. http://dx.doi.org/10.1177/1049732312461728.
37. Wolfe J, Hinds P, Sourkes B. Textbook of interdisciplinary pediatric palliative care. Philadelphia: Saunders Elsevier Health Sciences; 2011.
38. Field M, Behrman R, Institute of Medicine (US), Committee on Palliative and End-of-Life Care for Children and Their Families. When children die: improving palliative and end-of-life care for children and their families. Washington, DC: National Academy Press; 2003.
39. National Consensus Project for Quality Palliative Care. Clinical practice guidelines for quality palliative care. 3rd edition. 2013. Available at: http://www.nationalconsensusproject.org. Accessed April 22, 2014.
40. World Health Organization. Definition of palliative care. Available at: http://www.who.int/cancer/palliative/definition/en/. Accessed April 22, 2014.
41. American Academy of Pediatrics Committee on Bioethics and Committee on Hospital Care. Palliative care for children. Pediatrics 2000;106:351–7.
42. Walter J, Benneyworth B, Housey M, et al. The factors associated with high-quality communication for critically ill children. Pediatrics 2013;131(Suppl):S90–5. http://dx.doi.org/10.1542/peds.2012-1427k.
43. Feudtner C, Womer J, Augustin R, et al. Pediatric palliative care programs in children's hospitals: a cross-sectional national survey. Pediatrics 2013;132(6):1063–70. http://dx.doi.org/10.1542/peds.2013-1286.
44. Feudtner C, Blinman T. The pediatric surgeon and palliative care. Semin Pediatr Surg 2013;22(3):154–60.
45. Quill T, Abernethy A. Generalist plus specialist palliative care—creating a more sustainable model. N Engl J Med 2013;368(13):1173–5. http://dx.doi.org/10.1056/NEJMp1302093.
46. de Wit S, Donohue P, Shepard J, et al. Mother-clinician discussions in the neonatal intensive care unit: agree to disagree? J Perinatol 2012;33(4):278–81. http://dx.doi.org/10.1038/jp.2012.103.
47. Weeks J, Cook E, O'Day S, et al. Relationship between cancer patients' predictions of prognosis and their treatment preferences. JAMA 1998;279(21):1709–14. http://dx.doi.org/10.1001/jama.279.21.1709.
48. Weeks J, Catalano P, Cronin A, et al. Patients' expectations about effects of chemotherapy for advanced cancer. N Engl J Med 2012;367(17):1616–25. http://dx.doi.org/10.1056/NEJMoa1204410.
49. Wolfe J, Klar N, Grier H, et al. Understanding of prognosis among parents of children who died of cancer: impact on treatment goals and integration of palliative care. JAMA 2000;284(19):2469–75.
50. Christakis N. Extent and determinants of error in doctors' prognoses in terminally ill patients: prospective cohort study. BMJ 2000;320(7233):469–73. http://dx.doi.org/10.1136/bmj.320.7233.469.
51. Lamas D. Chronic critical illness. N Engl J Med 2014;370(2):175–7. http://dx.doi.org/10.1056/NEJMms1310675.

52. Mack J. Parent and physician perspectives on quality of care at the end of life in children with cancer. J Clin Oncol 2005;23(36):9155–61. http://dx.doi.org/10.1200/JCO.2005.04.010.

53. Mack J, Wolfe J, Grier H, et al. Communication about prognosis between parents and physicians of children with cancer: parent preferences and the impact of prognostic information. J Clin Oncol 2006;24(33):5265–70. http://dx.doi.org/10.1200/JCO.2006.06.5326.

54. Davis R, Genel M, Howe J, et al. Good care of the dying patient. JAMA 1996;275(6):474–8.

55. Institute of Medicine. Committee on the Crossing the Quality Chasm: Next Steps Toward a New Health Care System. Washington, DC: National Academy Press; 2004.

56. Connors A. A controlled trial to improve care for seriously ill hospitalized patients. JAMA 1995;274(20):1591. http://dx.doi.org/10.1001/jama.1995.03530200027032.

57. Durall A, Zurakowski D, Wolfe J. Barriers to conducting advance care discussions for children with life-threatening conditions. Pediatrics 2012;129(4):e975–82. http://dx.doi.org/10.1542/peds.2011-2695.

58. Rogers A, Karlsen S, Addington-Hall J. "All the services were excellent. It is when the human element comes in that things go wrong": dissatisfaction with hospital care in the last year of life. J Adv Nurs 2000;31(4):768–74.

59. Contro N, Larson J, Scofield S, et al. Family perspectives on the quality of pediatric palliative care. Arch Pediatr Adolesc Med 2002;156(1):14.

60. Lidz C. The weather report model of informed consent: problems in preserving patient voluntariness. Bull Am Acad Psychiatry Law 1980;8(2):152–60.

61. Covinsky K, Fuller J, Yaffe K, et al. Communication and decision-making in seriously ill patients: findings of the SUPPORT project. J Am Geriatr Soc 2000;48(Suppl 5):S187–93.

62. Hofmann J. Patient preferences for communication with physicians about end-of-life decisions. Ann Intern Med 1997;127(1):1–12. http://dx.doi.org/10.7326/0003-4819-127-1-199707010-00001.

63. Tulsky J, Fischer G, Rose M, et al. Opening the black box: how do physicians communicate about advance directives? Ann Intern Med 1998;129(6):441–9.

64. Diem S, Lantos J, Tulsky J. Cardiopulmonary resuscitation on television — miracles and misinformation. N Engl J Med 1996;334(24):1578–82. http://dx.doi.org/10.1056/NEJM199606133342406.

65. Lidz C, Appelbaum P, Meisel A. Two models of implementing informed consent. Arch Intern Med 1988;148(6):1385.

66. Jackson V, Jacobsen J, Greer J, et al. The cultivation of prognostic awareness through the provision of early palliative care in the ambulatory setting: a communication guide. J Palliat Med 2013;16(8):894–900. http://dx.doi.org/10.1089/jpm.2012.0547.

67. Bussmann S, Muders P, Zahrt-Omar C, et al. Improving end-of-life care in hospitals: a qualitative analysis of bereaved families' experiences and suggestions. Am J Hosp Palliat Care 2013. http://dx.doi.org/10.1177/1049909113512718.

68. Tamura-Lis W. Teach-back for quality education and patient safety. Urol Nurs 2013;33(6):267–71.

69. Williams M, Coleman E. Boosting the hospital discharge. J Hosp Med 2009;4(4):209–10. http://dx.doi.org/10.1002/jhm.525.

70. Rutherford P, Nielsen G, Taylor J, et al. How-to guide: Improving transitions from the hospital to community settings to reduce avoidable rehospitalizations. Cambridge (MA): Institute for Healthcare Improvement; 2012.

71. Thyen U, Kuhlthau K, Perrin JM. Employment, child care, and mental health of mothers caring for children assisted by technology. Pediatrics 1999; 103(6 Pt 1):1235–42.

72. Thyen U, Terres N, Yazdgerdi S, et al. Impact of long-term care of children assisted by technology on maternal health. J Dev Behav Pediatr 1998;19(4): 273–82.

73. Neff J, Sharp V, Muldoon J, et al. Profile of medical charges for children by health status group and severity level in a Washington State health plan. Health Serv Res 2004;39(1):73–90. http://dx.doi.org/10.1111/j.1475-6773.2004.00216.x.

74. Quinonez R, Garber M, Schroeder A, et al. Choosing wisely in pediatric hospital medicine: five opportunities for improved healthcare value. J Hosp Med 2013; 8(9):479–85. http://dx.doi.org/10.1002/jhm.2064.

75. Brumley R, Enguidanos S, Jamison P, et al. Increased satisfaction with care and lower costs: results of a randomized trial of in-home palliative care. J Am Geriatr Soc 2007;55(7):993–1000. http://dx.doi.org/10.1111/j.1532-5415.2007. 01234.x.

76. Gade G, Venohr I, Conner D, et al. Impact of an inpatient palliative care team: a randomized controlled trial. J Palliat Med 2008;11(2):180–90. http://dx.doi.org/ 10.1089/jpm.2007.0055.

77. Norton S, Hogan L, Holloway R, et al. Proactive palliative care in the medical intensive care unit: effects on length of stay for selected high-risk patients. Crit Care Med 2007;35(6):1530–5. http://dx.doi.org/10.1097/01.CCM.0000266533. 06543.0C.

78. Wu F, Newman J, Lasher A, et al. Effects of initiating palliative care consultation in the emergency department on inpatient length of stay. J Palliat Med 2013; 16(11):1362–7. http://dx.doi.org/10.1089/jpm.2012.0352.

79. Enguidanos S, Vesper E, Lorenz K. 30-Day readmissions among seriously ill older adults. J Palliat Med 2012;15(12):1356–61. http://dx.doi.org/10.1089/ jpm.2012.0259.

80. Bona K, Bates J, Wolfe J. Massachusetts' Pediatric Palliative Care Network: successful implementation of a novel state-funded pediatric palliative care program. J Palliat Med 2011;14(11):1217–23. http://dx.doi.org/10.1089/jpm.2011. 0070.

81. Catalyst Center. Care coordination in a statewide system of care: financing models and payment strategies. Boston (MA): Boston University School of Public Health; 2010.

82. Fisher E, McClellan M, Bertko J, et al. Fostering accountable health care: moving forward in Medicare. Health Aff 2009;28(2):w219–31.

83. Homer C, Patel K. Accountable care organizations in pediatrics: irrelevant or a game changer for children? JAMA Pediatr 2013;167(6):507–8. http://dx.doi.org/ 10.1001/jamapediatrics.2013.105.

84. Centers for Medicare and Medicaid Services. Medicare Hospital Quality Chartbook: Yale New Haven Health System Corporation Center for Outcomes Research and Evaluation; 2010.

85. Agency for Healthcare Research and Quality. Crosswalk of the first set of priorities for the Pediatric Healthcare Quality Measures Program Centers of Excellence with the CHIPRA Initial Core Measure Set. Available at: http://www.ahrq. gov. Accessed April 22, 2014.

86. Berry J. Pediatric Readmissions. Washington, DC: Center for Medicare and Medicaid Services Readmissions Summit; 2012.

Pediatric Palliative Care Consultation

Dominic Moore, MD, Joan Sheetz, MD*

KEYWORDS

- Pediatric palliative care • Elements of consultation • Referral criteria
- Barriers to referral • Value added benefits

KEY POINTS

- PPC consultation can benefit the patient, their family, and the healthcare team by aligning treatment goals with treatment plans, improving the experience of the patient and their family, and enhancing the cooperation of the healthcare team.
- PPC consultation is a process of getting to know a family's goals, values, hopes, priorities, and preferences. It can also include expert opinion and recommendations regarding prognosis, advance care planning, and resources along the continuum of care.
- Children should be referred to PPC at the time of diagnosis with a life-threatening illness or when there is a significant change in health status.
- Families benefit from PPC expertise in pain or other symptoms, spiritual or psychosocial crises, communication challenges, and discussions regarding goals of care.
- Clinicians can look to palliative care when treatment options are challenging or limited, if care invokes moral and emotional distress, or for end-of-life care recommendations.
- Challenges to effective PPC include misconceptions among families and clinicians, uncertainty about benefits and timing of referral, staffing shortages, and challenges in funding programs that save money rather than generate revenue.

INTRODUCTION

Pediatric palliative care (PPC) is a relatively new and quickly growing pediatric subspecialty. This article discusses PPC consultation with specific focus on the added value of PPC, elements of a PPC consultation, and challenges to and opportunities for PPC consultation. Ongoing research, current publication, expert opinion, and institutional experience were compiled for this article.

ADDED VALUE OF PPC

The core concepts of PPC have been present in the practice of many pediatricians for years. These skills are referred to as "primary palliative care," and should be a part of

Division of In-Patient Medicine, Pediatrics, Primary Children's Hospital, University of Utah, 100 North Mario Capecchi Drive, Salt Lake City, UT 84113, USA
* Corresponding author.
E-mail address: Joan.Sheetz@hsc.utah.edu

Pediatr Clin N Am 61 (2014) 735–747
http://dx.doi.org/10.1016/j.pcl.2014.04.007
0031-3955/14/$ – see front matter © 2014 Elsevier Inc. All rights reserved.
pediatric.theclinics.com

all pediatric education.[1] This section outlines the benefits of subspecialist PPC involvement as experienced by different participants in the healthcare interaction. Patient and family, physicians, support staff, and hospitals each benefit in a unique way. The additive result is an overall improvement in care.

Patient and Family

Children and families facing life-threatening conditions have many clinicians on their side. The PPC consultant generally adds support for the family and the team rather than assuming care.[2,3] Although PPC teams are each unique in composition they are usually a consistent group of clinicians that follow the patient longitudinally.[4] This continuous relationship over the course of an illness allows the PPC team to read-dress sensitive topics and significant decisions, such as advance care planning, which may also evolve over time. Often the most therapeutic intervention by PPC teams is impartial listening. A family's desire not to harm a relationship with the primary team may prevent expression of frustration, anger, and disappointment. The PPC team can clarify a family's perspective and help the family interpret medical realities in situations ripe for misunderstanding. Good communication also helps to assess the impact of illness on all members of the family. This information is useful in the process of helping parents navigate decisions and in aiding the family as they deal with their individual emotional, spiritual, and social reaction to the events that are unfolding.

The Primary Care Team

Pediatricians are caring for an increasingly complex group of children.[5] PPC consultation contributes to the care of these children with specialized knowledge of symptom management, familiarity with common life-limiting scenarios, teaching of primary palliative care, and support in difficult ethical and emotional situations. Life-threatening illness often brings a symptom burden that weighs heavily on children and families.[6] Attention to symptoms should be a top priority regardless of the goals of care. PPC teams specialize in assessment and treatment of pain, nausea, delirium, insomnia, anxiety, and the myriad of other symptoms common in sick children. Treatment includes pharmacologic and nonpharmacologic methods, with an emphasis on preserving quality of life. Specialized training and experience with uncommon illnesses allows the PPC clinician to be an asset in situations not often encountered by inpatient teams. PPC consultation service is a resource for trainees[7] and experienced clinicians to gain the PPC and pediatric hospice care (PPC-PHC) skill set recommended for all pediatricians (**Box 1**) by the American Academy of Pediatrics (AAP).[3(p970)] Every

---

Box 1
AAP recommended PPC-PHC skills

- Prevent, assess, and manage symptoms
- Communicate in clear, caring, and collaborative manner with patients and families
- Recognize when and how to consult with PPC-PHC specialists
- Communicate effectively the role PPC-PHC specialists play
- Ensure that patient care is consistent with best practices
- Maintain full engagement in well-coordinated care

Adapted from American Academy of Pediatrics. Pediatric palliative care and hospice care commitments, guidelines, and recommendations. Section on Hospice and Palliative Medicine and Committee on Hospital Care. Pediatrics 2013;132:966–7.

---

palliative care team is equipped to support the family and the primary team as they grapple with difficult ethical and moral decisions. PPC consultation does not take the place of an ethics consultation, but may offer experience and recommend formally involving the hospital ethics committee as appropriate. Physicians stand to gain expertise in symptom management, familiarity with common life-threatening scenarios, teaching, and support in ethically complex situations with a PPC consultation.

Medical assistants, respiratory therapists, nurses, and associated staff work at the bedside contributing to the often complex care that hospitalized children receive. They bear witness to the suffering that can occur despite the best efforts of the team. The AAP has specifically tasked PPC with support of hospital ancillary staff.[3(p970)] Involvement of a PPC team can use the knowledge of these team members, educate concerning end-of-life issues, and decrease the distress that is often a factor in burn out. In reporting their subjective and objective experience with the patient, staff distress regarding suffering can be channeled to help influence care in a productive way. PPC teams commonly include a nurse or nurse practitioner who may be well-positioned to connect with nursing staff or other clinicians at the bedside. Ethical and moral dilemmas faced by patients and their families lead to staff distress.[8–10] By establishing contact with members of the healthcare team, the PPC service can either address these issues on their own or suggest a way to help decrease the distress. Although the involvement of the PPC team does not automatically resolve any of these challenges, they have the potential to support, educate, and involve staff in such a way that staff satisfaction and retention are positively impacted.

Hospitals

Experience suggests that hospitals supporting PPC increase positive inpatient interactions, minimize negative experiences of especially vulnerable families, and keep up with industry standards. Emphasis on patient and family concerns, values, and understanding by PPC teams optimizes satisfaction. Word of mouth is the most powerful tool that a hospital can have on its side. One story of a positive patient experience, or conversely a negative experience, lives on in the discourse between friends and can be immortalized on public and private forums. Heightened emotions at the end of life put families and clinicians at a significant risk for miscommunication, a common factor in legal action taken against hospitals and clinicians.[11] The care and compassion shown by the healthcare team including PPC can create a bond of trust and potentially curtail litigious behavior. Focus on goals, symptom management, and communication by PPC can help a vulnerable family feel heard and valued. Although PPC services rarely generate the revenue to cover all involved expenses, the benefit to families and cost savings have led to 69% of pediatric hospitals recently surveyed having some form of a palliative care service.[4(p3)] The AAP recommends that "all large health care organizations serving children with life threatening conditions have dedicated interdisciplinary PPC-PHC teams."[3(p968)] In the era of measuring satisfaction and optimization of care, it behooves any hospital seeking to keep up with the standard of care to invest in their PPC service. This is a situation where doing the right thing for patients and families pays off for all involved parties.

ELEMENTS OF A CONSULTATION

PPC consultation is similar to yet different from other specialist consultations. As with other specialties, a pediatric clinician should consult palliative care in situations where the subspecialist palliative care skill set may be of added value. Unlike other types of consultations, however, palliative care involves not just a physician with special expertise but typically an entire interdisciplinary team, who consider not just the patient's needs but those of patient's circle of influence including parents, siblings, extended family, religious/spiritual community, and school. Goals of consultation vary from case to case. A review of PPC consultations from six pediatric centers showed most frequent goals were symptom management (58.1%), facilitating communication (48.5%) and decision making (42.1%), assisting with logistics or coordination of care (35.3%), assisting with transition to home (14.4%), and discussion of do-not-resuscitate orders (11.8%); in most cases, more than one goal was addressed.[12] Some palliative care programs offer inpatient consultation only, some also have an outpatient component, and some provide a palliative care unit or dedicated room.

Stakeholders

Palliative care is not limited to an organ or body system but rather is whole-person centered. Thus, palliative medicine consultations are perhaps more complex than other consultations, with multiple layers of stakeholders. Thorough consultation requires involving and meeting the needs of all appropriate stakeholders (**Box 2**). The elements of a PPC consultation are listed in **Box 3** and further detailed next.

The Referring Physician as Stakeholder

Determining the referring clinician's specific reasons for consultation at the outset allows the palliative consultation to best serve the clinician. Common reasons to obtain a palliative care consultation for a child include assistance with

- Establishing goals of care
- Developing a care plan that has the best likelihood of achieving the goals of care
- Assistance with medical decision making, including defining resuscitation wishes
- Pain and symptom management
- Prognostication
- Assistance with communication with the healthcare team

Box 2
Potential stakeholders in a pediatric palliative care consult

- Patient and parents
- Siblings
- Extended family
- Referring physician and housestaff
- Nurses
- Psychosocial clinicians: social work, psychology, child life
- Other consultants
- Primary care clinician
- Supportive services in hospital: occupational therapy, physical therapy, nutrition, education, interpretation, music therapy, chaplaincy, discharge planning and case management, pharmacy
- Supportive services in community: long-term care facilities, schools, houses of worship, early intervention clinician, home health and hospice, home therapists, volunteers
- Palliative care team

Box 3
Elements of pediatric palliative care consultation

1. Speak directly with the source of the referral to

   - Acknowledge the request

   - Ensure clarity around the nature of the request

   - Obtain important information that may not be available in the chart

   - Determine the family's understanding and expectations regarding palliative care

   - Delineate the nature and role of the PPC team as a consulting service

2. Prepare for the consultation

   - Meet the patient and family

   - Negotiate consultation participants (eg, will child be present at the initial consult?)

   - Logistics (eg, quiet, private space to meet; childcare for siblings)

   - Consider speaking with other clinicians caring for the child (eg, social worker) to gather additional information and delineate roles

3. Do the consultation

   a. Review the medical record, gather pertinent clinical data

   b. Meet with patient and family

   c. Examine patient

4. Document and follow-up

   a. Document the consultation promptly

   b. Speak directly with the source of the referral regarding findings and recommendations

   c. Follow-up with other clinicians and the family as indicated

---

- Assistance with communication among family members
- Assessment of spiritual or psychosocial distress
- Discharge or end-of-life planning

Additionally, palliative care consultation may be requested when ethical, spiritual, or emotional issues arise among staff.

Child, Parents, and Family as Stakeholders

The patient and parents may differ from the referring physician in their goals and expectations of the consult. PPC can help elicit a child's hopes, fears, understanding of their condition, and goals of care. In addition to choosing the best care for their ill child, parents often are concerned about the impact of a child's illness on siblings. The PPC team can offer advice on how and what to tell siblings, how to handle behavior issues, or just empathetically listen to parents' grief and concern about not being as available for siblings as they feel they should. Occasionally, extended family members may disagree with goals of care. Grandparents may suffer grief not only for their ill grandchild but also for their child, the parent. Palliative care teams are highly skilled at delicately drawing out these tender issues and helping a family problem-solve.

The Community of Medical Clinicians as Stakeholders

A medically complex child generally has a primary care physician and multiple specialists all contributing to their care plan. These care clinicians represent additional stakeholders, which a palliative care plan must include. A primary care physician manages care outside the hospital, and has valuable insights into a patient's condition and family dynamics acquired over the course of caring for the child. Any care plan developed should include their input and they should be fully aware of goals of care and the treatment plan developed to achieve those goals. All specialists involved in the care of a child with complex illness should have similar input and awareness. In academic settings, medical students and residents add the dimension of learners to the list of stakeholders. Palliative care consultation is an opportunity to provide education about generalist-level palliative care, which research has been demonstrated to be lacking in medical training.[13]

In the inpatient setting, the bedside nurse has intimate knowledge of the patient's care needs, family dynamics, and disease course that may differ from a physician's. Child life therapists, music therapists, occupational and physical therapists, speech therapists, and others all bring unique perspectives and knowledge to bear on a palliative assessment and care plan. Education specialists can help the palliative care team understand what supports may be available through the child's local school system, such as special education and physical, occupational, and speech therapies. Interpretation services provide not only language translation, but also cultural translation. Social workers are trained to gauge coping skills and families' strengths and challenges and serve as case managers in many institutions. They are uniquely trained to identify psychosocial needs and match them to available resources. Chaplains may have insight into a family's spiritual belief system that can be very helpful in developing advance care plans. Each family has a belief system about the meaning of health and illness, and may need help making sense of their experience from a spiritual perspective. In some PPC teams many of these staff are part of the formal team; in others, PPC actively seeks input from these valuable colleagues.

Palliative Illness and Symptom Assessment

A palliative care consultation involves a thorough and detailed history taking of the current illness, past medical history, and review of symptoms along with a comprehensive physical examination and review of medical records. A palliative care clinician focuses in depth on any symptoms that may be underrecognized or undertreated. Palliative care clinicians have expertise at diagnosing and treating persistent pain and other symptoms that do not respond to routine interventions. Sources of pain are investigated and classified by location and type (nociceptive vs neuropathic vs psychosomatic, acute vs chronic vs acute on chronic, mixed). The palliative consultation inquires about symptoms, such as nausea and vomiting, disturbed sleep, irritability, feeding intolerance, anxiety, delirium, dyspnea, and depression. PPC considers how emotional and spiritual distress interplay with physical distress, and may recommend integrative modalities to help reduce suffering, such as music therapy, play therapy, prayer, acupuncture or acupressure, massage, aromatherapy, and others as available.

The Family as the Unit of Care

Because palliative care focuses on the child and family individually and also as a unit, the interdisciplinary assessment includes the family. Members of the interdisciplinary palliative care team assess for coping, support systems, spiritual needs, and beliefs, and identify crises, such as family disruption, financial stress, transportation or housing issues, parental depression, parents' and patients' understanding of the medical condition, proposed treatments' risks and benefits, and attendant hopes and fears. Many siblings of ill children have unique needs of their own that the PPC team can help identify and support. Goals of care are discussed to enable creation of an advance care plan, which may be unlimited medical treatment, limited interventions, or cessation of medical interventions except those aimed at comfort.

Prognosis and Medical Decision Making

The palliative care team may aid medical decision making and advance care planning by helping the medical team to establish and communicate prognosis. Experienced palliative medicine specialists can offer prediction of illness trajectory when, as is frequently the case, evidence-based prognostic information is lacking. Advance care planning includes discussing and documenting advance directive plans, such as Do Not Attempt Resuscitation orders and Physician Orders for Life Sustaining Treatment, and also other treatment and end-of-life preferences, such as preferred site of care, goals hoped for before death, and preferred location of death.

Recommendations, Advance Care Planning, and Continuum of Care

Because PPC considers the family holistically, interventions may be recommended for the child and family. Medical management suggestions for pain and other distressing symptoms may be given, including the use of opioids and sedatives; integrative medicine strategies, such as aromatherapy, acupuncture, and hypnosis; and other modalities as available. When patient or sibling distress is identified, child life therapy may be recommended. Music therapy can often be helpful in achieving specific goals, such as reducing procedural pain, developmental stimulation, relaxation, and grief therapy. PPC teams are uniquely positioned to know what resources are available and how to pull them in to help maximize daily quality of life and ease suffering for children with life-threatening illness and their families.

A family meeting between the parents, the child if appropriate and willing, the palliative care team, and other caregivers as indicated can be very valuable. Guided discussion can allow the patient's story to unfold, along with their hopes and fears. Asking about the family's and patient's understanding of the illness or condition can lead to a conversation about prognosis, goals of care, and advance directives. This conversation can also reveal a family's coping strengths, and shine light on areas where they may be struggling. The goal of these conversations is to help the care team give the right care at the right time.

Palliative care teams can discuss hospice services with patients and families and assist with making a hospice referral at the appropriate time. Although PPC programs vary in scope, increasingly PPC teams provide outpatient follow-up and home visits, and most are able to provide telephone support.[4(p3)] When a child is discharged home, the PPC team can continue providing expert advice to the primary care pediatrician and hospice agencies as needed. Should the patient be readmitted for further treatment, acute exacerbations of illness, or symptom management the PPC team can provide consistency, a comforting presence, and unique insights into previously helpful medical management, successful coping strategies, and the family's communication preferences. Because of the longitudinal relationship the palliative care team often has with a patient and family, they have a deep understanding of the medical course, psychosocial strengths and vulnerabilities, and history of decision-making and serve as a repository of this information.

OPPORTUNITIES FOR CONSULTATION

Since 2000, the AAP has recommended palliative care be integrated from the time of diagnosis of a life-threatening illness, and continued throughout the illness experience, whether cure, life-extension, or comfort is the outcome.[14] It is recommended that all pediatricians should have basic competencies in treating pain and distressing symptoms when caring for children with life-threatening illnesses and complex chronic conditions.[3(p968)] They should also be able to recognize who and when to refer for palliative care consultation. However, uncertainty in prognosis can make knowing who and when to refer challenging.

Determining Who to Refer

Although more data are accumulating to provide better prognostic information, diagnoses can help make determinations of which children to refer and when during their illness trajectory. Certain diagnoses carry a high likelihood of death during childhood. One practical approach is to consider referral based on diagnosis of a complex chronic condition.[15] Categories of complex chronic condition and some examples of each include the following:

- Neuromuscular (eg, brain and spinal cord malformations, central nervous system diseases, cerebral palsy)
- Cardiovascular (eg, congenital heart disease, conduction abnormalities, cardiomyopathies)
- Respiratory (eg, cystic fibrosis, chronic respiratory diseases, malformations)
- Renal (eg, chronic renal failure, anomalies)
- Gastrointestinal (eg, chronic liver failure, congenital anomalies)
- Hematology and immunodeficiency (eg, sickle cell disease, hereditary anemias, HIV)
- Metabolic (eg, disorders of amino acid, carbohydrate or lipid metabolism, storage disorders)
- Other congenital or genetic defect (eg, chromosomal anomalies, bone and joint anomalies, diaphragm and abdominal wall anomalies, and other congenital anomalies)
- Malignancy

Another paradigm for determining which children should be referred for palliative care based on prognosis and illness trajectory has been proposed by Together for Short Lives, a UK organization that supports children with life-threatening illness and their families. Four illness trajectories are described[16]:

- Category 1: Life-threatening conditions for which treatment is available but may fail, such as cancer or irreversible kidney failure
- Category 2: Conditions wherein premature death is inevitable but treatment may prolong life, such as cystic fibrosis or Duchenne muscular dystrophy
- Category 3: Progressive conditions without curative treatment options, such as muccopolysaccharidoses and Batten disease
- Category 4: Irreversible but nonprogressive conditions causing severe disability, health complications, and risk of premature death, such as severe cerebral palsy, some brain or spinal cord injuries.

When to Refer for Palliative Care Consultation

It may be useful to consider situations and changes in patient status in addition to diagnosis to trigger palliative care referral.[17] Examples include a child with a chronic, complex, or life-threatening illness or condition who experiences

- An increase in frequency or duration of hospitalizations
- Accelerated symptoms that are not readily managed
- Evidence of disease progression

- Decision-making around adoption of new technology, such as enteral feeding tube, tracheostomy, dialysis, total parental nutrition, invasive or noninvasive ventilation
- Extended intensive care unit stay for acute illness, injury, or exacerbation of a chronic condition

Referral to palliative care may be delayed for a variety of reasons, but research has shown that bereaved parents whose child received palliative care services were very satisfied with the experience and many reported they wished they had been referred to palliative care earlier in their child's illness.[18]

OVERCOMING CHALLENGES TO PPC CONSULTATION

Although it is difficult to fully assess the reasons PPC consultations are not made, looking at obstacles to timely referrals is important. This section examines the common challenges inherent in certain roles and suggests methods for overcoming them. Challenges for patients and their families, PPC specialists, referring physicians, hospital staff, and hospitals are addressed individually, although there is overlap between the groups.

Patients and Families

Experience indicates that involvement early in the illness trajectory can be beneficial. Patients often harbor a strong desire to please or at least avoid disappointing a trusted and loved physician.[19] Some worry that requesting a PPC consultation might displease their doctor or bring up issues that they wish to avoid. Families dealing with the complexities of the medical system may hesitate to involve yet another clinician. It may be helpful to normalize involvement of PPC with such explanations as, "We find it helpful to involve a team called palliative care in children with Mary's condition. They are an extra layer of support for our team and your family. Please let me know if you feel we would benefit from their help." In this statement and those listed in **Box 4** the practice of PPC referral by providers is normalized, the role of PPC as a consultant to the primary clinician or team is clarified, and the family is given permission to request consultation if they desire. PPC teams work to tailor their conversations and care to the needs of the family. By listening to the ways the referring physicians and family believe they can be most helpful the PPC team can optimize their initial involvement and find the best way for their role to evolve over time. A trusting relationship built through effective symptom management may expand to include other PPC services as illness and time progress.

Box 4
Useful phrases for introducing palliative care to families

- "It seems that these symptoms are becoming very severe." (Allow response) "I think that it would be helpful to have the help of palliative care to think about the best way to control these symptoms."

- "I would like to expand the team of people helping you to include palliative care. They will help me with____."

- "Often the people I take care of in this situation have found palliative care to be helpful for____. I would like to have them involved."

- "Since ____ has changed, it seems like now would be a good time to get palliative care on board to help us give you the best care possible."

Palliative Care Clinicians

Challenges PPC services may face in integrating into the healthcare environment include succinctly describing their multifaceted role, addressing misperceptions about palliative care, and earning the trust required to be involved in delicate situations. Palliative care is an accepted term in the medical community, but is still not widely understood by clinicians or the general public.[20] This term, from the Latin "palliare" or "to cloak," is not quite as descriptive as "gastroenterology" or "cardiology." It is the task of the PPC physician to have a clear, concise explanation of what they do. Popular culture thrives on "sound bites" that give a brief indication of why someone should pay attention to a message. An "elevator pitch" has been described as a prepared explanation that can "quickly and simply define a person, profession, product, service, organization or event and its value proposition" during a short elevator ride.[21] PPC clinicians need to be prepared to describe their work with a brief, clear, and accurate message that can be tailored to the audience (**Box 5**).

The definition of PPC recently published in *Pediatrics* is a good source for crafting such an explanation. This document states the goal of PPC is to "relieve suffering, improve quality of life, facilitate informed decision-making, and assist in care coordination between clinicians and across sites of care."[3(p966)]

If a person is interested in hearing more, PPC advocates might choose to address one of the "Top 10 Things Palliative Care Clinicians Wished Everyone Knew About Palliative Care" (**Box 6**) noted by Dr Strand and his colleagues[22] at Mayo Clinic.

Palliative care in its modern form began with the hospice movement led by Dame Cicely Saunders and has evolved to mean much more than end-of-life care. PPC involvement may stretch over years of a life-threatening illness with waxing and waning periods of need. Through experience, time, and education misconceptions about palliative care will resolve. Showing respect is the best way for earning the trust of family, staff, and referring physicians. Sincerely eliciting experience and expertise, acknowledging the intellect and emotion of those involved, and validating the suffering that has been experienced can build trust and mutual respect, which are essential to effective collaboration. By carefully setting precedent of partnership and developing a track record of collaboration long-held misconceptions and apprehensions may be overcome.

The Primary Care Team

Some clinicians worry about referring to PPC too soon, denying families hope, or being seen as abandoning their patients. Meeting families and patients early allows for more reasoned advance care planning and keeps difficult decisions from interfering with the experience at the end of life. Trigger criteria may help clinicians considering PPC consultation. Careful explanation of the referral and an assurance of continued

---

Box 5
Palliative care "elevator pitches"

- "We provide an extra layer of support for patients, families, and clinicians."
- "We work for the best life possible, no matter how long that life may be."
- "Our goal is to help make very day as good as it can be."
- "We support you along your journey, wherever it may take you."
- "Our goal is to provide the child with the best possible quality of life."

Box 6
Top 10 things palliative care clinicians wished everyone knew about palliative care
1. Palliative care can help address the multifaceted aspects of care for patients facing a serious illness
2. Palliative care is appropriate at any stage of serious illness
3. Early integration of palliative care is becoming the new standard of care for patients with advanced cancer
4. Moving beyond cancer: palliative care can be beneficial for many chronic diseases
5. Palliative care teams manage total pain
6. Patients with a serious illness have many symptoms that palliative care teams can help address
7. Palliative care can help address the emotional impact of serious illness on patients and their families
8. Palliative care teams assist in complex communication interactions
9. Addressing the barriers to palliative care involvement: patients' hopes and values equate to more than a cure
10. Palliative care enhances healthcare value

involvement by their well-known clinician can help to avoid any feelings of deflation or abandonment. See **Box 4** for phrases helpful in discussions with families being referred. PPC consultants are present at the request of the primary physician. It is up to the primary physician to determine the role that the palliative care team will play. Sometimes primary clinicians wish to hold the responsibility for goals of care conversations, symptom management, or other aspects of care. The consulting PPC team should recommend interventions or services, unless it is the wish of the primary team to transfer certain management decisions, such as advanced symptom management, completely to the palliative care team.

Other hospital staff including social work, nursing, and child life may also have concerns with involving palliative care. Common worries include interruption in a close connection to a patient or family, unnecessary duplication of services, and a concern that goals are shifting in a way that the staff member disagrees with. Staff and the palliative care team should address these issues by clearly defining roles and striving to succeed in their own realm while supporting and encouraging colleagues to succeed. This can be difficult when emotions and dedication run high. The task is made somewhat easier when lines of communication remain open and respectful between members of the care team. This allows clinicians to maintain the focus on providing best care for the child, regardless of who specifically is providing the care. Shifting goals and plans for a child facing a life-threatening diagnosis can make families and staff uncomfortable. This is partly caused by the unpredictable nature of disease course. It is also a result of the struggle that most parents and clinicians have between medical understanding and the hope for cure or survival. The family's wishes may not seem clear or constant, but the palliative care team may play an important role in maintaining focus on the long-held values of the family so that ultimately they are honored even if they are not in line with the values and goals of those caring for them.

Hospitals

Challenges for hospitals seeking to effectively incorporate PPC include organizing a PPC team when trained clinicians are scarce, budgeting funds for a service likely to generate cost savings rather than revenue, and planning for growth. Those seeking to establish a palliative care service may be surprised to find how much of their existing staff is interested in the field. Administration can use appropriate channels to gauge interest in necessary staff (physicians, nurse practitioners, nurses, social work, and chaplaincy). This initial assessment can involve and empower those interested in palliative care. Even if they are not a part of the final team, it is important to have broad-based support within an institution.[23] A common pitfall in developing a palliative care service is relying on team members to start to plan and/or see patients without any full time equivalent allocation. This practice leads to difficulty providing care, false starts in implementation, and burning out dedicated physicians and staff.[24] The Center for the Advancement of Palliative Care is a rich source of information for building a successful palliative care program (www.capc.org). Although funding sources, such as billing and philanthropy, are important, the best way to ensure consistent, quality palliative care is for the team to be in the operating budget of the hospital. Financially insecure teams have difficulty operating well, and team members in such organizations are likely to be in demand for employment elsewhere in the growing field of palliative care. Planning for staff, cost, and operations should involve much more than what the first few months of the service will look like. It is also important to consider the trajectory over years and consider what volume will necessitate more staff. Building a successful PPC service is an attainable goal for any hospital, but requires careful planning and willingness to adequately support the necessary staff.

PPC continues to grow as a subspecialty in pediatric medicine. The important role that it currently plays is largely because of the added value in healthcare interactions. Elements of a PPC consult described in this article remain important to ensuring the highest quality of care for children with life-threatening illness. As healthcare teams use PPC consultation and overcome obstacles to appropriate PPC they will benefit patients, professionals, and systems of healthcare delivery.

REFERENCES

1. Quill TE, Abernethy AP. Generalist plus specialist palliative care: creating a more sustainable model. N Engl J Med 2014;368(13):1173–5.
2. American Academy of Pediatrics; Committee on Bioethics and Committee on Hospital Care. Palliative care for children. Pediatrics 2000;106(2 Pt 1):351–7.
3. Pediatric palliative care and hospice care commitments, guidelines, and recommendations. Section on Hospice and Palliative Medicine and Committee on Hospital Care. Pediatrics 2013;132:966–72. http://dx.doi.org/10.1542/peds.2013-2731.
4. Feudtner C, Wormer J, Augustin R, et al. Pediatric palliative care programs in children's hospitals: a cross-sectional national survey. Pediatrics 2013;132:1–8.
5. Simon TD, Berry J, Feudtner C, et al. Children with complex chronic conditions in inpatient hospital settings in the United States. Pediatrics 2010;126(4):647–55.
6. Wolfe J, Grier HE, Klar N, et al. Symptoms and suffering at the end of life in children with cancer. N Engl J Med 2000;342(5):326–33.
7. Sahler OJ, Frager G, Levetown M, et al. Medical education about end-of-life care in the pediatric setting: principles, challenges, and opportunities. Pediatrics 2000;105(3):575–84.
8. Mekechuk J. Moral distress in the pediatric intensive care unit: the impact on pediatric nurses. Int J Health Care Qual Assur Inc Leadersh Health Serv 2006; 19(4–5):i–vi.

9. Montagnino BA, Ethier AM. The experiences of pediatric nurses caring for children in persistent vegetative state. Pediatr Crit Care Med 2007;8(5):440–6.

10. Cavaliere TA, Daly B, Dowling D, et al. Moral distress in neonatal intensive care unit RNs. Adv Neonatal Care 2010;10(3):145–56.

11. Hickson GB, Clayton EW, Githens PB, et al. Factors that prompted families to file medical malpractice claims following perinatal injuries. JAMA 1992;267(10): 1359–63.

12. Feudtner C, Kang TI, Hexem KR, et al. Pediatric palliative care patients: a prospective multicenter cohort study. Pediatrics 2011;127(6):1094–101. http://dx. doi.org/10.1542/peds.2010-3225.

13. Sheetz MJ, Bowman MA. Pediatric palliative care: an assessment of physicians' confidence in skills, desire for training, and willingness to refer for end-of-life care. Am J Hosp Palliat Care 2008;25:100–5.

14. Nelson RM, Botkin JR, Kodish ED, et al. Palliative care for children. Pediatrics 2000;106(2):351–7.

15. Feudtner C, Hays RM, Haynes G, et al. Deaths attributed to pediatric complex chronic conditions: national trends and implications for supportive care services. Pediatrics 2001;107(6):E99.

16. Available at: https://www.togetherforshortlives.org.uk/assets/0000/4121/TfSL_A_ Core_Care_Pathway__ONLINE_.pdf.

17. Friebert S, Osenga K. Pediatric palliative care referral criteria. Center to Advance Palliative Care; 2009. Available at: http://www.capc.org/old-tools-for-palliative-care-programs/clinical-tools/consult-triggers/pediatric-palliative-care-referral-criteria. pdf. Accessed November 6, 2013.

18. Sheetz MJ, Sontag Bowman MA. Parents' perceptions of a pediatric palliative program. Am J Hosp Palliat Care 2013;30:291–6. http://dx.doi.org/10.1177/ 1049909112449376.

19. Adams JR, Elwyn G, Legare F, et al. Communicating with physicians about medical decisions: a reluctance to disagree. Arch Intern Med 2012;172(15):1184–6.

20. Thompson LA, Knapp C, Madden V, et al. Pediatricians 'perceptions of and preferred timing for pediatric palliative care. Pediatrics 2009;123(5):777–82.

21. Pincus A. The perfect (elevator) pitch. Businessweek 2007.

22. Strand JJ, Kamdar MM, Carey EC. Top 10 things palliative care clinicians wished everyone knew about palliative care. Mayo Clin Proc 2013;88(8):859–65.

23. Duncan J, Spengler E, Wolfe J. Providing pediatric palliative care: PACT in action. MCN Am J Matern Child Nurs 2007;32(5):279–87.

24. Dev R, Del Fabbro E, Miles M, et al. Growth of an academic palliative medicine program: patient encounters and clinical burden. J Pain Symptom Manage 2013;45(2):261–71.

Improving Quality of life in Hospitalized Children

 CrossMark

Adam Rapoport, MD, FRCPC, MHSc*, Kevin Weingarten, MD, FRCPC, MHSc

KEYWORDS

- Palliative care • Children • Hospital • Distress • Quality of life

KEY POINTS

- There are many ways to add to children's quality of life within the hospital environment.
- Inpatient settings offer both opportunities and challenges with respect to providing care to children with life-threatening illnesses.
- The barriers to pediatric palliative care (PPC) on hospital wards, as with those in other settings, frequently stem from misconceptions. However, some barriers are intensified by characteristics of acute inpatient centers.
- The wealth of human resources and the availability of unique interventions within the inpatient setting facilitate creative ways for improving quality of life and easing distress of hospitalized children and their families.

CASE: PART 1

Eight year-old Koby was born with hypoplastic left heart syndrome for which he underwent a series of cardiac surgeries beginning shortly after birth. These interventions were done to relieve symptoms from his underlying defect; they were never intended to fix the problem. Immediately following his initial surgery Kobe had a cardiac arrest that resulted in permanent neurologic impairment, including mild global developmental delay, behavioral issues, and a learning disability.

Over the past several years Koby has lived at home, but he has required frequent outpatient visits and admissions. The cardiology team recently shared with Koby's family that he is now in end-stage heart failure and that only a heart transplant could significantly extend his life expectancy.

Koby has been in hospital for the past month while undergoing transplant assessment and to optimize medical therapy for his heart failure. Staff have noticed changes in his mood and general demeanor; Koby was always outgoing and happy, but he now seems more introverted and quiet.

Paediatric Advanced Care Team (PACT), The Hospital for Sick Children, 555 University Avenue, Toronto, Ontario M5G 1X8, Canada
* Corresponding author.
E-mail address: adam.rapoport@sickkids.ca

Pediatr Clin N Am 61 (2014) 749–760
http://dx.doi.org/10.1016/j.pcl.2014.04.010
0031-3955/14/$ – see front matter © 2014 Elsevier Inc. All rights reserved.

MAXIMIZING QUALITY OF LIFE IN THE INPATIENT SETTING

The primary goal of palliative care is to maximize the quality of life of the child and the family.[1] This is often accomplished in parallel with efforts to prolong life. Despite the centrality of this goal in pediatric palliative care (PPC), few studies have rigorously investigated methods of assessing quality of life or potential interventions to improve it in children with life-threatening illnesses.[2,3] There is a dearth of research in this area, in part because quality of life is highly individualized and current tools fail to recognize its subjectivity.[4] With this in mind, and absent a universal definition of the term, perhaps the most practical way of understanding and maximizing the quality of life of patients and families is by asking them directly and regularly what would make their lives a little better.

Although any one patient might provide numerous responses to this question at any given moment, ways of improving quality of life can usually be placed into one of 2 categories: things that increase the good and those that decrease the bad.[5] Decreasing the bad in the hospitalized patient usually involves reducing distressing symptoms (primarily addressed later in this article) and, for many, being discharged home. When discharge from hospital is desired by the patient and family, and when the child's condition and the available community resources offer adequate support, efforts to ensure that the inpatient stay is no longer than absolutely necessary are generally appreciated. Nonetheless, sometimes the right place of care for a child with a life-threatening illness is in the hospital, and during those times clinicians can help maximize quality of life by focusing on increasing the good things each day (**Table 1**).

There are many ways to add to a child's quality of life within the hospital environment. Simple things like decorating a patient's room to make it feel more like home can help, and might include having a parent bring a child's blanket, pillow, or favorite stuffed animal, or putting up posters or artwork in the room. Photographs of family and friends can make a hospital room feel more personal and can become a welcome topic of conversation, and visits from family and friends may also brighten a child's day. Recent technological advances have resulted in new modalities for hospitalized patients to have virtual visitors: texting, video chatting, blogging, and posting to social media sites, are just a few of the ways that children and parents can stay connected with family and friends.

Finding ways to incorporate a child's daily routine and normal activities can be helpful. Continuing with school during hospitalization, whenever possible, is another way to bring normalcy to an otherwise abnormal environment. Formal educational services have been shown to improve coping in hospitalized children.[6] Participation in school

Table 1	
Strategies for improving quality of life for patients in hospital	
Strategy	**Example**
Create familiar environment	Bring in toys, pictures, mementos, decorations
Leverage technology	Video chat, social media, music, video and other multimedia
Continue routines	School, tutoring, music lessons
Use therapists and specialists	Physiotherapy, occupational therapy, clown, music, massage, child life specialists, art
Think broadly	Expressive art, meditation, hypnosis, aroma therapy, Reiki
Legacy creation	Photos, hand/foot molds, journaling, blogging
Companionship	Family, friends, volunteers, pets

may be achieved through on-site tutoring or sometimes through videoconferencing with the child's classroom. When not engaged in other activities, having familiar faces come to visit may be helpful. However, it may not always be possible for someone known to the child to be present, but trained volunteers can offer a welcome distraction while providing welcome respite to families.

Although lacking an extensive body of rigorous data, empirical evidence suggests that a variety of therapists can be instrumental in efforts to improve quality of life in the hospitalized child. Child life specialists,[7] pet therapy,[8] and therapeutic clowns[9] can engage the child and help reduce boredom, provide distraction, and allay anxiety, and also help family members find ways to get involved (**Fig. 1**). Child life specialists may also arrange special moments: spa days, visits from local celebrities and athletes, screenings of plays and movies, and marking special occasions such as birthdays. Music therapy has been shown to have positive effects such as decreasing various symptoms in children, including pain[10] and anxiety,[11,12] and increasing their ability to cope with stress.[13] Qualitative and quantitative studies on the effects of music therapy in PPC have shown its ability to improve communication between parent and child.[14] Bereaved parents have also reflected that music therapy helped to form lasting positive memories (**Fig. 2**).[15] Massage therapy results in modest reductions in pain and a variety of other symptoms in adults receiving palliative care[16]; it may also reduce pain and induce relaxation in hospitalized children with chronic illness.[17] Although art therapy may also improve quality of life in patients with life-threatening conditions,[18] it can also serve as a tool for hospitalized children to express their thoughts and feelings, which in turn may identify ways to improve overall well-being.[19] Regardless of the evidence to support these and other forms of integrative and expressive therapies,

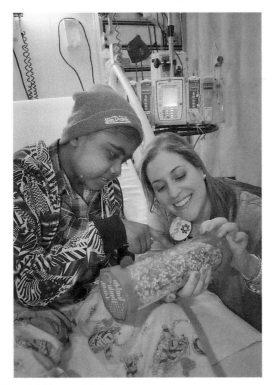

Fig. 1. Patient with child life specialist.

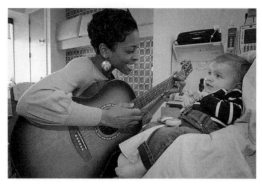

Fig. 2. Patient with music therapist.

whether or how a particular intervention may benefit an individual child varies. When available, these and other interventions to improve quality of life should be offered, and, if accepted, their effects should be regularly assessed.

Although these and other good experiences in hospital may inadvertently create positive memories for bereaved parents, the hospitalization of a child with a life-threatening condition can be a time for intentional legacy creation as well. Children, like adults, want to be remembered when they die; creating personal messages, art, and other keepsakes for family and friends can help assure a dying child that their memory will live on while providing their loved ones with gifts that will be treasured. Photographs, hand/foot molds and prints, and journaling (written, audio, or video) are just a few examples of activities in which children can engage as inpatients and that many pediatric hospitals support.[20]

CHALLENGES TO INTRODUCING PPC IN THE HOSPITAL SETTING

Many children with life-threatening conditions spend long periods in hospital for diagnostic purposes, medical or surgical treatments, or perhaps for end-of-life care. Although increasing efforts are being made to shift the care of children with complex chronic conditions into the home and the community,[21] dedicated pediatric health centers remain a primary setting in which these patients visit their subspecialists, undergo tests and procedures, and ultimately are where patients may feel most comfortable turning for their acute care needs. For this reason, the inpatient setting remains the most common location for PPC introduction.[22] The central role of the hospital for a child with a life-threatening illness makes it an important location for the integration of palliative care services. However, unique challenges exist to integrating palliative care within the pediatric hospital setting (a more thorough discussion regarding factors that affect referral to PPC is provided elsewhere in this issue).

The barriers to PPC on the hospital wards, as with those in other settings, frequently stem from misconceptions about PPC. However, some barriers are intensified by specific characteristics of acute inpatient centers. Although the presence of palliative care services has grown considerably within pediatric hospitals,[23] the overarching goal of inpatient care is to help children to recover from illness. Apart from patient rooms or units designated for palliative care, the ubiquitous glow of vital sign monitors and the overhead buzzers and bells of the hospital environment serve as a reminder that care in the inpatient setting is intended ultimately to fix medical problems or at the least prevent deterioration. Despite endorsements for its early integration by both general pediatric[1] and subspecialty[24] bodies, many health care providers continue to view palliative care as an option reserved only for when all curative therapies have been exhausted.[25–27] Until it is widely recognized that palliative care and curative care need not be mutually exclusive, the goal of medical care in the inpatient hospital setting may be at odds with palliative care.

Beyond the fix-it mentality that families expect and providers espouse within the pediatric inpatient setting, the nature of the highly subspecialized care that occurs there may also impede palliative care. Most PPC services work in a consultative model[22]: patients are referred to them by other services or clinicians when involving palliative care might be beneficial. Guidelines recently published by the American Academy of Pediatrics recommend that all physicians be able to inform patients and families about PPC.[28] However, many subspecialists, particularly those who do not regularly collaborate with palliative care, may not possess the knowledge and language to adequately convey to families what palliative care involvement might add. If palliative care is perceived by most families as giving up,[29] then it must be introduced by individuals who can confidently dispel these and other myths in order to achieve timely integration. It is paradoxical that the availability of an inpatient PPC service may exacerbate the problem by unintentionally sending the message that palliative care requires the expertise of a subspecialty team. Efforts to promote palliative care as an essential competency for all health care providers caring for children with life-threatening illness remain essential.

DISTRESSING EFFECTS OF HOSPITALIZATION ON THE CHILD AND FAMILY UNIT

Several challenging and distressing effects are associated with hospitalization, including sleep, emotional, and behavioral disturbances. Hospitalization often affects the entire family unit as well (symptoms in children receiving palliative care are discussed elsewhere in this issue).

The impact of hospitalization on the emotional well-being of children has long been recognized. More than 60 years ago Moncrieff said, "The emotional needs of the sick child need as much consideration as his food or drug therapy."[30] More recently, work has been done to determine those factors that place children at greater risk for difficulty coping while in hospital.[31] These include, but are not limited to, age between 0.5 and 4 years, prolonged admission, more severe trauma or illness, length of time since diagnosis, and the child's previous experience(s) in hospital.[31,32] Many of these factors can be seen in the PPC population and create difficulties for children merely because they are admitted, regardless of their diagnosis and concurrent symptoms. Two suggested methods to help children cope with hospitalization are preparation techniques and cognitive coping strategies.[33] The preparation techniques include using reading material or videos before procedures and introduction to new areas of the hospital (eg, intensive care unit, operating suite). Cognitive coping strategies, including relaxation, distraction, and cognitive restructuring, may also be helpful in the hospital environment.[34]

However, the effects of prolonged hospitalization are not isolated to the patient: siblings and parents are also affected. Siblings can have feelings of abandonment, guilt, jealousy, confusion, or resentment.[32] Regarding parents, a recent review showed how critical illness (specifically admission to the pediatric intensive care unit [ICU]) affected parents in many ways: physical and emotional fatigue, changed routines, lower quality of life, and increased physical symptoms.[35] Parents also have stress-related symptoms and difficulties with family functioning as long as 6 months after a child's admission to the ICU.[36] Divorce rates may be increased secondary to stress and prolonged hospitalization; however, studies examining this issue have yielded conflicting results.[37] There is anecdotal evidence that many providers think that stressful situations accentuate preexisting qualities of relationships and do not in themselves increase separation rates.

One of the most important and impaired aspects of daily living in the hospital is sleep. Even in hospitals where private rooms are the norm, constant noise, disturbances (both for necessary and accidental reasons), and the continuous vigilance of nurses and family members can be expected.[38] These factors, among others, create an environment that is not conducive to normal sleep and may exacerbate sleep disturbance and fatigue related to their underlying condition. Physiologic changes caused by sleep disturbance may result in impaired natural host defenses and inhibition of growth hormone secretion.[39,40] In addition, sleep deficits have behavioral and cognitive effects such as decreased attention and concentration, and increased irritability, depression, and impulsivity.[41] One study even showed that sleep disturbance may lead to increased feelings of depression and hopelessness,[42] which for PPC patients and their families could compound existing hardships. Efforts should be made to reduce nighttime noise and frequency of vital sign monitoring, in addition to restructuring medication schedules in inpatient units.[41] In addition, simple interventions such as decreasing nighttime intravenous fluid rates can decrease wakings and improve sleep in the hospital setting.[43] Individual sleep hygiene tips, such as those published by Seattle Children's hospital, can also be helpful, even for the hospitalized child (**Table 2**).[44]

CASE: PART 2

The hospital palliative care team met Koby and his family to discuss goals of care in light of his end-stage heart failure. Koby, his family, and the palliative care team think that efforts should be focused on blending life-prolonging measures with measures that would maximize quality of life, including keeping Koby out of hospital as much as possible. However, intensive measures designed to prolong his life, such as cardiopulmonary resuscitation and ICU admission, no longer fit with their goals. Koby was discharged from the hospital with palliative care support in the community, his congestive heart failure (CHF) medications optimized, and a Do Not Resuscitate order implemented.

A few months later, Koby presented to the emergency room with significant increased work of breathing, cyanosis, and hypoxia. He had been more irritable recently with significant abdominal pain. Investigations suggested worsening CHF as the likely cause of these changes but the cardiology team thought that all therapeutic interventions to maximize heart function had been exhausted. The palliative care

Table 2 Individual sleep hygiene tips	
Sleep schedule	Have regular bedtimes and wake times
Bedtime routine	Do the same things each night (charts can help)
Bedroom	Dark, cool, and quiet rooms are preferred
Set limits	For books, electronics, even scheduled worry time
Naps	Be aware of their impact on nighttime sleep
Security object	Can be of particular use in hospital
Sleep diary	Can help identify problems

Adapted from Mindell JA, Owens JA. A clinical guide to pediatric sleep: diagnosis and management of sleep problems. 2nd edition. Philadelphia: Lippincott Williams & Wilkins; 2010.

team suggested starting an opioid to relieve the dyspnea and abdominal pain, which was thought to be ischemic. However, the cardiac team was reluctant to prescribe opioids to a child with hypoxia.

CONSIDERATIONS ABOUT SYMPTOM MANAGEMENT IN THE HOSPITAL SETTING

The inpatient setting offers unique advantages to help address particularly challenging situations. Among the most obvious is that inpatients have around-the-clock access to expert staff and other resources, which allows rapid symptom assessment, investigation, and management. Furthermore, ready access to PPC specialists in the inpatient setting has increased significantly over the past 2 decades.[22] These additional resources in the inpatient pediatric setting not only promote timely initiation of therapy but they may also result in faster symptom control. Close patient observation by nursing staff and continuous electronic monitoring may permit more rapid titration of medication than would normally be attempted in the outpatient setting.[45]

The unique resources available in the inpatient setting may also allow both novel and targeted therapies, resulting in improved symptom management with fewer adverse effects than might be experienced in the outpatient setting. For example, it would be reasonable to treat new-onset dyspnea in a child at home with lung metastases using opioids. However, if an investigation in hospital determined that the cause of the dyspnea were an effusion, an indwelling tunneled catheter might result in symptom resolution without the adverse effects associated with regular systemic opioids. This innovative approach has been shown to offer advantages compared with needle thoracentesis and therapeutic pleurodesis. These traditional techniques are associated with pain, reaccumulation, loculation, and the potential for multiple procedures.[46] They also can be associated with prolonged hospitalization, which an indwelling tunneled catheter has been shown to avoid (albeit in small studies).[46,47] So far, these catheters have been easy and safe to insert, and have been easy for families to manage at home.[46,47]

The initiation of indwelling tunneled catheters is just one example of a procedure done in hospital but that can ultimately ease distress by helping a patient return to a preferred location of care. Another such intervention, particularly relevant for Kobe in the case described earlier, is the initiation of continuous inotropic therapy.[48] In the context of CHF it is usually used to maintain relative health while awaiting cardiac transplantation. However, it has also been used in patients who are no longer candidates for transplantation, in an attempt to maintain quality and longevity of life at home. In either case, early results show that it is not only safe but also cost-efficient, and it improves family dynamics by avoiding prolonged hospitalization.[48]

Other procedures that are initiated in hospital but may facilitate transition to a preferred location include central neuraxial infusions (ie, epidural and intrathecal), peripheral nerve and plexus blocks, and implantable pumps (eg, baclofen, opioids, local anesthetics).[49,50] These therapies have the potential to increase pain control, decrease spasticity (ie, baclofen), and decrease systemic medication use. With necessary supports in place these therapies can be maintained outside the hospital as well.[50,51] Data for the safety of these procedures suggest that they are safe, although the data are still mainly limited to case reports and series.[49]

These and other interventions, such as noninvasive ventilation, are now being used in PPC in an attempt to take full advantage of in-hospital resources. At the same time, these procedures and treatments are attempting to improve quality of life and give patients and their families the option for home as the location of care. Although early indications are positive, caution is needed before considering any of these to be standards of care. The PPC population is vulnerable, and as such goals of care must be made clear before embarking on the use of any intervention carrying significant risks.

EDUCATING AND SUPPORTING TRAINEES AND TEAM MEMBERS

The team approach to PPC is discussed elsewhere in this issue. PPC is almost impossible to practice well in isolation. Health care providers across several disciplines and levels of training are needed to implement PPC effectively and prepare future generations for the task. However, providing care to children with life-threatening conditions, and end-of-life care in particular, can take its toll on frontline staff. To create an environment in which PPC can thrive, it is therefore necessary to support health care providers and their trainees as they are tasked with easing distress in the hospitalized patient.

Hospitalization, and the distress associated with it, presents an opportunity for pediatric trainees to learn PPC skills. Two issues that have been gaining attention lately are trainee preparedness and education in PPC.[52–57] One survey of pediatric residents throughout their 3 years of training showed that residents think that pediatricians should have an important role in providing PPC.[56] However, the same residents reported minimal training, experience, competence, and comfort in most areas of PPC. In addition, these issues did not improve between the first year of training and the third, suggesting that this educational program had no impact on perceived PPC competence. An argument might be made that an area of pediatrics more frequently exposed to death, such as oncology, might provide a more robust training in this area. Roth and colleagues[52] surveyed pediatric oncology fellowship directors in the United States and almost all respondents thought that it was very/extremely important for fellows to learn about PPC during their training. However, most of the programs did not have a palliative care curriculum and lacked significant formal education in end-of-life care.[52]

Workshops are an educational tool used to enhance PPC. However, they may not produce lasting improvement in knowledge, which was found in an intense 1-day workshop for oncology fellows.[53] Many fellows thought that ongoing, integrative education and experience in PPC is needed in order to crystallize knowledge, comfort, and competency.[52,56,57] It could therefore be argued that by having PPC exposure throughout any training process (eg, physician, nurse, social work, occupational therapy, physical therapy), trainees would develop lifelong appreciation for the art of PPC.

Although education and training are intended to prepare those exposed to PPC, support is also needed for the grief and moral distress generated from that exposure.[58,59] Although this is elaborated on elsewhere in this issue, it is important to emphasize how grief and moral distress can affect the care of children in PPC. Conflicts between staff (or between staff and family members) regarding end-of-life decision making can lead to moral distress.[58] Grief can be a prominent feature both during and after experiences in PPC.[59] It therefore follows that there is a need for more emotional support for those involved in such care. This support might lead to positive reinforcement and less compassion fatigue among caregivers, resulting in a better experience for all involved. It therefore seems clear that it is in everyone's best interest to support all staff involved in the care of children and their families receiving PPC.

CASE: PART 3

The palliative care and cardiology teams worked together to optimize Koby's comfort, in line with the family's goals of care. A continuous milrinone infusion was initiated by the cardiology team in an attempt to help Koby spend more time at home. The palliative care team worked with the cardiology service, Koby, and his family to intro-duce additional methods of ameliorating distressing symptoms. Opioids and oxygen were titrated to achieve comfort, and massage therapy techniques were taught to Koby's mother once they were found to be helpful. While these measures were being optimized, Koby met with the hospital music therapist and worked on a song that he dedicated to his family. The palliative care team facilitated several opportunities for voicing concerns and feelings, out of recognition that the cardiology staff may be struggling with the impending death of a patient whom they had loved and cared for over many years.

The inpatient setting offers both opportunities and challenges with respect to providing care to children with life-threatening illnesses. Additional resources and unique capabilities found within pediatric hospitals offer important ways to improve the quality of life of these patients and their families. However, health care providers should be mindful of the detrimental effects of hospitalization and look for ways to ease distress wherever possible.

REFERENCES

1. American Academy of Pediatrics. Committee on Bioethics and Committee on Hospital Care. Palliative care for children. Pediatrics 2000;106(2 Pt 1):351–7.
2. Huang IC, Shenkman EA, Madden VL, et al. Measuring quality of life in pediatric palliative care: challenges and potential solutions. Palliat Med 2010;24(2): 175–82.
3. Knapp C, Madden V, Revicki D, et al. Health status and health-related quality of life in a pediatric palliative care program. J Palliat Med 2012;15(7):790–7.
4. Carr AJ, Higginson IJ. Are quality of life measures patient centred? BMJ 2001; 322(7298):1357–60.
5. Feudtner C. Collaborative communication in pediatric palliative care: a founda-tion for problem-solving and decision-making. Pediatr Clin North Am 2007; 54(5):583–607, ix.
6. Ratnapalan S, Rayar MS, Crawley M. Educational services for hospitalized chil-dren. Paediatr Child Health 2009;14(7):433–6.
7. Wilson JM. Child life services. Pediatrics 2006;118(4):1757–63.
8. Kaminski M, Pellino T, Wish J. Play and pets: the physical and emotional impact of child-life and pet therapy on hospitalized children. Child Health Care 2002; 31(4):321–35.
9. Linge L. Joyful and serious intentions in the work of hospital clowns: a meta-analysis based on a 7-year research project conducted in three parts. Int J Qual Stud Health Well Being 2013;8:1–8.
10. Hartling L, Newton AS, Liang Y, et al. Music to reduce pain and distress in the pediatric emergency department: a randomized clinical trial. JAMA Pediatr 2013;167(9):826–35.
11. Colwell CM, Edwards R, Hernandez E, et al. Impact of music therapy interven-tions (listening, composition, Orff-based) on the physiological and psychosocial behaviors of hospitalized children: a feasibility study. J Pediatr Nurs 2013;28(3): 249–57.
12. Goldbeck L, Ellerkamp T. A randomized controlled trial of multimodal music ther-apy for children with anxiety disorders. J Music Ther 2012;49(4):395–413.
13. Treurnicht Naylor K, Kingsnorth S, Lamont A, et al. The effectiveness of music in pediatric healthcare: a systematic review of randomized controlled trials. Evid Based Complement Alternat Med 2011;2011:464759.

14. Knapp C, Madden V, Wang H, et al. Music therapy in an integrated pediatric palliative care program. Am J Hosp Palliat Care 2009;26(6):449–55.

15. Lindenfelser KJ, Grocke D, McFerran K. Bereaved parents' experiences of music therapy with their terminally ill child. J Music Ther 2008;45(3):330–48.

16. Ernst E. Massage therapy for cancer palliation and supportive care: a systematic review of randomised clinical trials. Support Care Cancer 2009; 17(4):333–7.

17. Cotton S, Luberto CM, Bogenschutz LH, et al. Integrative care therapies and pain in hospitalized children and adolescents: a retrospective database review. J Altern Complement Med 2014;20(2):98–102.

18. Rhondali W, Lasserre E, Filbet M. Art therapy among palliative care inpatients with advanced cancer. Palliat Med 2013;27(6):571–2.

19. Wikstrom BM. Communicating via expressive arts: the natural medium of self-expression for hospitalized children. Pediatr Nurs 2005;31(6):480–5.

20. Foster TL, Dietrich MS, Friedman DL, et al. National survey of children's hospitals on legacy-making activities. J Palliat Med 2012;15(5):573–8.

21. Law J, McCann D, O'May F. Managing change in the care of children with complex needs: healthcare providers' perspectives. J Adv Nurs 2011;67(12): 2551–60.

22. Feudtner C, Womer J, Augustin R, et al. Pediatric palliative care programs in children's hospitals: a cross-sectional national survey. Pediatrics 2013;132(6): 1063–70.

23. Morrison RS, Maroney-Galin C, Kralovec PD, et al. The growth of palliative care programs in United States hospitals. J Palliat Med 2005;8(6):1127–34.

24. Smith TJ, Temin S, Alesi ER, et al. American Society of Clinical Oncology provisional clinical opinion: the integration of palliative care into standard oncology care. J Clin Oncol 2012;30(8):880–7.

25. Thompson LA, Knapp C, Madden V, et al. Pediatricians' perceptions of and preferred timing for pediatric palliative care. Pediatrics 2009;123(5):e777–82.

26. Dalberg T, Jacob-Files E, Carney PA, et al. Pediatric oncology providers' perceptions of barriers and facilitators to early integration of pediatric palliative care. Pediatr Blood Cancer 2013;60(11):1875–81.

27. Docherty SL, Miles MS, Brandon D. Searching for "the dying point:" providers' experiences with palliative care in pediatric acute care. Pediatr Nurs 2007; 33(4):335–41.

28. American Academy of Pediatrics. Section on Hospice and Palliative Medicine and Committee on Hospital Care. Pediatric Palliative Care and Hospice Care Commitments, Guidelines, and Recommendations. Pediatrics 2013;132(5): 966–72.

29. Knapp C, Thompson L. Factors associated with perceived barriers to pediatric palliative care: a survey of pediatricians in Florida and California. Palliat Med 2012;26(3):268–74.

30. Prugh DG, Staub EM, Sands HH, et al. A study of the emotional reactions of children and families to hospitalization and illness. American Journal of Orthopsychiatry 1953;23(1):70–106.

31. Wright MC. Behavioural effects of hospitalization in children. J Paediatr Child Health 1995;31:165–7.

32. Children's Specialized Hospital. Effects of hospitalization on siblings. Available at: http://www.childrens-specialized.org/Programs-Services/Specialty-Programs/Recreational-Therapy-and-Child-Life/About-Child-Life/Sibling-Support/Effect-of-Hospitalization-on-Siblings.aspx. Accessed April 9, 2014.

33. Peterson L, Shigetomi C. The use of coping techniques to minimize anxiety in hospitalized children. Behav Ther 1981;12:1–14.
34. Hildenbrand AK, Clawson KJ, Alderfer MA, et al. Coping with pediatric cancer: strategies employed by children and their parents to manage cancer-related stressors during treatment. J Pediatr Oncol Nurs 2011;28(6):344–54.
35. Shudy M, Lihinie de Almeida M, et al. Impact of pediatric critical illness and injury on families: a systematic literature review. Pediatrics 2006;118:S203.
36. Board R, Ryan-Wenger N. Long-term effects of pediatric intensive care unit hospitalization on families with young children. Heart Lung 2002;31(1):53–66.
37. Syse A, et al. Does childhood cancer affect parental divorce rates? A population-based study. Clin Oncol 2009;28:872–7.
38. Hinds PS, Hockenberry MJ, Rai SN, et al. Nocturnal awakenings, sleep environment interruptions, and fatigue in hospitalized children with cancer. Oncol Nurs Forum 2007;34:393–402.
39. Irwin M. Effects of sleep and sleep loss on immunity and cytokines. Brain Behav Immun 2002;16:503–12.
40. Irwin M, Wang M, Campomayor CO, et al. Sleep deprivation and activation of morning levels of cellular and genomic markers of inflammation. Arch Intern Med 2006;166(16):1756–62.
41. Linder LA, Christian BJ. Nighttime sleep characteristics of hospitalized school-age children with cancer. J Spec Pediatr Nurs 2013;18:13–24.
42. Mystakidou K, et al. Does quality of sleep mediate the effect of depression on hopelessness? Int J Psychol 2009;44(4):282–9.
43. Boonstra L, et al. Sleep disturbances in hospitalized recipients of stem cell transplantation. Clin J Oncol Nurs 2010;15(3):271–6.
44. Hilt R. Sleep hygiene for children. Patient and Family Education, 2011. Available at: www.seattlechildrens.org/pdf/PE1066.pdf. Accessed April 9, 2014.
45. Mercadante S, Villari P, Ferrera P, et al. Rapid titration with intravenous morphine for severe cancer pain and immediate oral conversion. Cancer 2002;95(1):203–8.
46. den Hollander BS, Connolly BL, Sung L, et al. Successful use of indwelling tunneled catheters for the management of effusions in children with advanced cancer. Pediatr Blood Cancer 2014;61(6):1007–12.
47. Schiff D, Meixel A. PleurX! Catheter placement for palliation of pediatric patients with symptomatic malignant effusions. J Pain Symptom Manage 2012;43(2):439–40.
48. Berg AM, Snell L, Mahle WT. Home inotropic therapy in children. J Heart Lung Transplant 2007;26(5):453–7.
49. Rork JF, Berde CB, Goldstein R. Regional anesthesia approaches to pain management in pediatric palliative care: a review of current knowledge. J Pain Symptom Manage 2013;46(6):859–73.
50. Anghelescu DL, Faughnan LG, Baker JN, et al. Use of epidural and peripheral nerve blocks at the end of life in children and young adults with cancer: the collaboration between a pain service and a palliative care service. Paediatr Anaesth 2010;20:1070–7.
51. Krames E. Implantable devices for pain control: spinal cord stimulation and intrathecal therapies. Best Pract Res Clin Anaesthesiol 2002;16(4):619–49.
52. Roth M, Wang D, Kim M, et al. An assessment of the current state of palliative care education in pediatric hematology/oncology fellowship training. Pediatr Blood Cancer 2009;53:647–51.
53. Gerhardt C, et al. Longitudinal evaluation of a pediatric palliative care educational workshop for oncology fellows. J Palliat Med 2009;12(4):323–8.

54. Amery J, Rose CJ, Byarugaba C, et al. A study into the children's palliative care educational needs of health professionals in Uganda. J Palliat Med 2010;13(2): 147–53.

55. Sahler OJZ, Frager G, et al. Medical education about end-of-life care in the pediatric setting: principles, challenges, and opportunities. Pediatrics 2000; 105(2):575–84.

56. Kolarik RC, Walker G, Arnold RM. Pediatric resident education in palliative care: a needs assessment. Pediatrics 2006;117:1949.

57. Yang CP, et al. Pediatric residents do not feel prepared for the most unsettling situations they face in the pediatric intensive care unit. J Palliat Med 2011; 14(1):25–30.

58. Klein SM. Moral distress in pediatric palliative care: a case study. J Pain Symptom Manage 2009;38(1):157–60.

59. Lee KJ, Dupree CY. Staff experiences with end-of-life care in the pediatric intensive care unit. J Palliat Med 2008;11(7):986–90.

Transitions to and from the Acute Inpatient Care Setting for Children with Life-Threatening Illness

Savithri Nageswaran, MBBS, MPH[a],*,
Andrea Radulovic, RN, BSN, MPH[b], Aura Anania, MSW, BSW[a]

KEYWORDS

- Children • Life-threatening illness • Hospitalization • Transition

KEY POINTS

- Hospitalizations may be associated with changes in health status and care needs of children with life-threatening illnesses (LTI).
- Challenges in transitioning children with LTI to and from acute care settings are many.
- Strategies to improve transitional care exist and include improving communication between clinicians across clinical settings, anticipating medication problems, and preparing families for the transition.
- Pediatric palliative care teams can play an important role in transitional care of children with LTI.

Dr S. Nageswaran's work on this project is supported by the Pilot Project Support Grant from the National Palliative Care Research Center, Healthy Tomorrow's Partnership for Children Program Grant from the Health Resources and Services Administration (H17MC11228), and Integrated Community Systems for CSHCN Grant from the Health Resources and Services Administration (D70MC23061).
Ms A. Anania's work on this project is supported by Healthy Tomorrow's Partnership for Children Program Grant from the Health Resources and Services Administration (H17MC11228) and Integrated Community Systems for CSHCN Grant from the Health Resources and Services Administration (D70MC23061).
Case examples presented in this article are actual clinical cases the authors encountered in clinical practice, but clinical details have been slightly modified to protect anonymity.
[a] Department of Pediatrics, Wake Forest School of Medicine, 1 Medical Center Boulevard, Winston-Salem, NC 27157, USA; [b] Brenner Children's Hospital, Wake Forest Baptist Health, Winston-Salem, NC 27157, USA
* Corresponding author.
E-mail address: snageswa@wakehealth.edu

Pediatr Clin N Am 61 (2014) 761–783
http://dx.doi.org/10.1016/j.pcl.2014.04.008
0031-3955/14/$ – see front matter © 2014 Elsevier Inc. All rights reserved.

pediatric.theclinics.com

INTRODUCTION

There has been a recent focus in reducing hospital readmissions in the United States, especially among Medicare beneficiaries, as a way to reduce health care costs.[1] This has resulted in increased attention to the quality of transitional care–delivery of care that involves seamless transitions of patients from acute inpatient care settings to the community to other clinical care settings.[1,2] Most quality-improvement activities and research in transitional care target hospitalized adults. Readmissions rates, however, have more recently been included as a quality measure of pediatric health care,[3] and quality-improvement efforts aimed at transitional care for hospitalized pediatric patients are emerging.[4,5]

Seamless transitional care involves smooth transition of all aspects of care of patients from one clinical setting to another by maintaining continuity of care. When patients do not receive seamless transitional care, they are at risk of not receiving appropriate medical care that is needed in the setting to which they are transitioned.[6,7] Poor transitional care of patients results in new problems, such as an adverse event from medication error or worsening of existing problems due to lack of adequate follow-up medical care.

IMPORTANCE OF TRANSITIONAL CARE IN CHILDREN WITH LIFE-THREATENING ILLNESSES

As described in the article by Bogetz and colleagues elsewhere in this issue, children with life-threatening illness (LTI) account for greater proportions of hospitalizations and hospital days of all children, compared to a decade ago;[8] and a large proportion of readmissions to children's hospitals in the United States.[9,10] Children with LTIs are living longer compared with those a few decades ago.[11] Although these children were cared for in congregate settings in the past, since the 1950s there has been a strong movement toward deinstitutionalization and providing care for children with LTIs in the community. These factors have resulted in a steady increase in the number of children with LTIs receiving complex medical care at home.[12]

The American Academy of Pediatrics (AAP) developed the concept of a "medical home," a model of care that is compassionate, continuous, family-centered, coordinated, and delivered by primary care providers (PCPs).[13] The Agency for Healthcare Research and Quality (AHRQ), as an extension of the medical home model, introduced the concept of the "medical neighborhood" and defined it as a patient's medical home, with all specialists and community agencies serving the patient.[14] The models in **Fig. 1** represent the medical neighborhood for children by adapting a model proposed by another AHRQ white paper to represent medical complexity and care coordination needs.[15] Using the AHRQ model, circles are used to represent the providers and entities involved in an individual's health care. As seen in **Fig. 1**A, for a child with no underlying health condition, the medical neighborhood consists of the medical home and the dentist. For a child with a non–life-threatening condition, such as seizure disorder, the medical neighborhood may in addition consist of a neurologist and a pharmacy (see **Fig. 1**B). For a child with LTI, however, who is likely to have impairment of multiple organ systems and significant functional limitations and use assistive technology, the medical neighborhood has many more entities (see **Fig. 1**C). Case example 1, a child with LTI who is hospitalized, illustrates the enormous medical complexity of children with LTIs.

> **Case Example 1**: A 1-year-old girl with Dandy-Walker malformation, seizure disorder, and respiratory failure was hospitalized for 132 days in a tertiary care medical center. During this hospitalization, she received 187 laboratory draws, 76 radiographs, 16 neurophysiologic evaluations, 5 CT scans, 2 MRIs, and 9 different surgical procedures. She received care from 20 different specialty health care teams in addition to the primary team of physicians and nurses. She received supportive care from pastoral care, palliative care, and child-life therapy. At the time of discharge home, she had new medical needs, a tracheostomy through which she received oxygen, and a gastrostomy tube and received 15 different medications. In the 6 months after her discharge, she had 18 specialty clinic appointments and was hospitalized thrice.

Because children with LTIs are hospitalized more often, have multiple clinicians and agencies involved in their care in the community and in the hospital, and have complex medical care needs at home, transitional care is more complex for this population with a greater opportunity for problems.

TYPES OF TRANSITIONS INVOLVING ACUTE CARE SETTING

In this article, the term, *hospital*, refers to the acute inpatient care setting and *caregivers* refers to parents and other informal caregivers of children with LTIs. There are different types of transition that can occur during hospitalization in an acute care setting. These are described in **Box 1**. Most children with LTIs transition from the hospital to home. Less commonly, children can be transitioned from the hospital to other facilities, such as long-term care, rehabilitation, or hospice facilities, and other hospitals.

COMMON CHALLENGES AND OPPORTUNITIES IN PROVIDING TRANSITIONAL CARE TO CHILDREN WITH LTIS

In addition to a change in clinical setting, hospitalization involves change in clinicians and teams delivering care to a child with LTI resulting in discontinuity in care delivery. Moreover, during hospitalization, a child's health condition can change significantly. The change in health condition of a child with LTI during hospitalization often leads to changes in the medications, technology, nutrition, specialist care, tests and procedures, support services, and home care services that the child receives. Case example 2 shows how a common illness resulting in hospitalization changed the health condition of a child with LTI.

> **Case Example 2**: A 10-month-old child with Down syndrome, congenital heart disease that was repaired, and pulmonary hypertension was receiving medical care from her primary care physician and 3 specialists and did not receive home health nursing services. She was hospitalized for respiratory syncytial virus bronchiolitis. At the time of admission, she had a gastrostomy tube for nutrition and medication administration and nasal cannula oxygen and received 5 medications (furosemide, enalapril, pantoprazole, inhaled albuterol, and corticosteroid). She had a complicated 6-month hospital course. At the time of discharge, her health care needs had increased significantly. She had a tracheostomy tube through which she received supplemental oxygen; she received continuous feeds through the gastrostomy tube, 17 different medications, home health nursing services, and follow-up with 10 specialist services.

Many barriers to transitioning children with LTIs across clinical settings exist. Over the past several decades, there has been a shift in how health care is delivered. For example, the introduction of the hospitalist model of care delivery has resulted in

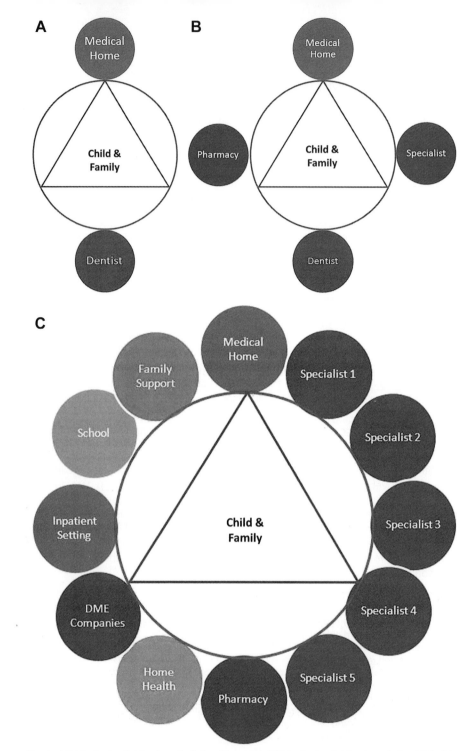

Fig. 1. (*A*) Medical neighborhood of a healthy child. (*B*) Medical neighborhood of a child with a chronic condition. (*C*) Medical neighborhood of a child with an LTI or complex medical condition. (Adapted with permission from "Fig. 1. Care Coordination Ring." In: McDonald KM, Schultz E, Albin L, et al. Care Coordination Measures Atlas, Version 3. (AHRQ Publication No. 11-0023-EF). Rockville (MD): Agency for Healthcare Research andQuality; 2010. p. 7.)

> **Box 1**
> **Types of transitions across clinical settings for children with LTIs**
>
> *Transition out of the acute care setting (hospital)*
> - Home: transitioning involves transitioning to community clinicians or entities
>   - PCPs
>   - Specialist physicians
>   - Home health
>   - Home hospice
>   - DME companies
>   - Pharmacy
>   - Emergency medical services
>   - Physical therapy, occupational therapy, and other therapy services
>   - School
>   - Other special services for children with LTIs, such as Medicaid waiver programs and early intervention services.
> - Inpatient hospice facility
> - LTCF
> - Rehabilitation facility
> - Other hospitals
>
> *Transition into the acute care setting (hospital)*
> - Home
> - Other facilities (eg, inpatient hospice facility or LTCF)
> - Other hospitals

different clinicians providing care for children in the hospital and the community.[16] Second, advances in technology, medications, and testing have increased the complexity of medical care, creating greater opportunities for errors during transitions across clinical settings. Third, there has been a steady increase in complex medical care delivered at home and a shift toward delivering medical care at home rather than in the hospital.

There are barriers to transitional care at the clinician level as well. Hospital and community-based clinicians report not having adequate time to perform tasks related to transitional care.[17] Moreover, there is not clear assignment of responsibility of roles about who performs the tasks related to transitional care.[16,18] Until recently, quality of transitional care has not been a focus of the US health care system. As such, the health care system is not organized for delivering optimal transitional care.

In the following sections, various challenges in transitional care are identified and strategies that facilitate seamless transitions across settings are provided.

Communication with Clinicians and Other Agencies

Communication is the most important aspect of transitioning children with LTIs. As children with LTIs are transitioned from the hospital to the community, there should be effective communication between hospital-based clinicians and community-based clinicians. A systematic review showed that communication and information problems at the time of discharge are common and result in potential harms to patients discharged to the community.[6]

Clinicians report several barriers in communicating with other clinicians during transition of children across clinical settings.[17–19] Some of these barriers are listed.

Clinicians' perceived barriers to communication across clinical settings
- Lack of time
- Lack of reimbursement
- Lack of agreement between clinicians about information to be communicated
- Lack of knowledge about the best method of communication
- Difficulty accessing clinicians in other clinical settings

Communication with primary care providers

PCPs play a major role in the care of children with LTIs in the community and often serve as the primary resource for caregivers and other community clinicians, such as home health nurses. It is imperative that there is effective communication between hospital-based clinicians and PCPs.

Over the past 10 years, increasingly hospital-based physicians rather than PCPs provide medical care for children with LTIs when they are hospitalized. One of the concerns of this model of care delivery is the lack of continuity of care during transitions to and from the hospital.[20] The AAP describes communication with PCPs as one of the responsibilities of hospital-based clinicians.[21] Communication between hospital-based physicians and PCPs is, however, not optimal.[17–19]

In 2011, a survey of PCPs of children (pediatricians, family physicians, and midlevel clinicians) was conducted in northwest North Carolina that inquired about their preferences for and experiences with communication of hospital-based clinicians.[22] Of the 123 respondents, a large proportion reported need for communication during hospitalization, but their communication needs were largely unmet (**Table 1**). These observations were similar to other reports on this topic.[18,19]

When inquired specifically about discharge summaries, 97% of PCPs in the North Carolina survey reported that they needed discharge summaries. Only 76% reported, however, receiving discharge summaries consistently and 33% received discharge summaries before the first follow-up visit with their patients. Only 56% rated the completeness of discharge summaries as excellent or very good. PCPs' preference for information to be included in the discharge plan were discharge medication (99%), discharge diagnoses (98%), issues to follow-up (94%), hospital course (81%), radiology reports (76%), laboratory results (76%), and consult notes (76%).

Strategies to improve communication between hospital-based clinicians and PCPs Accuracy and thoroughness of discharge summaries are critically important for effectively transitioning children with LTIs from the hospital. Discharge summaries should have accurate information about medications, nutrition, and details about technology used by a child with LTI. Discharge summaries should also include information

Table 1
Communication preferences and experiences of primary care providers

Communication Type	Preference for Receipt of Information (Yes)	Receipt of Information (Usually/Always)
Notification about child's hospitalization	96%	58%
Updates during hospitalization	87%	43%
Discharge plan	98%	58%

about follow-up appointments with specialist physicians and other clinicians and other issues to follow-up after discharge. The discharge summary should be sent to the PCP in a timely fashion preferably before the first postdischarge follow-up. Other pertinent records that help facilitate continuation of care of a child with LTI in the community should be shared with the PCP as well.

Experience suggests that direct phone communication with PCP prior to discharge of a child with LTI is valuable in communicating pertinent information to the PCP to continue care in the community. Communication by phone, however, is not the most preferred method of communication for both hospital-based and PCPs.[18] This is likely due to time constraints and logistical difficulties.

In addition to communication prior to discharge, PCPs should be notified at the time of hospitalization and when major changes in clinical condition of a child with LTI occur. In the survey of PCPs, 61% of the respondents said that they usually/always visit their patients hospitalized at the children's hospital. Many PCPs have long-standing relationships with children with LTIs and their families. PCPs' perspectives on children and the caregivers, which are often formed in the context of a longitudinal relationship over several years, are helpful for hospital-based clinicians, who may or may not know a child and family well. PCPs' perspective is especially valuable in situations where major decisions, such as use of life-sustaining treatments, are made.

Communication with home health nurses

Home health nursing is skilled nursing care at home that is either intermittent (nursing visits) or continuous (private duty nursing [PDN]). PDN is continuous, complex nursing services provided by a licensed nurse at a recipient's home.[23] The demand for pediatric home health care services (including home health nursing) has grown substantially,[24] and the number of children with LTIs receiving care at home from home health nursing agencies has steadily increased.[12]

Home health nursing services are not uniformly available. It may be difficult to find a home health agency that serves some geographic areas, especially those that are rural. Even if a home health agency is available, home health nurses with expertise in caring for children with LTIs may not be available.

In 2012, a focus group of stakeholders involved in transitioning children with LTIs from the hospital to the community conducted in northwestern North Carolina. In this focus group, home health nurses reported that they value accurate home health orders when children with LTIs are discharged. They reported that changes made to the orders at the last minute prior to discharge are problematic. Home health nurses found direct communication with hospital-based nurses about children with LTIs prior to discharge valuable.

Strategies to improve communication with home health nursing agencies Typically, home health agencies develop a plan of care for their clients based on the home health orders written by physicians. Discharge home health orders should be detailed and accurate to help home health agencies develop this plan of care. Physicians should avoid generic "resume home health" discharge orders because the home health nursing needs prior to hospitalization may not be the same as after hospitalization. Clinicians should remember that home health nursing agencies need orders for all medications, including vitamins, supplements, and nutrition, if they are to be administered by home health nurses. So, if medications or nutrition change during hospitalizations, home health nursing orders should reflect these changes. Discharge home health orders should be aligned with caregiving at home and hence could be different from orders for care in the hospital. Children with LTIs can have many home health orders;

hence, changes to existing home health orders should be identified clearly and specifically.

Communication with hospice clinicians

Children with LTIs with a life expectancy of 6 months or less could be transitioned to hospice care. Some children with LTIs are transitioned to an inpatient hospice facility. More commonly, children with LTIs receive hospice services at home. The Affordable Care Act mandates that children are eligible to receive hospice care concurrently with cure-directed therapy (described in the article by Bogetz and colleagues elsewhere in this issue).

The availability and extent of hospice services for children are often limited and vary by geographic region.[25] Hospice agencies serve many geographic areas, but pediatric expertise in most hospice agencies is also often limited or lacking.[25] Hospital-based clinicians should, therefore, understand the extent of pediatric services and expertise held by the hospice agencies to which they refer. Referral to hospice often involves a collaborative working relationship between pediatric clinicians and hospice clinicians to care for children with LTIs. Pediatric clinicians can be a valuable resource for hospice clinicians (see Case example 3). Pediatric palliative care teams in tertiary care hospitals can serve as resources for hospice agencies with limited pediatric expertise. Some hospice agencies have pediatric expertise and can also be a resource for those with less pediatric expertise.

When a child is transitioned to hospice care, it is important for hospital-based clinicians to communicate with hospice clinicians about the child's clinical information, goals of care, plan of care especially with regard to symptom management and advance directives, and family characteristics. Hospital-based palliative care clinicians are valuable in facilitating this communication between hospital-based clinicians and hospice clinicians.

Case Example 3: A 3-month-old girl with inoperable glioma of the brain with extensive cerebral and spinal metastasis was discharged home with hospice care. Symptom management was offered by the oncologist at the tertiary care children's hospital, and emotional and other support services were provided by the community hospice agency. The oncologist, the pediatric palliative care team, the pharmacy of the children's hospital, and the community hospice agency worked collaboratively to provide palliative and end-of-life care to the infant. She died peacefully at home 5 weeks after discharge from the hospital.

Communication with emergency medical service providers

Another important agency to communicate with when a child is discharged from the hospital is the emergency medical service (EMS). It may be helpful to contact the nearest EMS to update them about a child with LTI. Care plans (**Fig. 2**) are helpful in communicating the plan for emergency care about children with LTIs to EMS providers.

In cases of emergency out of the hospital, EMS providers need clear orders for resuscitation or life-sustaining treatments for a child with LTIs. EMS providers are required to provide resuscitation in the event of cardiac arrest and life-saving interventions in the event of an emergency unless there is a physician order stating otherwise. Although a physician's orders to not resuscitate or to forgo life-sustaining treatments placed in a child's medical chart are sufficient when a child is hospitalized, these orders are not sufficient for EMS providers when responding to a child at home or in the community. Hence, specific do-not-resuscitate (DNR) forms or medical orders for life sustaining treatments (MOLST) forms are helpful in these situations to clarify the goals of care for children with LTIs. The DNR order form helps clarify resuscitation goals to

EMS providers in the event of cardiac arrest. MOLST forms, implemented in many states,[26] provide greater clarification about patients'/caregivers' goals about life-sustaining treatments in emergency situations. In a survey of EMS providers, Waldrop and colleagues[27] identified several barriers when providing emergency care to seriously ill patients, including lack of education of EMS providers about advance directives and lack of education of other healthcare clinicians and families about EMS providers' scope of practice.

Families of children with LTIs should be prepared for what to expect when an EMS system is activated. Hospital-based clinicians should anticipate situations where out-of-hospital resuscitation orders may be necessary. Pediatric palliative care clinicians can guide hospital-based clinicians in preparing families for out-of-hospital emergencies, completing the DNR/MOLST forms to align with family goals, and communicating the emergency plan to EMS providers.

Communication with other community clinicians and agencies

Durable medical equipment (DME) companies are important entities in the medical neighborhood of children with LTIs. To address all their needs, some children with LTIs are served by more than one DME company because there is a lot of variability in the services provided by DME companies. Lack of availability of DME companies that provide ventilator care at home may cause substantial delay in discharging children with LTIs from the hospital or limit the option of discharging these children home. Communication with representatives of the DME companies is especially critical for children receiving tracheostomy or chronic mechanical ventilation.

In the transition stakeholder focus group (described previously), DME company representatives mentioned that they do not receive discharge summaries but that discharge summaries would be helpful. They also mentioned that they need more notification time to order special supplies (eg, specific tracheostomy tube) prior to discharge. DME clinicians preferred to be notified of changes in equipment, changes in settings, the rationale for the equipment, and specifics about the equipment (eg, size of tube). It may not be logistically possible to obtain or use equipment and supplies used in the hospital (eg, equipment for oxygen delivery) for use in a home setting. This problem can be addressed if hospital-based clinicians work collaboratively with DME providers prior to discharge of a child with LTI.

As described in Case example 2, change in a child's health condition leading to hospitalization can significantly alter the need for services, such as specialist care, school, and other health care services, compared with before the hospitalization. These specialist physicians and other clinicians should be notified about the child's hospitalization especially when there is a change in health condition. Children with LTIs who are hospitalized may acquire new services, such as physical, occupational, and speech therapy and other services (see Case example 4), that need to be continued after discharge.

> **Case Example 4**: A 10-year-old girl was hospitalized for profound myopathy from vitamin deficiency from malabsorption. She was receiving physical therapy 3 times a week during her hospitalization. Outpatient physical therapy was arranged. Because the inpatient and outpatient systems are different, she did not receive physical therapy for 10 days postdischarge. This gap in service was identified during the postdischarge follow-up and the problem was rectified.

Medication Management

Medication management is a huge challenge as children are transitioned to and from the hospital.[28] Children with LTIs receive multiple medications and, hence, are at greater risk for harm due to medication errors. Children's health conditions may change during hospitalization and their medications at discharge may be different from what they were getting at home. Children with LTIs need rare medications that may not be readily available in the pharmacy. In addition, many medications may need to be compounded for use in children. Home health orders should reflect these changes to prevent confusion when a child with LTI is transitioned home.

Prior research has shown that children who are given prescriptions at the time of discharge are at greater risk of harm from medication errors than while they are in the hospital.[29] At the time of discharge of a child with LTI, caregivers are often handed prescriptions without appropriate patient education about proper administration, side effects, drug interactions, need for monitoring drug levels, and obtaining refills. Also, health care clinicians do not anticipate problems in obtaining medications, such as delay in obtaining unusual medication by a community pharmacy, family's inability to fill prescriptions due to lack of insurance or problems with insurance coverage, and lack of supplies to administer medications. Problems in prescription medications may result in serious complications for children with LTIs who are discharged home and may cause rehospitalizations.

Medication management is particularly a challenge for non–English-speaking caregivers (see Case example 5). Misunderstanding and miscommunication occur because pharmacies do not usually have interpreters for non–English-speaking families. Caregivers may not understand instructions given and may not be able to express questions or concerns that they may have, including those potentially involving an error. Sometimes, when prescription medications are not available, the pharmacy may provide medications for a few days and ask caregivers to come back to get the entire prescription. Non–English-speaking caregivers have mentioned that they did not understand that they had to come back and instead assumed that the prescription was a short period of time. For example, when a 90-day supply of diuretics was prescribed to a child, the pharmacy erroneously provided only a 30-day supply. The non–English-speaking caregiver could not communicate with the pharmacy about the error.

Case Example 5: A 2-month-old infant was discharged home after treatment for group B streptococcal meningitis that resulted in cerebral damage and a seizure disorder. At the time of discharge he had a ventriculoperitoneal shunt and gastrostomy tube and received multiple seizure medications. The caregiver spoke only Spanish and did not receive education about medication in Spanish. Three days after discharge, the child's caregiver found him very sleepy. The caregiver was concerned that the medications she filled after discharge might be causing the sleepiness and sought emergency care for the child. It was found that the child was receiving 10 times the dose of levetiracetam and 3 times the dose of phenytoin. He was rehospitalized until he clinically improved.

Strategies to reduce medication errors during transitions

Medication reconciliation is important to prevent medication errors during transition.[16,29] Caregivers should be educated about medication use by creating medication charts and medication calendars. For non–English-speaking families, these materials should be translated. It is important that medications are filled by the pharmacy for home use prior to discharging a child from the hospital so that there is no discontinuity in medication use when the child goes home from the hospital.

Policies and Regulations Regarding the System of Care for Children with LTIs

It is important for clinicians to understand the policies and regulations regarding the system of care of children with LTIs especially as it relates to transitioning care from the hospital to home. Children with LTIs may qualify for Supplemental Security Income or Medicaid waiver programs. Medicaid waiver programs (1915[c] waivers) allow for the provision of long-term care for children with LTIs in home and community-based settings by paying for wraparound services, including personal care services, respite care, home modifications, care coordination, and other services.[30] The Medicaid waiver programs vary from one state to another. Often, the application process for these programs is cumbersome. Because hospital-based clinicians have the clinical information necessary to complete these application forms, they can assist families with these applications.

Many children with LTIs need home health nursing services, either PDN or skilled nursing services. Approval from an insurance company is necessary before home health nursing services can be initiated. Health insurance companies may require letters of medical necessity to approve new or increased services. In addition, some types of equipment for use at home, such as cough assist devices or chest physiotherapy vests, require special authorization. Because the insurance approval process can take time, paperwork requesting authorization should be initiated as soon as possible during a child's hospitalization so that delays in discharge can be avoided.

Many children with LTIs receive Medicaid insurance. Although Medicaid pays for most health services, some nursing supplies, such as saline and heparin flushes, are not covered. Also, vitamins and supplements are not paid for by Medicaid. Families have to pay out of pocket for these supplies and medications. Clinicians should be aware that there are also limitations on the number of suction catheters, tracheostomy, and gastrostomy tubes that may be covered. For example, according to North Carolina Medicaid policy, gastrostomy tubes are limited to 1 tube per quarter. This policy does not allow for additional gastrostomy tube in cases of tube malfunction, necessitating emergency care when a gastrostomy tube malfunctions and a replacement is needed. Such policies make it difficult for children with LTIs to receive appropriate care that they need and caregiving at home substantially more difficult.[31] Letters of medical necessity are often required to prove the need for exception to these rules. These can be time consuming and burdensome.

Although according to the Affordable Care Act, children can receive hospice care concurrently with cure-oriented care (discussed in the article by Bogetz and colleagues elsewhere in this issue), this law has not been fully implemented. Hence, children with LTIs may lose PDN services when transitioned to hospice care or may forgo hospice care in order to continue to receive PDN services. Involvement of hospice changes the agency that provides supplies from the DME company to the hospice agency, making the system more difficult for caregivers to navigate (Case example 6).

Case Example 6: A 3-month-old girl who had private health insurance was discharged to hospice care. The private insurance had different rules regarding hospice care than the typical hospice benefit, which provides coverage for all expenses related to the primary condition. Hence, the hospice agency, which typically provides all medications related to their patients, was unable to provide intravenous pain medications. This necessitated obtaining the medication and a patient-controlled analgesia (PCA) pump from another agency. The hospice personnel were not trained to use the PCA pump supplied by the other agency. The agencies negotiated about which PCA to be used, but this process resulted in delays in managing the child's pain.

Language barriers are particularly problematic for caregivers of children with LTIs when policies and regulations change. For example, as of 2012, in North Carolina, people picking up opioid prescriptions from pharmacies are required to show valid photo identification. This resulted in confusion for non–English-speaking families because they did not understand why they suddenly were not able to pick up prescriptions for their child.

Strategies to understand the system of care for children with LTIs

The policies and regulations pertaining to insurance and the system of care of children with LTIs are many and keep changing. Working collaboratively with partners, such as home health agencies, hospice, DME companies, and representatives from Medicaid waiver programs help in understanding these policies and regulations. Because pediatric palliative care teams have established collaborations with other community agencies, they are a valuable resource for hospital-based clinicians to understand the system of care for children with LTIs.

Transportation Issues During Transitions

Transportation is a major issue requiring attention with regard to transitioning children with LTIs. Some caregivers of children with LTIs do not have access to a private vehicle for transportation. This makes it difficult for caregivers to visit their child with LTI in the hospital, which in turn hampers their preparation for discharge. It is important for clinicians to ask caregivers of children with LTIs about their transportation availability. In cases of families lacking transportation, arrangements should be made for nonemergency medical transportation from the hospital to home and from home to clinic appointments in the future. Arranging medical transportation can be cumbersome due to insurance approval and can delay discharge of a child from the hospital. Medical transport attendants may not have the training or the equipment (eg, car seat) needed to transport children with LTIs. Often an adult family member has to ride with a child and siblings are not allowed. All these factors add to the challenges of transporting a child with LTI even by nonemergency medical transportation. Even if private transportation is available, the private vehicle may not be equipped to meet the transportation needs of a child with LTI (**Box 2**). Equipment and vehicle modifications are often not covered by health insurance but paid by waiver programs for children with LTIs. Transportation issues should be considered well in advance of discharge of a child with LTI from the hospital and a plan for transportation developed.

Box 2
Transportation issues related to transitioning children with LTIs to and from acute care hospitals

- Lack of private vehicle
  - Need for insurance approval for medical transport
  - Lack of training of medical transport attendants
  - Lack of equipment (eg, car seat) in medical transport vehicle
- Child's condition makes transportation in private vehicle impossible
- Lack of equipment for safe transportation (eg, car seats with optimal head and back support for children with neuromuscular disorders)
- Lack of adaptations to accommodate equipment, such as wheelchair

Preparing Caregivers for Home Care

Preparing caregivers for transitioning to home is important and depends on whether a child has a new condition, an established condition with no change from before hospitalization, or an established condition with change in clinical condition during hospitalization. Families face challenges, especially if new to caregiving for children with LTIs. Caregivers often do know what to expect about caring for children with LTIs at home, especially in the first few months at home, and about the impact of caregiving children with LTIs on families.

Preparing caregivers of children with LTIs transitioned to home involves educating them about using and caring for technology, such as ventilator, tracheostomy or gastrostomy tube, or other technology, and education about medication use (described in Section C2). Preparation of families also involves educating them about what is involved in home care, availability of community resources, rules and systems, who to ask for help, and handling difficult situations (eg, lack of availability of qualified nurses and how to advocate for their child with LTI). Examples of resources for caregivers or clinicians who wish to prepare caregivers about care of children with LTIs are listed:

- Complex Child E-Magazine www.complexchild.com
- Family Voices www.familyvoices.org
- **Resources about specific conditions**
  - Muscular Dystrophy Association www.mda.org
- **Regional resources**
  - Exceptional Children's Assistance Center www.ecac-parentcenter.org

In some children with LTIs, there may be social complexity in the family (Case example 7) or medical complexity in the caregiver (Case example 8). These additional complexities may add to the challenges of caring for a child with LTI. Clinicians should assess caregivers' ability to provide care for children with high medical complexity at home and make necessary plans to obtain additional supports to the family.

Case Example 7: An infant with prematurity, ventricular septal defect, and severe pulmonary hypertension. Her clinical condition was so severe that she spent most of the first year of her life in an intensive care setting. She was discharged home with a tracheostomy for chronic mechanical ventilation, a gastrostomy tube for nutrition, and a central line for medication administration. Her caregiver was a single mother who worked full time, had a 4-year-old child, and had no family support for caregiving. The PPC team crafted a letter of medical necessity reflecting the medical and social complexity and the need for additional home health nursing support. As a result, she received adequate home health nursing services to meet her needs.

Case Example 8: A 6-month-old infant was diagnosed with muscular dystrophy. His condition required frequent suctioning. His mother had muscular dystrophy as well. Mother's condition made her unable to let go of the suction catheter when suctioning the child with LTI. Identifying mother's medical problem during the child's hospitalization enabled clinicians to write a letter of medical necessity to the insurance company and recommend additional nursing care services.

In some situations, children with LTIs may be transitioned to a new foster home. Clinicians need to remember that it may take a considerably long time to identify a foster parent willing to provide care for a child with LTI. Even if foster parents have the expertise in caring for other children with LTIs, they may not be familiar with the specific technology or care needed for a child with LTI being transitioned home. Foster parents of children with LTIs may need additional training (eg, tracheostomy change and gastrostomy feeding) before receiving the child. Foster parents may not have the opportunity to know the child, the child's health condition, and the child's care needs. So, children with LTIs discharged to foster homes need close follow-up and the foster parents should be supported during the transition.

Clinicians should know that a small group of children among children with LTIs survive despite a prognosis of imminent death or significantly longer than prognosticated by clinicians and are referred to as "unexpected survivors."[32] Clinicians should recognize this possibility in children with LTIs who are given a prognosis of imminent death and develop plans for all possible options, including short-term and long-term survival. Close follow-up with the family and community-based clinicians help keep the goals of care and the supports provided well aligned as a child's condition changes.

Strategies to prepare caregivers for transition

Nursing staff caring for children with LTIs in the hospital can train families of children receiving gastrostomy tube, tracheostomy tube, and other aspects of home care during a child's hospitalization. Caregivers should also be provided with written information about use of technology. Caregivers report that they learn home care from nurses in the hospital and that training helps them learn about caregiving of children with LTIs and subsequently help them teach home health nurses. Discharge planning should include preparation and training of caregivers of children with LTIs by hospital-based clinicians prior to discharge of children with LTIs from the hospital.

One strategy to prepare caregivers of children with LTIs who are newly discharged home is to provide a care notebook, a notebook that is individualized and contains both specific information regarding a child's condition—use of technology and equipment, such as gastrostomy, gastro-jejunostomy, or tracheostomy tube; contact information of clinicians; follow-up appointment information; a medication chart—and general information about community resources. Experience suggests that care notebooks serve as a resource for caregivers for home care. One parent using the care notebook provided the following feedback: "I wanted to make sure to let you know this [care notebook] was extremely helpful going home from the hospital with…*this document really helps, we're using it every day.*" For non–English-speaking families, all education materials (medication chart and technology care guidelines) should be translated.

Issues Surrounding Transition to Other Facilities

In some situations, children with LTIs may be transitioned to other hospitals, rehabilitation centers, long-term care settings, or inpatient hospice facilities. Rehabilitation centers and long-term care facilities that provide care to children are few. Even if long-term facilities serve pediatric patients, they may not serve children with high medical complexity (eg, those with chronic mechanical ventilation). Case example 9 is an illustration of the problem of lack of long-term facilities caring for children with LTIs. Similarly, inpatient mental health facilities that can handle complex medical conditions are not easily accessible. Lack of facilities that serve children can considerably delay discharge from the acute care inpatient setting.

> **Case Example 9**: A neonate with prematurity, pulmonary hypertension, subglottic stenosis, and dysphagia had a gastrostomy tube, and a tracheostomy for chronic mechanical ventilation. His family had limited social support and the home environment was not conducive for caring for a child with LTI. Plans were made to transfer this child to a long-term care facility (LTCF). His clinical condition changed with need for additional respiratory support. This increase in need for additional medical care delayed his transfer and his place at the LTCF was filled. Alternate options for transition including medical foster care were then considered.

All the considerations surrounding transitioning children with LTIs, including attention to communication, medication management, policies and regulations, and preparedness of families and staff at the receiving facility, also apply to transitioning children to other facilities.

Communication is critically important especially when a child is transitioned from a hospital to another facility. A copy of all pertinent medical records, imaging studies, pathology slides, and other relevant information should be sent to the hospital. Sharing of information may prevent duplication of services. In addition, clinicians should communicate medical information directly with the clinicians in the receiving facility.

When children with LTIs are transitioned to other facilities (rehabilitation facilities, long-term facilities, and hospice), caregivers need to be prepared about these facilities of care. Caregivers should be offered a tour of the facility if possible and arrangements made for caregivers to speak with the facility staff directly. Sharing experiences of other families with children who have received care in the facility helps as well.

When referring children with LTIs to outside facilities (especially for out-of-state facilities), it is important to understand the policies and regulations regarding such referral. For example, before a child can be transferred to a facility outside the state, North Carolina Medicaid requires proof that none of the other facilities within the state provides that specific service.

Challenges Associated with Transition into a Hospital

Transitioning children to a hospital from home or other facilities also presents challenges. Although transition from a hospital to the community has been the main focus of many quality-improvement activities, the transition into a hospital has received less attention.

Most hospitalizations of children with LTIs are for acute issues, such as intercurrent illness, and as such are not planned.

Communication between clinicians in the community and hospital settings is critical as children are transitioned into the hospital. Hospital-based clinicians may not be familiar with a child's clinical condition, goals of care, advance directives, and long-term plan of care. In addition to communication about clinical condition, hospital-based clinicians need to be made aware of unique characteristics and needs of children with LTIs. For example, children with LTIs may express distress in a certain way or comforted by certain techniques. Strategies to communicate knowledge about these subtle characteristics of children with LTIs using tools, such as an *All about Me* book or sign posted in the room, are helpful to prevent or manage distressing symptoms. Because pediatric palliative care clinicians have longitudinal relationships with children with LTIs and are familiar with children with LTIs and their caregivers, they are a valuable resource for hospital-based clinicians when children with LTIs are transitioned into the hospital.

There is a high risk for medication errors, especially omissions, when children receiving multiple medications are hospitalized.[28] When medication changes that happen in the outpatient setting are not reflected in a child's medical record, then medication errors are likely to occur at the time of hospitalization (see Case example 10). A system to reconcile medications for all hospitalized children may reduce such errors.

Case Example 10: A 10-year-old boy with severe neurologic impairment, cerebral palsy, dystonia, and gastrostomy tube dependence was discharged home on lorazepam, methadone, trihexyphenidyl, primidone, baclofen and levetiracetam. Because of persistent symptoms, lorazepam and methadone were increased in the outpatient setting. When he was rehospitalized a few months later, clinicians who were not aware of the changes made to this boy's medications in the outpatient setting prescribed a lower dose of lorazepam and methadone than what he had been getting. He developed withdrawal symptoms due to the medication error. Review of the medication list with the child's caregiver at the time of admission may have averted this error.

Similar to medication errors, there are errors in continuing nursing services from home. Often the orders for nursing services that children with LTIs receive at home are not carried forward during hospitalization. For children with LTIs, existing home health nursing orders should be reviewed carefully at the time of hospitalization.

In some cases, hospitalizations are scheduled for procedures, further evaluation, or de-escalation of therapy and can be anticipated. In cases of scheduled hospitalizations, experience suggests that having a plan ahead of time is helpful in coordinating procedures, avoiding duplication of services and limiting the duration of hospitalization (Case examples 11 and 12). For such anticipated hospitalizations, palliative care teams can develop plans of care for hospitalization that are aligned with the goals of care for a child with LTI.

Case Example 11: A 4-year-old girl with myelomeningocele, rib and vertebral anomalies, and multiple other congenital deformities was hospitalized at a facility not familiar with her for rib expansion surgery. She had failure to thrive. Anticipating that she would need help for nutritional support in the future, her procedures were coordinated such that the gastrostomy tube placement was performed at the same time as the rib expansion surgery. Prior to this hospitalization, measures were taken to facilitate a successful admission, such as sending pertinent medical records to the outside hospital, obtaining Medicaid approval for gastrostomy tube placement in an out-of-state facility, arranging for transportation, and finding resources for this non–English-speaking family. After surgery, her care was coordinated by obtaining medical records from the hospital and reconnecting the child back to clinicians locally.

Case Example 12: A 3-year-old child with severe immunodeficiency, pancytopenia, and failure to thrive of unknown cause needed evaluation for failure to thrive. She was at high risk for acquiring secondary infections during hospitalization. The authors' team coordinated a conference of clinicians representing 6 different specialties and the PCP, developed a detailed plan for hospitalization, including test and procedures to be performed; and helped implement the plan during her hospitalization.

GENERAL STRATEGIES TO IMPROVE TRANSITIONAL CARE

Specific challenges in transitional care and strategies to address those challenges are discussed previously. Some general strategies to improve transitional care for children are described.

Leveraging Existing Resources

Transitioning children with LTIs is a complex process and cannot be achieved by an individual clinician or a health care team. Resources within the institution should be leveraged to maximize transitional care to children with LTIs. In some hospitals, care coordinators or case managers may help the primary medical team by identifying home health nursing services or DME companies and provide other transitional services. Members from the pharmacy can assist caregivers in medication education. A child's primary nurses are helpful in educating caregivers about technology and other aspects of caregiving for the child with LTI. Primary nurses can also serve as a resource to home health nurses by providing specific clinical information about managing a child with LTI (eg, how to problem solve in a child who has recurrent episodes of desaturations and bradycardia). Palliative care clinicians are valuable not only in developing plans of care, establishing goals of care, and advance-care planning for children with LTIs but also communicating these plans to PCPs and other community clinicians. These communications may be especially important if the health status of a child with LTI had changed during the hospitalization.

Creating Systems to Improve Transitional Care

Transitional care for children with LTIs offers tremendous opportunity for creating systems to improve quality of care. An example of such a system is creation of a systematic process at the time of discharge (eg, a discharge checklist). Harlan and colleagues[4] showed significant improvement in timeliness of transfer of discharge information after instituting a quality-improvement project to improve communication with PCPs. Another quality-improvement opportunity is to create a medication reconciliation program at the time of hospitalization and prior to discharge. Prior studies have shown that such systems improve transitional care.[28] There is a rapid growth of knowledge in transitional care of adults.[1] Models of care delivery from the adult literature can be adapted to improve quality of transitional care for children with LTIs.

Another system-level intervention is to schedule interdisciplinary discharge planning meetings. Such meetings could occur at defined transition points, such as a day before discharge. It is important that during these meetings, roles and responsibilities for various transition tasks are assigned to team members.[6,16] Pediatric palliative care clinicians are valuable members of these discharge planning meetings. Pediatric palliative care clinicians can help with transitional care activities related to communication with community clinicians, such as hospice providers; ensure that the discharge plan is aligned with the overall goals of care for the child; and maintain longitudinal follow-up of children with LTIs after discharge from the hospital.

Developing Care Plans

One of the strategies to improve communication among entities in the medical neighborhood involves health information exchange and management.[14] The care plan is an important tool to enhance collaboration between clinicians.[15,33,34] As described previously, the change in health status of children with LTIs that results in hospitalization can change their health care needs, such as technology use, clinicians' involvement (specialist physicians and services), medications, and planned follow-up tests and procedures. Care plans can help ensure that services from before hospitalization are continued during hospitalization as appropriate and that new care needs are met on discharge. Case example 13 shows how preparing a care plan helped in the care of a child with LTI.

Patient Name: _____ MR#: _____ DOB: _____ Date of Care Plan: _____

Diagnoses: _____

Problems/Symptoms: _____

Immunizations: _____ Allergies: _____

Weight w/date: _____ Height w/date: _____

Family Information
Mother's Name: _____ Cell #: _____ Home #: _____ Email: _____

Father's Name: _____ Cell #: _____ Home #: _____ Email: _____

Other Guardian's Name/Relationship: ___ _____ _____ Cell #: _____ Home #: _____

Address of Child: _____

Transportation (check each one that is YES)
☐Utilizes public transport   ☐Long distance travel required
☐Gas and car repair concerns   ☐Requires medical transport

Social Information
Siblings' names and ages: _____

How does the child communicate? _____

Things that the child enjoys/what makes the child happy/smile/laugh:_____
_____

Faith beliefs or value beliefs of family: _____
Other social information: _____

Additional Notes
Insurance Co: _____

Goals of Care/Quality of Life discussions: _____

Advance Care Planning: _____

Resuscitationstatus discussions: _____

Other issues (Anesthesia, ED etc.)_____

MEDICATIONS	Dose	Route	Instructions

Pharmacy Name & Address: _____ Phone: _____ Fax: _____

Nutrition
Last nutritional assessment: _____ Formula name: _____

Methods by mouth: ☐ no restriction   ☐ with restriction   Type of foods: _____

Other methods: ☐ NG   ☐ GT   ☐ TP   ☐ GJ   ☐ JT

Tube feeding frequency: ☐Continuous 24 hr/day vs X hrs/day   ☐Bolus + continuous nighttime feedings or bolus only

Check all that are YES:
☐ Difficulty swallowing   ☐Ferrel bag   ☐ TPN (check for most recent order and labs)
☐ Concern for aspiration   ☐Nissen-fundoplicatin in place   ☐ Supplements: Protein or Caloric
☐ GT venting   ☐Nissen-fundoplicatin intact   ☐ Thickener

HOSPITALIZATIONS & ED VISITS

Circle type of visit	Admission Date	Admission Dx	Discharge Date	Discharge Dx	Notes
HOSPTLZTN / ED					
HOSPTLZTN / ED					
HOSPTLZTN / ED					
HOSPTLZTN / ED					

BRENNER SUB-SPECIALISTS	Provider	Last seen	Next appt	Problems	Procedures/ Studies/OR	Plan	Comments

Fig. 2. Care plan. Completed by nurse clinician and/or social worker and reviewed by the physician of the pediatric palliative care team. Care plan is placed in child's medical records. Updated when there are major changes to clinical condition.

CARE PROVIDERS & SERVICES	Name/Contact Person	Address	Phone/Fax	Preferred Method of Contact	Other
Primary Care Provider					
Home Health Nursing					
CDSA					
CC4C					
CAP-C					
Medicaid or Social Services					
Financial					
Family Support					
School					
Other					

HOME CARE ORDERS/ INSTRUCTIONS

Type	Technology	Orders/Nursing Interventions	Comments
Respiratory			
Gastrointestinal			
Central Line			
Neurology			
Renal			
Skin			
Orthopedic			
Endocrine			
Other			

EMERGENCY PLAN OF CARE

Type	Emergency Plan
Respiratory	
Gastrointestinal	
Central Line	
Neurology	
Renal	
Skin	
Orthopedic	
Endocrine	
Other	

Fig. 2. (*continued*)

Case Example 13: A 7-month-old child with trisomy 13 with complex congenital heart disease and ventriculomegaly was discharged from the hospital. A nurse clinician summarized the recommendations from all clinicians involved and developed a care plan. During this process, the nurse identified neurologist's recommendation to obtain a follow-up MRI of the brain under sedation. This enabled the MRI to be coordinated with the replacement of the child's gastojejunostomy tube under sedation. Thus an additional sedation was avoided and burden on family was decreased by avoiding another trip to the hospital.

A sample care plan that can be used in clinical practice is provided in **Fig. 2**. Care plans are developed by a clinician in collaboration with the caregiver of a child with LTI by summarizing clinical information in a structured format and communicated with all health care providers involved in the care of a child with LTI. There are many resources for developing care plans[34–36] and an extensive list of care plan templates is available at the AAP Web site.[37] The electronic medical record can be leveraged to create and maintain care plans for children with LTIs. Pediatric palliative care teams, because of their focus on holistic care of children with LTIs by interdisciplinary clinicians, are well suited to develop and maintain care plans for children with LTIs. Because pediatric palliative care clinicians have longitudinal relationships with children with LTIs, they are valuable in implementing the care plan when new information about prognosis or management is available after discharge from the hospital.

Creating Relationships with Other Clinicians and Agencies Serving Children with LTIs

It is important for hospital-based clinicians to work closely with pediatric palliative care clinicians in the care of children with LTIs. Pediatric palliative care clinicians can be a resource to hospital-based clinicians to maintain continuity of care because pediatric palliative care teams have longitudinal relationships with children with LTIs and their families. Collaboration with palliative care clinicians is particularly important when goals of care need to be communicated and clinical decisions need to be made after discharge from the hospital.

Because children with LTIs receive care from multiple clinicians within the medical neighborhood, it is important for hospital-based clinicians to develop collaborative relationships with other clinicians, such as PCPs, home health agencies, hospice agencies, and DME companies. Agencies that participate in community coalitions—groups of agencies that worked toward a common cause—are more likely to collaborate with one another in the care of children with LTIs, showing that such coalitions may be important in fostering collaborations between clinicians.[38] Collaborations with community-based clinicians can also inform hospital-based clinicians about community-based services for children with LTIs. Pediatric palliative care teams, because of their availability in inpatient and outpatient settings, have established relationships with other community agencies and can be valuable for hospital-based clinicians in developing these relationships.

Education of Clinicians

Hospital-based clinicians, especially resident physicians, need to be educated about the importance of creating an accurate and timely discharge summary and communication at the time of discharge. It is encouraging that of the 54 chapters in the recently published core competencies for pediatric hospital medicine, several chapters—on hospice and palliative care, technology-dependent children, and communication and health information systems—pertain to transitional care of children with LTIs.[39]

Training resident physicians in appropriate skills in pharmacotherapy principles, such as establishing and evaluating therapeutic goals, providing patient education, and considering the use of complementary and alternative medicine,[40] could potentially decrease the problems associated with medication errors in children with LTIs. Similar to education about medications, clinicians also need training on writing accurate home health orders. A survey of primary care resident physicians showed significant lack of knowledge about medication management among resident physicians.[41] Recognizing the need for structured instruction in pharmacotherapy, the Society of Teachers of Family Medicine Group on Pharmacotherapy has developed guidelines for a pharmacotherapy curriculum for family medicine residents.[40]

Children with LTIs are living much longer than before and receive care for their chronic critical illnesses at home. Clinicians who are primarily hospital based may not have the awareness about how critical care is delivered outside of the hospital and the burdens of caregiving at home. Because pediatric palliative care teams have broader experiences about children with LTIs beyond the hospital setting, they can be helpful to hospital-based teams in providing their perspectives about caring for children with LTIs beyond hospital settings. Palliative care clinicians can also help educate trainees about care of children with LTIs in settings outside of the hospital.

Advocacy in Transitioning Children to the Community

Children with complex medical conditions are being cared for at home and the complexity of care delivered at home is increasing. Caregivers of children with LTIs may face social difficulties, such as poverty, difficulties accessing insurance, language barriers, and lack of family support. Although health insurance pays for medical care, wraparound services are not paid for by health insurance and instead paid by Medicaid waiver programs. These waiver programs are not universally available, however, and are highly variable. Moreover, there is often a long waiting list prior to being enrolled in these programs. These factors should be considered as children with LTIs are transitioned to home. Clinicians should advocate for optimal supports for families to care for children with LTIs at home because lack of such supports substantially increases the burden of caregiving for families of children with LTIs. In several states, pediatric palliative care teams in academic medical centers have joined together with hospice agencies and other agencies serving children with LTIs to form coalitions to advocate for improving services for children with LTIs and their families.

SUMMARY

Transitioning children with LTIs is a complex and difficult process. This article highlights some of the key components of transitional care applicable to children with LTIs, which include communication with other clinicians, medication management, policies and regulations in the system of care of children with LTIs, transportation issues, and preparation of caregivers. Strategies to improve transitional care and, thereby, improve clinical outcomes of children with LTIs do exist, however, and include leveraging existing resources to improve communication across clinical settings, preparing caregivers, understanding policies and regulations, educating clinicians about the care of children with LTIs, and creating systems to deliver transitional care. Pediatric palliative care teams may play a key role in transitional care by serving as a resource for hospital-based clinicians in facilitating communication between clinicians, educating clinicians, and advocating for children with LTIs and their families.

Research about models of transitional care delivery for adults is rapidly growing.[1,2] Although many of the strategies from the adult literature can be adapted for pediatric practice, future research should focus on testing on models of transitional care delivery to children, especially those with LTIs.

REFERENCES

1. Osei-Anto A, Joshi M, Audet AM, et al. Health care leader action guide to reduce avoidable readmissions. 2010. Available at: http://www.jhartfound.org/images/uploads/resources/Health_Care_Leader_Readmission_Guide.pdf. Accessed December 1, 2013.
2. Kim CS, Flanders SA. In the Clinic. Transitions of care. Ann Intern Med 2013; 158(5 Pt 1). ITC3-1.
3. Dougherty D, Schiff J, Mangione-Smith R. The Children's Health Insurance Program Reauthorization Act quality measures initiatives: moving forward to improve measurement, care, and child and adolescent outcomes. Acad Pediatr 2011; 11(Suppl 3):S1-10.
4. Harlan GA, Nkoy FL, Srivastava R, et al. Improving transitions of care at hospital discharge–implications for pediatric hospitalists and primary care providers. J Healthc Qual 2010;32(5):51-60.
5. Value in Inpatient Pediatrics (VIP) Network Projects. Available at: http://www.aap.org/en-us/professional-resources/practice-support/quality-improvement/Quality-Improvement-Innovation-Networks/Pages/Value-in-Inpatient-Pediatrics-Network-Projects.aspx. Accessed November 30, 2013.
6. Kripalani S, LeFevre F, Phillips CO, et al. Deficits in communication and information transfer between hospital-based and primary care physicians: implications for patient safety and continuity of care. JAMA 2007;297(8):831-41.
7. Spehar AM, Campbell RR, Cherrie C, et al. Seamless Care: Safe Patient Transitions from Hospital to Home. Advances in Patient Safety: Volume 1. Rockville (MD): Agency for Healthcare Research and Quality; 2005.

8. Simon TD, Berry J, Feudtner C, et al. Children with complex chronic conditions in inpatient hospital settings in the United States. Pediatrics 2010; 126(4):647–55.

9. Berry JG, Hall DE, Kuo DZ, et al. Hospital utilization and characteristics of patients experiencing recurrent readmissions within children's hospitals. JAMA 2011;305(7):682–90.

10. Berry JG, Toomey SL, Zaslavsky AM, et al. Pediatric readmission prevalence and variability across hospitals. JAMA 2013;309(4):372–80.

11. Feudtner C, Christakis DA, Zimmerman FJ, et al. Characteristics of deaths occurring in children's hospitals: implications for supportive care services. Pediatrics 2002;109(5):887–93.

12. Johnson CP, Kastner TA. Helping families raise children with special health care needs at home. Pediatrics 2005;115(2):507–11.

13. American Academy of Pediatrics Medical Home Initiatives for Children With Special Needs Project Advisory Committee. Policy statement: Organizational principles to guide and define the child health care system and/or improve the health of all children. Pediatrics 2004;113(Suppl 5):1545–7.

14. Taylor E, Lake T, Nysenbaum J, et al. Coordinated care in the medical neighborhood: critical components and available mechanisms. White Paper (Prepared by Mathematica Policy Research under Contract No. HHSA290200900019I TO2). AHRQ Publication No. 11–0064. Rockville (MD): Agency for Healthcare Research and Quality; 2011. Available at: http://pcmh.ahrq.gov/portal/server.pt/community/pcmh__home/1483/pcmh_home_v2. Accessed December 1, 2011.

15. McDonald KM, Schultz E, Albin L, et al. Care coordination atlas version 3. AHRQ Publication No. 11-0023-EF. Rockville (MD): Agency for Healthcare Research and Quality; 2010. Available at: http://www.ahrq.gov/professionals/systems/long-term-care/resources/coordination/atlas/care-coordination-measures-atlas.pdf. Accessed November 30, 2013.

16. Greenwald JM, Denham C, Jack BW. The hospital discharge: a review of high risk care transition with highlights of a reengineered discharge process. J Patient Saf 2007;3:97–106.

17. Gupta VB, O'Connor KG, Quezada-Gomez C. Care coordination services in pediatric practices. Pediatrics 2004;113(Suppl 5):1517–21.

18. Ruth JL, Geskey JM, Shaffer ML, et al. Evaluating communication between pediatric primary care physicians and hospitalists. Clin Pediatr (Phila) 2011;50(10): 923–8.

19. Harlan G, Srivastava R, Harrison L, et al. Pediatric hospitalists and primary care providers: a communication needs assessment. J Hosp Med 2009;4(3): 187–93.

20. Bellet PS, Wachter RM. The hospitalist movement and its implications for the care of hospitalized children. Pediatrics 1999;103(2):473–7.

21. Lye PS. Clinical report–physicians' roles in coordinating care of hospitalized children. Pediatrics 2010;126(4):829–32.

22. Murphy KL, Kobayashi D, Golden SL, et al. Rural and nonrural differences in providing care for children with complex chronic conditions. Clin Pediatr (Phila) 2012;51(5):498–503.

23. Controlling the Cost of Medicaid Private Duty Nursing Services. Final Report to the Joint Legislative Program Evaluation Oversight Committee. Report Number 2008-12-05. Available at: www.ncleg.net/PED. Accessed January 15, 2012.

24. Committee on Child Health Financing, Section on Home Care, American Academy of Pediatrics. Financing of pediatric home health care. Committee on Child

Health Financing, Section on Home Care, American Academy of Pediatrics. Pediatrics 2006;118(2):834–8.

25. Varela AM, Deal AM, Hanson LC, et al. Barriers to hospice for children as perceived by hospice organizations in North Carolina. Am J Hosp Palliat Care 2012;29(3):171–6.

26. Physician Orders for Life Sustaining Treatment. 2012. Available at: www.polst.org. Accessed March 30, 2014.

27. Waldrop DP, Clemency B, Maguin E, et al. Preparation for frontline end-of-life care: exploring the perspectives of paramedics and emergency medical technicians. J Palliat Med 2014;17(3):338–41.

28. Stone BL, Boehme S, Mundorff MB, et al. Hospital admission medication reconciliation in medically complex children: an observational study. Arch Dis Child 2010;95(4):250–5.

29. Johnson KB, Butta JK, Donohue PK, et al. Discharging patients with prescriptions instead of medications: sequelae in a teaching hospital. Pediatrics 1996;97(4):481–5.

30. Waivers. Available at: http://www.medicaid.gov/Medicaid-CHIP-Program-Information/By-Topics/Waivers/Waivers.html. Accessed March 30, 2014.

31. Golden SL, Nageswaran S. Caregiver voices: coordinating care for children with complex chronic conditions. Clin Pediatr (Phila) 2012;51(8):723–9.

32. Hurst CE, Radulovic A, Nageswaran S. Unexpected Survivors: Caring for Children with Uncertain Prognoses. Pediatric Academic Societies Annual Meeting. Washington, DC, May 4, 2013.

33. American Academy of Pediatrics Council on Children with Disabilities. Care coordination in the medical home: integrating health and related systems of care for children with special health care needs. Pediatrics 2005;116(5):1238–44.

34. Antonelli R, Stille C, Freeman L. Enhancing collaboration between primary and subspecialty care providers for children and youth with special health care needs. Washington, DC: Georgetown University Center for Child and Human Development; 2005.

35. Adams S, Cohen E, Mahant S, et al. Exploring the usefulness of comprehensive care plans for children with medical complexity (CMC): a qualitative study. BMC Pediatr 2013;13:10.

36. Stille CJ, Fischer SH, La Pelle N, et al. Parent partnerships in communication and decision making about subspecialty referrals for children with special needs. Acad Pediatr 2013;13(2):122–32.

37. Care Delivery Management: Care Plans. Available at: http://www.medicalhomeinfo.org/how/care_delivery/#care. Accessed March 20, 2013.

38. Nageswaran S, Golden SL, Easterling D, et al. Factors associated with collaboration among agencies serving children with complex chronic conditions. Matern Child Health J 2013;17(9):1533–40.

39. Stucky ER, Ottolini MC, Maniscalco J. Pediatric hospital medicine core competencies: development and methodology. J Hosp Med 2010;5(6):339–43.

40. Bazaldua O, Ables AZ, Dickerson LM, et al. Suggested guidelines for pharmacotherapy curricula in family medicine residency training: recommendations from the Society of Teachers of Family Medicine Group on Pharmacotherapy. Fam Med 2005;37(2):99–104.

41. Adcock BB, Byrd DC, O'Neal MR. Evaluation of primary care residents' knowledge of pharmacotherapy. South Med J 1999;92(9):882–5.

Adolescents and Young Adults with Life-Threatening Illness

Special Considerations, Transitions in Care, and the Role of Pediatric Palliative Care

Jennifer S. Linebarger, MD, MPH[a],*, Toluwalase A. Ajayi, MD[b],*,
Barbara L. Jones, MSW, PhD[c]

KEYWORDS

- Pediatrics • Young adults • Adolescents • Palliative care • Transition of care
- Life-threatening illnesses

KEY POINTS

- Medical advancements have led to an increased prevalence of children with life-threatening illnesses who are also surviving longer.
- Adolescents and young adults (AYAs) with life-threatening illness experience unique vulnerabilities, complex health concerns, and, unfortunately, barriers to assessing health care.
- Many pediatric and adolescent patients with life-threatening illnesses age into adult care; thus, it is recommended that pediatric palliative care teams make timely transitions of care to appropriate young adult or adult services.
- Owing to the parent/family and patient attachment to pediatric providers, there may be feelings of reluctance and fear to leave behind health care providers who may have cared for years.
- Training can be 1 avenue for increasing providers' comfort in working with AYAs with life-threatening illnesses.

INTRODUCTION

Adolescents and young adults (AYAs) represent a distinctive group of young people who are either experiencing, or have recently experienced a period of accelerated growth and change that bridges the complex transition from childhood to adulthood.

[a] Pediatric Palliative Care Team, The Children's Mercy Hospital, 2401 Gillham Road, Kansas City, MO 64108, USA; [b] Palliative Care, Rady Children's Hospital, Scripps Mercy Hospital San Diego, 4077 5th Avenue, MER 35, San Diego, CA 92103, USA; [c] The Institute for Grief, Loss and Family Survival, School of Social Work, University of Texas at Austin, 1925 San Jacinto Boulevard, MS D3500, Austin, TX 78712, USA
* Corresponding authors.
E-mail addresses: jslinebarger@cmh.edu; Ajayi.Toluwalase@scrippshealth.org

Pediatr Clin N Am 61 (2014) 785–796
http://dx.doi.org/10.1016/j.pcl.2014.05.001   pediatric.theclinics.com
0031-3955/14/$ – see front matter © 2014 Elsevier Inc. All rights reserved.

It is often an unsettling period characterized by rapid hormonal changes, physical maturation, and cognitive and emotional development. The patterns of behavior AYAs adopt during this time may have long-term consequences for their health and quality of life. When the challenges that accompany a life-threatening illness are added to this already tumultuous developmental stage, the problem of transitioning from pediatric medical homes to adult medical homes becomes even more crucial. AYAs with life-threatening illness experience unique vulnerabilities, complex health concerns, and, unfortunately, barriers to accessing health care. For them, the process of transitioning from a pediatric medical home to an adult medical home is increasingly complex. The transition of AYAs with life-threatening illnesses is fraught with difficulties, and in some cases these difficulties lead to increased mortality during the transition period.[1–4] This mortality is linked to a poor transition process. At the time of transition, patients struggle to form a relationship with members of their new medical home. Meanwhile, care plans and routine surveillance are disrupted by the lack of bridging communication from 1 medical home to the next.

In order to understand the scope of the nuances and challenges that come with caring for AYAs with life-threatening illness, it is important to begin with the parameters that define this group and the transition of health care. The Centers for Disease Control and Prevention (CDC) and the World Health Organization define adolescents as young people between the ages of 10 and 19 years. The CDC takes a step further and defines young adults as ages 20 to 24 years. Yet, professionals within oncology state that this age group actually includes individuals up to 39 years of age.[5,6] With these ambiguities in the parameters that delineate this group of patients, the challenges that come with caring for them become clearer, especially with regard to transitioning their health care. Taking these definitions together, caring for AYAs with life-threatening illness consists of caring for a patient population that spans nearly 3 decades.

Transition of health care, has been defined as "the purposeful, planned movement of adolescents and young adults with chronic physical and medical conditions from child-centered to adult-oriented health care systems."[7] When caring for a patient population that spans 3 decades, the problem of transitioning their care can seem insurmountable. AYAs with life-threatening illness have unique developmental and psychosocial considerations. Often caught between pediatrics and adult medicine, they have specific needs for support, communication, and involvement with their care that is rooted in their developmental, cognitive, and psychosocial needs.[8]

Currently the medical community does not have either a defined method, or a systematic way to care for this patient population. Learning the developmental considerations and psychosocial needs and understanding the tools to transition to adult medical homes may help create such a system. Other considerations to help transition in this care period include introducing team members who are skilled in caring for children and young adults with life-limiting illness. The palliative care team may be especially useful in ensuring smooth transitions.

DEVELOPMENTAL CONSIDERATIONS

According to the American Academy of Pediatrics (AAP), palliative care for children, adolescents, and young adults should be patient centered and family engaged, offering a respectful partnership that is concerned about quality, access, and equity.[9] Specifically, the AAP recommends that the pediatric palliative care (PPC) team be committed to offering care across the age spectrum and life span. As many pediatric and adolescent patients with life-threatening conditions age into adult care, the AAP recommends that the PPC team make timely transitions of care to appropriate young adult or adult services.[9] Transitions should take into account the unique developmental and familial needs of the patients and occur seamlessly so that the patient remains safely cared for. When AYA patients cannot be transitioned to adult care, the pediatric team must continue to provide care that respects the unique needs of these emerging young adults.[9]

DEVELOPMENTAL TASKS

Adolescents and young adults with life-threatening illness encounter unique challenges as they face the developmental tasks of physical changes, autonomy, identity, cognition, and spirituality (**Table 1**).

Adolescents with chronic illness may experience delays in physical and sexual development of puberty. There may also be changes in body shape and function because of the illness or treatments for the illness (eg, hair loss, weight gain or loss, muscle weakness, disability/deformations, fatigue, shortness of breath). Such alterations may impact body image, may lead to concerns about sexual activity, and may directly or indirectly lead to sexual dysfunction.

With regard to autonomy, adolescents with a life-threatening illness may have increased dependence on their family when compared with their peers. Some will exert themselves to regain a sense control (such as through treatment nonadherence),[17] while others with long-standing illness may have a degree of learned passivity.[18] In response, some providers find it best to take a more authoritative approach, determining what is essential for health and for which there should be no compromise, and allow negotiation for issues that are not critical.

Identity formation is a critical part of adolescent and young adult development, and facing a life-threatening illness significantly impacts the emerging identity of AYAs. AYAs with cancer report a paradox of identity as they struggle to reconcile their previously known self with their "cancer identity."[17] This identity paradox can be seen when some adolescents become defined by their illness, and their identity shifts to that of a patient rather than of a teen who has an illness/condition.

Cognitively, even among healthy adolescents and adults, the capability for abstract thinking is strongly impacted by health status. And for the most ill of the adolescents, their future is determined by limitations rather than possibilities. By about the age of 9 years, an adult understanding of death is achieved.[19] Death is defined by irreversibility, nonfunctionality, universality, and causality. With the development of abstract thinking, adolescents question the existential implications of death. Adolescents often continue to speak and plan as if there is no understanding of the reality of prognosis, and having survival goals is common (eg, wish trips, graduation, school dances, or other social functions). Providers should be aware and understanding of this psychological dynamic and not label it as pathologic.

Spiritually, recent literature suggests that AYAs with cancer struggle to make meaning and generate understanding of the spiritual aspects of their life-threatening condition.[17] AYAs do exhibit evidence of personal growth, benefit-finding, and spiritual enhancement as they face their life-threatening conditions.[17,20,21]

ISOLATION

Adolescents often experience significant isolation from their family members and peer group because of lengthy hospital stays or intensive treatment protocols. Isolation and alienation can cause significant emotional distress.[22] This isolation may only increase if the adolescent needs to transition to a new care team as he or she ages out of pediatrics. AYAs need support and strategies to reinforce and enhance relationships with

Table 1
Developmental tasks of adolescence

	Physical (Tanner)[10]	Autonomy (Gilligan)[11]	Identity (Erikson)[12]	Cognition (Piaget[13]; Elkind[14])	Spirituality (Fowler[15]; Puchalski[16])
Early (10–14 y)	Onset and tempo of pubertal changes vary Physical changes can lead to self-consciousness, embarrassment, or anxiety	Dependence	Am I normal? Comparing self to others, and evolving sense of self esteem	Concrete operational (black and white thinking), with a developing use of logic	Mythical/literal; Extrinsic religiosity Literal meaning is given to religious symbols and stories; follow the religious belief system around them (family)
Middle (15–16 y)	Females mature before males Being an early developer or a late bloomer can have psychological impacts	Independence A stage of experimentation that may include limit testing and risk-taking behavior	Who am I? Forming a sense of self– what one wants to do or be	Transitional stage in which one may see: • Personal fable–belief that no one has the thoughts or experience I do…which can lead to feelings of invincibility • Imaginary audience– belief that everyone is paying attention to me	Synthetic/conventional Conformity to the same religious authority shared by family or peers
Late (17–19 y)	Adult physical appearance	Interdependence A growing recognition of reliance on and responsibility toward others	Who am I in relation to others? Asking this question leads to a sense of commitment, safety and care within relationships	Formal operational– abstract or hypothetical thinking	Intrinsic religiosity May have deeper reflection (even questioning) about their religious belief system

Ages based on classifications from the World Health Organization.
Data from Available at: http://www.who.int/maternal_child_adolescent/topics/adolescence/dev/en/. Accessed April 11, 2014.

family, peers, and health professionals to reduce this isolation.[22] D'Agostino and colleagues[23] recognized that a salient aspect of AYA autonomy and identity development is the importance placed on peer group acceptance and peer relationships, and AYAs need to sustain a sense of connection to their peers when faced with difficult diagnoses and their associated treatment. In 1 study, AYAs with cancer (aged 16–22 years) identified social support (friends and health care providers) as their major coping strategy to deal with cancer, whereas family support was identified as their important source for emotional support.[24]

Peer support programs assist AYA patients in establishing and maintaining relationships with their normal peers as well as with other AYAs with cancer, offer opportunities to achieve age-related developmental tasks (building interpersonal and problem-solving skills), and promote positive psychosocial growth.[25,26] Peer support also provides AYAs with an opportunity to address some of their concerns, such as coping with uncertainty about the future, establishing autonomy while being increasingly dependent on family and friends, sexual identity, and infertility, thereby reducing feelings of social isolation.[25] Studies of AYA patients have indicated that their needs for peer support remain unmet.[26]

ADVANCE PLANNING, COMMUNICATION, AND DECISION MAKING

With the development and maturation of adolescence comes an increased role in health care decision making. According to the AAP, PPC clinicians should "facilitate clear, compassionate, and forthright discussions with (pediatric) patients and families about therapeutic goals and concerns, the benefits and burdens of specific therapies, and the value of advance care planning."[9] When adolescents and young adults are facing advance care decisions, they may need interventions that are geared toward their developmental needs. Based upon their growing autonomy and independence, AYAs may prefer more informed control in decisions about their care, having structured dialogues with their family and health care team about medical decisions, and opportunities for expression of spiritual concerns.[27–29] Specific tools such as *Voicing my Choices* have been developed to assist AYAs, their families, and health care providers to think through options for care and for AYAs to communicate their preferences.[28] Unlike the affiliated document *Five Wishes*, *Voicing my Choices* is not a legally binding document. However, it does encourage the AYA to choose a health care agent, which is especially important once the AYA turns 18. More information on these tools is available on these and other tools at https://www.agingwithdignity.org/.

Decision making may be complicated by issues with competency and capacity. The distinction between the two are outlined in **Table 2**.

The elements required for capacity include
- The patient has adequate awareness (understanding and appreciation) of disease and treatment options.
- The patient uses reasoning to make a choice.
- The patient makes a choice and communicates wishes.
- The choice is consistent with the patient's goals and values.

Capacity does not mean agreeing with the medical team. It is important to honor the patient's preferences, which may include deferring decision making to the parents. Nevertheless, AYAs need the opportunity to fully understand of their medical condition and prognosis in order to participate in decisions about their care. Therefore, it is critically important to provide the AYA patient with informed control, honest disclosure of his or her medical information, and supported guidance in medical decision making.[5,17,22]

Table 2 Adolescent and young adult decision-making: competency and capacity	
Competency	Legal term • In the United States it begins at the age of majority, 18 y Based on the ethical value of autonomy Implies the ability to consent • Consent: to make independent personal, medical, and financial decisions
Capacity	Functional competency • Not necessarily related to age • Impacted by developmental stage, conditioning and experience, and cultural influences • Also impacted by disease state (it can be partially or temporally impaired by pain, medications, neurologic injury, or psychiatric illness) Implies having the skills to make an informed decision

TRANSITIONING MEDICAL HOMES

Medical advancements have led to an increased prevalence of children with medical complexity as well as increased life expectancy.[30] As these children are living into adolescence, young adulthood, and even beyond, the need for a transition from pediatric to adult medical care has evolved. According to a 2011 report from the AAP, the American Academy of Family Physicians, and the American College of Physicians, the goal of a planned health care transition is to maximize lifelong functioning and well-being for all youth.[31]

The AAP defines the medical home as a model of care that is "accessible, family-centered, continuous, comprehensive, coordinated, compassionate and culturally effective."[32] The value of such a medical home model has proven beneficial to those with special health care needs as well as healthy children.[33,34] Internal medicine has adapted this model as the patient-centered medical home or PCMH (a term also now used within pediatrics), which "seeks to meet the health care needs of patients and to improve patient and staff experiences, outcomes, safety, and system efficiency."[35,36] Within the PCMH framework, experts have identified important quality measures within general health care, chronic illness care, coordination of care, and the transition of care.[37]

THE TRANSITION PROCESS

The 2011 clinical report from the AAP includes several algorithms outlining the transition process. The process starts with engaging AYAs in a developmentally appropriate manner while they are in the pediatric medical home, ideally around the age of 12 years.[31]

Key elements of a discussion about transitioning to adult care includes are outlined in **Box 1**.

Box 1 Discussions for adult transitioning
• Expectations for vocation
• Independent living
• Guardianship
• Reproduction
• Life expectancy

Assessing Transition Readiness

There is currently at least 1 validated tool that assesses transition readiness,[38] and there are several examples of patient and parent surveys are available through the Center for Health Care Transition Improvement (www.gottransition.org). Some centers use checklists based on the shared management model depicted in **Table 3**.[39]

These checklists vary based on the patient's age and developmental state, and clarify the skills and tasks that will facilitate movement through the model. At one Midwestern institution, there are three checklists that place increasing responsibility on the patient as they age (**Table 4**).

By the end of the transition process, an AYA should be able to describe his or her health condition and health care needs as well as the health care resources and support people available to him or her (**Fig. 1**). Many programs utilize a health passport document. General and disease-specific passports are available through the Good2Go transition program at Toronto's Sick Kids (www.sickkids.ca/good2go and www.sickkids.ca/myhealthpassport/).

Not all AYAs have the developmental or cognitive capability to summarize their health care history. For these patients, the health care provider and guardian can create a summary that includes details such as those in **Box 2**.

TRANSITION CHALLENGES

Although the transition process seems streamlined, the actual transition to adult health care is not necessarily so straightforward. Research has demonstrated greater hurdles for those patients who have comanagement by a primary care physician and medical subspecialists, which is common for many adolescents with medical complexity. Some centers have disease-specific programs that help guide the subspecialty transfer, but they are not universally available. There is evidence that those with more complex conditions or with conditions affecting the nervous system appear to have less good transitions.[40]

Owing to parent/family and patient attachment to pediatric providers, there may be feelings of reluctance and fear to leave behind health care providers who may have cared for the patient for years. Transition may affect parents' perception of their child's health-related quality of life more than child's actual health-related quality of life.[41] Lugasi and colleagues[42] proposed clarifying the meaning given to the transition and the expectations (hopes/fears) regarding the move to adult health care. They also suggested enhancing the level of patients' knowledge and skills, being clear in the transition planning, and having a supportive environment.

There is also a noted culture gap between pediatric-oriented and adult-oriented health care. In part, this gap is outlined in the shared management model; the internist anticipates patients who supervise their own health condition while the pediatrician typically embraces a family-centered model. At the same time, the internists may be asked to oversee a health condition to which they have had little exposure. Most

Table 3 Assessing transition readiness			
Time	Provider	Parent/Family	Young Person
↓	Major responsibility	Provides care	Receives care
	Support to parent/family and young person	Manages	Participates
	Consultant	Supervisor	Manages
	Resource	Consultant	Supervisor

Table 4
Phases associated with pediatric to adult health care transition

Phase	Age	Definition
Investigating phase	Envisioning the future (12–14 y)	This is a time to plant the seeds about future transition to adult health care providers. Patients of this age should be expected to name their disease.
Coaching phase	Age of responsibility (15–17 y)	By this age, patients should become independent in the daily disease management needed. Providers and parents can coach them to explain their disease and past medical history as well as their current medication and management.
Launching phase	Age of transition (18–21 y)	Patients will ideally transition to adult health care providers at this age. Helping them know when to ask for help with disease or when they need to seek medical attention is an important skill at this age.

families and youth feel that adult-oriented providers lack training, up-to-date knowledge, and interest, and this creates anxiety for them.[43] Similarly, a survey of internists found transition to be a double-edged sword; they feared well-informed parents/families not staying involved, but also that the families would have high expectations for the internists' time.[44]

The study of internists also found anxiety about the need to face disability and end-of-life issues at an early age and early in the doctor–patient relationship. The authors proposed 2 solutions: (1) improved communication between pediatricians and internists may help internists cope with an unexpected or early death by allowing providers to share their grief, and (2) resources to assist providers in dealing with young adult patient loss.[44]

THE ROLE OF PALLIATIVE CARE

Given its interdisciplinary approach, palliative care is uniquely poised to help address the challenges to caring for the seriously ill adolescent and young adult. The PPC team is experienced in caring for children and young adults with complex

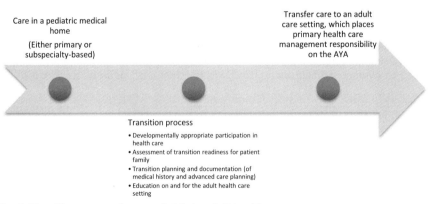

Care in a pediatric medical home

(Either primary or subspecialty-based)

Transfer care to an adult care setting, which places primary health care management responsibility on the AYA

Transition process
- Developmentally appropriate participation in health care
- Assessment of transition readiness for patient family
- Transition planning and documentation (of medical history and advanced care planning)
- Education on and for the adult health care setting

Fig. 1. Transition process from pediatric to adult health care.

Box 2
Details for health care providers and guardians in summarizing AYA health care history

Baseline functional and neurologic status

Cognitive status, including formal tests results when possible

Condition-specific emergency treatment plans and contacts

Health education history and assessment of the patient's understanding regarding his or her health condition

Prognosis, with particular attention to entry into adult life

Information about advance directives should include identification of the decision maker proxy or guardian and any history of advance directive planning

medical conditions. In addition to complex symptom management, this team is trained to facilitate communication between multiple caregivers and different medical teams.

During the past decade, an increasing number of children's hospitals have created dedicated palliative care services to address the needs of children and young adults with advanced life-threatening conditions, placing specific emphasis on symptom relief, logistics and care coordination, and psychosocial and decision-making support.[45] In 2011, a multicenter study was published that looked at the demographics of patients referred to PPC teams at 6 major pediatric centers in the United States and Canada. This study found that 10% to 16% of pediatric palliative referrals were 19 years of age.[46] Another study surveyed 226 children's hospitals and related institutions in the United States. Of the 162 respondents, 112 indicated that their institution has a PPC program. Of the hospitals with a PPC program, 74.1% provided consultations for adult patients being cared for in their hospitals.[47] Taking these 2 sets of data together, it can be extrapolated that an increasing percentage of PPC teams are participating in the care of a significant number of AYAs with life-threatening illness. The reasons for this are likely multifactorial. Reasons include the fact that there are some patients within this population in which transition is not appropriate because of the nature of disease, or simply because there are not adult medical homes that are comfortable in caring for these patients without pediatric consultation or assistance.

It is part of the expertise of this team to facilitate communication between multiple caregivers and different medical teams. Embedding a member of the palliative care team as part of the medical home early in the course of the patient's disease allows the patient and the family to become familiar with the palliative care team and build the same level of trust as they would have with any member of the medical home. The palliative care team works together with members of the primary medical team creating an interdisciplinary team that can follow the patient on an inpatient and outpatient basis. Having members of the team that can follow them into the adult world helps lower the anxiety and feelings of abandonment that families often have when the topic of transition is broached. Similarly, having a medical professional who has been involved in the child's care since early in the course of the illness helps reduce the discomfort of the new medical team. It ensures that medical information gets transferred more efficiently and reliably. It provides an easy foundation for the patient, the family, and the new medical team to start building trust and ensure optimal communication, which will not only result in better care but also a better quality of life for the patient.

SUMMARY

There is currently a gap in the health care system for AYAs with life-threatening illnesses. PPC is in position to help fill that gap. Working together with the medical homes, the components of the multidisciplinary PPC team can assist the primary team early in the course of the life-threatening illness. As the child graduates from the pediatric model of care, the palliative care team can then serve as the bridge between the existing care model and the future one.

The palliative care provider often takes a big picture assessment of each patient they meet, looking beyond a single organ system at the whole person as well as beyond the individual to include his or her support network. PCC clinicians also hold expertise in conversations about the goals of care and advance care planning. Such conversations are always important to document, but especially as a patient is moving from 1 health care setting to another (such as from pediatric to adult health care); the palliative care team is uniquely positioned to help.

To best support adolescents and young adults transition to adult care, practitioners must partner with the patient and family to understand both their developmental and psychosocial needs. Specifically when working with AYAs, health care practitioners must work diligently to earn and maintain trust and to respond to their feelings of fear and uncertainty.[5] Some patients may wish to remain in pediatric care but would like to be treated with the autonomy and respect often reserved for adult patients. In these situations, consulting with an adult palliative care team might be appropriate. Others may specifically want to work with an AYA or adult team but retain the level of relationship they enjoyed with their pediatric team. Good assessment begins with listening to the patient with an attitude of respect, candor, and collaboration. Build trust; be upfront about confidentiality as well as the importance of members the health care team sharing information with each other.

ACKNOWLEDGMENTS

Authors thank Ann C. Modrcin, Division Director of Rehabilitation Medicine at Children's Mercy Hospital for her concept development of **Table 4**.

REFERENCES

1. Gurvitz M, Valente AM, Broberg C, et al. Prevalence and predictors of gaps in care among adult congenital heart disease patients (The Health Education and Access Research Trial: HEART-ACHD). J Am Coll Cardiol 2013;61(21):2180–4.
2. Tuchman LK, Schwartz LA, Sawicki GS, et al. Cystic fibrosis and transition to adult medical care. Pediatrics 2010;125:566.
3. Lewis K. All grown up: moving from pediatric to adult diabetes care. Am J Med Sci 2012;345(4):278–83.
4. DeBaun MR, Telfair J. Transition and Sickle cell disease. Pediatrics 2012;130(5): 926–35. http://dx.doi.org/10.1542/peds.2011-3049.
5. Wein S, Pery S, Zer A. Role of palliative care in adolescent and young adult oncology. J Clin Oncol 2010;28:4819–24.
6. Ferrari A, Thomas D, Franklin AR, et al. Starting an adolescent and young adult program: some success stories and some obstacles to overcome. J Clin Oncol 2010;28:4850–7.
7. Rosen DS, Blum RW, Britto M, et al, Society for Adolescent Medicine. Transition to adult health care for adolescents and young adults with chronic conditions: position paper of the Society for Adolescent Medicine. J Adolesc Health 2003;33(4):309–11.

8. Rosenberg A, Wolfe J. Palliative care for adolescents and young adults with cancer. Clinical Oncology Adolescents Young Adults 2013;3:41–8.
9. American Academy of Pediatrics Section on Hospice and Palliative Medicine and Committee on Hospital Care. Pediatric palliative care and hospice care commitments, guidelines and recommendations. Pediatrics 2013;132(5):966–72.
10. Katzman K, Gordon C, Woods ER, et al. In: Neinstein LS, editor. Adolescent health care: a practical guide. 5th edition. Lippincott Williams & Wilkins; 2007.
11. Gilligan C. In a different voice: psychological theory and women's development. Cambridge (MA): Harvard University Press; 1982.
12. Erikson EH. Childhood and society. 2nd edition. New York: Norton. W.W. & Company, Inc; 1993.
13. Piaget J, Inhelder B. The psychology of the child. 1st edition. Basic Books; 1972.
14. Elkind D. Egocentrism in adolescence. Child Development 1967;38:1025–34.
15. Fowler JW. Stages of faith: The psychology of human development. HarperCollins; 1981.
16. Puchalski CM, Ferrell B. Making health care whole: integrating spirituality into patient care. West Conshohocken (PA): Templeton Press; 2010. p. 126–7.
17. Jones B, Parker-Raley J, Barczyk A. Adolescent cancer survivors: identity paradox and the need to belong. Qual Health Res 2011;21(8):1033–40.
18. Conrad P. The noncompliant patient in search of autonomy. Hastings Cent Rep 1987;17(4):15–7.
19. Linebarger JS, Sahler OJ, Eagan KA. Coping with death. Pediatr Rev 2009;30: 350–6.
20. Hendricks-Ferguson V. Hope and spiritual well-being in adolescents with cancer. West J Nurs Res 2008;30(3):385–401.
21. Turner-Sack AM, Menna R, Setchell SR. Posttraumatic growth, coping strategies, and psychological distress in adolescent survivors of cancer. J Pediatr Oncol Nurs 2012;29(2):70–9.
22. Pritchard S, Cuvelier G, Harlos M, et al. Palliative care in adolescents and young adults with cancer. Cancer 2011;117(S10):2323–8.
23. D'Agostino NM, Penney A, Zebrack B. Providing developmentally appropriate psychosocial care to adolescent and young adult cancer survivors. Cancer 2011;117(S10):2329–34.
24. Kyngäs H, Mikkonen R, Nousiainen EM, et al. Coping with the onset of cancer: coping strategies and resources of young people with cancer. Eur J Cancer Care 2001;10(1):6–111.
25. Zebrack B, Bleyer A, Albritton K, et al. Assessing the health care needs of adolescent and young adult cancer patients and survivors. Cancer 2006;107(12):2915–23.
26. Zebrack B, Block R, Hayes-Lattin B, et al. Psychosocial service use and unmet need among recently diagnosed adolescent and young adult cancer patient. Cancer 2012;119(1):201–14.
27. Jones B. Companionship, control and compassion: a social work perspective on the needs of children with cancer and their families at the end of life. J Palliat Med 2006;9(3):774–88.
28. Wiener Z, Battles B, Ballard H, et al. Allowing adolescents and young adults to plan their end of life care. Pediatrics 2012;130:897–905.
29. Bluebond-Langner M, Belasco JB, Wander MD. I want to live, until I don't want to live anymore": involving children with life-threatening and life-shortening illnesses in decision making about care and treatment. Nurs Clin North Am 2010;45:329–43.
30. Burns KH, Casey PH, Lyle RE, et al. Increasing prevalence of medically complex children in US hospitals. Pediatrics 2010;126:638–46.

31. American Academy of Pediatrics, American Academy of Family Physicians, American College of Physicians. Clinical report – supporting the health care transition from adolescence to adulthood in the medical home. Pediatrics 2011;128: 182–200.

32. Medical Home Initiatives for Children With Special Needs Project Advisory Committee, American Academy of Pediatrics. The medical home. Pediatrics 2002; 110:184–6.

33. Homer CJ, Klatka K, Romm D, et al. A review of the evidence for the medical home for children with special health care needs. Pediatrics 2008;122:e922–37.

34. Long WE, Bauchner H, Sege RD, et al. The value of the medical home for children without special health care needs. Pediatrics 2012;129:87–98.

35. Jackson GL, Powers BJ, Chatterjee R, et al. The patient-centered medical home: a systematic review. Ann Intern Med 2013;158(3):169–78.

36. Stange KC, Nutting PA, Miller WL, et al. Defining and measuring the patient-centered medical home. J Gen Intern Med 2010;25:601–12.

37. Chen AY, Schrager SM, Mangione-Smith R. Quality measures for primary care of complex pediatric patients. Pediatrics 2012;129:433–45.

38. Sawicki GS, Lukens-Bull K, Yin K, et al. Measuring the transition readiness of youth with special healthcare needs: validation of the TRAQ—Transition Readiness Assessment Questionnaire. J Pediatr Psychol 2011;36(2):160–71.

39. Kieckhefer GM, Trahms CM. Supporting development of children with chronic conditions: from compliance toward shared decision management. Pediatr Nurs 2000;26(4):354–63.

40. Bloom SR, Kuhlthau K, Van Cleave J, et al. Health care transition for youth with special health care needs [review]. J Adolesc Health 2012;51:213–9.

41. Geerts E, van de Wiel H, Tamminga R. A pilot study on the effects of the transition of paediatric to adult health care in patients with haemophilia and their parents: patient and parent worries, parental illness-related distress and health-related quality of life. Haemophilia 2008;14:1007–13.

42. Lugasi T, Achille M, Stevenson M. Patients' perspectives on factors that facilitate transition from child-centered to adult-centered health care: a theory integrated metasummary of quantitative and qualitative studies. J Adolesc Health 2011; 48:429–40.

43. Reiss JG, Gibson RW, Walker LR. Health care transition: youth, family, and provider perspectives. Pediatrics 2005;115:112–20.

44. Peter NG, Forke CM, Ginsburg KR, et al. Transition from pediatric to adult care: internists' perspectives. Pediatrics 2009;123:417–23.

45. Field MJ, Behrman RE, Institute of Medicine (US), Committee on Palliative and End-of-Life Care for Children and Their Families. When children die: improving palliative and end-of-life care for children and their families. Washington, DC: National Academy Press; 2003.

46. Feudtner C, Kang TI, Hexem KR, et al. Pediatric palliative care patients: a prospective multicenter cohort study. Pediatrics 2011;127(6):1094–101. http://dx.doi.org/10.1542/peds.2010-3225.

47. Feudtner C, Womer J, Augustin R, et al. Pediatric palliative care programs in children's hospitals: a cross-sectional national survey. Pediatrics 2013;132(6): 1063–70.

Pediatric Palliative Care for Children with Complex Chronic Medical Conditions

Scott Schwantes, MD*, Helen Wells O'Brien, MDiv, MEd, BCC

KEYWORDS

- Children with complex chronic conditions • Dysautonomia • Neuroirritability
- Feeding intolerance • Spiritual care

KEY POINTS

- Children with complex chronic conditions and life-threatening conditions benefit from a dynamic pediatric palliative care team to adapt to the child and family's evolving needs throughout their illness trajectory.
- Children with complex chronic conditions and life-threatening conditions have a subset of distressing symptoms, which can be managed through careful diagnosis and treatment.
- Ongoing dialogue with families of children with complex chronic conditions can prepare for anticipated forks in the road throughout the child's disease trajectory.
- The spiritual and psychosocial care of children with complex chronic conditions and their families takes on special dimensions given the lifelong nature of the child's life-threatening condition.

INTRODUCTION

Children with complex chronic conditions (CCC) use a significant degree of health care, including hospitalizations, admissions to intensive care units, surgical interventions, ongoing involvement of multiple subspecialty services and providers, and death in the hospital and emergency department.[1–11] This population is also expected to continue to increase with progress in advanced medical care.[6] Pediatric palliative care (PPC) serves a critical role in the lives of children with CCC and their families to ensure that the child's medical care can intersect meaningfully with the family's goals and values as well as identified quality of life for their child.[12–16]

Throughout the life of the child, PPC interfaces with ongoing restorative care as the child's needs fluctuate over the illness trajectory.[3,17] PPC provides important services throughout this journey, with many of the members of PPC playing different roles of

Disclosure: The authors have nothing to disclose.
Department of Pediatrics, Gillette Children's Specialty Healthcare, Regions Hospital, 200 University Avenue East, St Paul, MN 55101, USA
* Corresponding author.
E-mail address: sschwantes@gillettechildrens.com

Pediatr Clin N Am 61 (2014) 797–821
http://dx.doi.org/10.1016/j.pcl.2014.04.011   pediatric.theclinics.com
0031-3955/14/$ – see front matter © 2014 Elsevier Inc. All rights reserved.

varying prominence, exercising the full nature of a well-integrated interdisciplinary team to meet these goals.[18]

The tenets of sound PPC apply to the care of children with CCC, who represent a high proportion of all children with life-threatening illness. In this article, some of the subtle yet important ways of crafting a philosophy of care to help develop models of care for these patients and their families are explored. In addition, specific distressing symptoms common in this population are highlighted. Areas for management are proposed for these children with lifelong life-threatening conditions, using anticipated forks in the road as an analogy for charting future complex decision making.

PHILOSOPHY OF CARE
Caregiver Role in Lifelong Life-Threatening Condition

Children with CCC have a lifelong life-threatening condition. This reality focuses the holistic care of the child and their family to identify opportunities to thrive despite this life-threatening condition.[19,20] The underlying conditions of these children can be rare and frequently poorly understood (eg, serious neurologic illness, neurodegenerative disorder). Throughout the course of the child's life, the parents and caregivers become the experts on their child and have a deeper understanding of their day-to-day needs than many medical professionals. Although many may find the medical care of their child a means of expressing love and value, their role as parent/family member must also be preserved.[21–23]

Many clinicians are comfortable with the role of expert, manifest by educating parents and family members about the child's underlying condition. Within this population, it is not uncommon to find the roles reversed as the clinician learns about the child from their experts: the family.

Balancing Restorative Medicine with Palliative Care

Throughout the child's trajectory, PPC supports families and teams as they assess the benefits and burdens of proposed interventions to aid in the development of the child's medical plan of care. This equation changes throughout the child's trajectory, and what may have been deemed beneficial at 1 point in their life may become burdensome, depending on how that intervention affects the child's life at that moment.[17] The PPC team involved in the care of the child with CCC serves as a resource not only to the patient and family but also to the community physician and subspecialists involved in the patient's care.[3,6,11,24–26]

Focus on Living and Thriving in Home Community

One role of PPC is to help patients and their families thrive despite the life-threatening condition. By working with the families and their communities to develop strategies to thrive in their home and community, PPC can help prevent repeated and prolonged hospitalizations.[1–3]

This help may involve the allocation of additional community resources (eg, consumer-directed waivers) as well as the role for personal care attendants or skilled nursing to support the child at home.[12,24,27] Partnering with schools and other community organizations to help prepare the community for a child with CCC aids the child and family to thrive in their home community.[3,21,24,28–31]

As the child's condition advances, their care tends to increase in complexity and frequency.[1] PPC plays a strong role in ensuring that these interventions continue to offer benefit to the child without undue burden.[27] Even routine clinic visits may elicit significant burden in the child with CCC. It is important to recognize when the child's conditions or the family's goals and values diverge from previously beneficial paths. In these scenarios, it is incumbent on the PPC team, in coordination with the child's medical team, to develop novel approaches to minimize disturbances to their quality of life.

UNIQUE DISTRESSING SYMPTOMS

Although this section addresses physical symptoms commonly experienced by children with CCC, care must be taken to address other sources of concomitant or contributing distress, including psychological, social, and spiritual issues, which are discussed in more detail later.

Assessing distress in the child with CCC and concomitant intellectual developmental delay who may also be nonverbal is challenging and potentially anxiety provoking for clinicians.[32] Tools including the Non-Communicating Children's Pain Checklist–Revised[33] and the revised Face Legs Activity Cry and Consolability[34] can aid the clinician in identifying pain and distress in the nonverbal, cognitively impaired child. The Disability Distress Assessment Tool[35] has been developed to better distinguish pain from distress among individuals with communication limitations.

Polypharmacy

Polypharmacy is common in the medical regimens of children with CCC. Such polypharmacy contributes to the complexity of their care, and may at times have adverse effects that cause distress. When a child prescribed multiple medications presents with distressing symptoms, a pharmacist can perform a polypharmacy check to look for potential adverse reactions or interactions as a source of distressing symptoms. In addition, the pharmacist can also help during admission and discharge, another risk factor for medical error in children with CCC.[36]

Complex Pain Management

Many children with CCC undergo a greater number of painful procedures than their typical counterparts. In addition, many of their underlying conditions can cause significant pain.[37–42] This situation is further complicated because the child may also have intellectual and developmental disabilities.[37,39,43] When approaching pain in the child with CCC, it is helpful to recall the different types of pain (nociceptive/somatic, inflammatory, neuropathic, central/psychogenic) as well as the components of the pain pathway (transduction, conduction, transmission, perception, modulation).

When working with patients experiencing ongoing pain, the aforementioned processes and types of pain must be considered when developing a treatment option. This goal is accomplished through careful history taking, noting what works (even partially) and what has been unsuccessful. Plotting the types of pain and physiology of pain in a matrix with attempted interventions can identify gaps in therapy and opportunities to address uncontrolled pain (**Table 1**).

Table 1 Complex pain management matrix					
	Transduction	Conduction	Transmission	Perception	Modulation
Nociceptive	X	X	X	—	—
Inflammatory	X	—	—	—	—
Neuropathic	—	—	X	—	—
Central	—	—	—	X	X

Through this context, management including nonpharmacologic and pharmacologic interventions for the child can be derived. Through the use of sound and established pain management concepts, a good quality of life with pain not limiting activities of daily living or inhibiting goals can be achieved for patients with CCC.

Acute or breakthrough pain

Children with CCC experience acute episodes of pain (eg, postoperative pain, acute pain after pathologic fracture).[38] During these times, continue their long-standing medications with the introduction of acute management medications consistent with the intervention undergone. If they have been exposed to opioids on a long-standing basis, and have developed tolerance to opioids, higher doses may be needed to control their acute pain.

Neuroirritability

Sometimes thought of as central neuropathy, neuroirritability can be challenging to diagnose and equally challenging to treat. Irritability in nonverbal children with CCC can frequently be perceived as pain. Caregivers identify pain with higher frequency in these children.[38] Often, this discomfort is attributed to nociceptive pain, and a path to identify the source should rightfully be undertaken.[39] If a thorough investigation has been executed, yet no identifiable source has been found, neuroirritability should be diagnosed and treated (**Box 1**).

Box 1
Cause of pain and irritability in a nonverbal neurologically impaired child

Head, eyes, ears, nose, throat (HEENT)

   Acute otitis media, sinusitis, pharyngitis, dental abscess, tooth eruption, corneal abrasion, ventricular shunt malfunction

Chest

   Pulmonary aspiration pneumonitis/pneumonia, esophagitis, supraventricular tachycardia, pericardial effusion, costovertebral tenderness

Abdomen

   Gastrointestinal: gastroesophageal reflux, gastritis, gastric/duodenal ulcer, appendicitis, intussusception, constipation, impaired gut motility, visceral hyperalgesia

   Liver/gall bladder: hepatitis, cholecystitis, cholelithiasis

   Pancreas: pancreatitis

   Renal: urinary tract infection, nephrolithiasis, neuropathic bladder pain

   Genitourinary: inguinal hernia, testicular/ovarian torsion, hair tourniquet, menstrual cramps

Skin

   Pressure/decubitus ulcer

Extremities

   Pathologic fracture, hip subluxation, osteomyelitis, spasticity, hair tourniquet

Psychosocial

   Change in home environment, nonaccidental trauma, loss of caregiver

General

   Medication toxicity, sleep disturbance

While diagnosing a child with neuroirritability, it is also helpful to identify signs or symptoms of hyperalgesia and allodynia. These symptoms help to support the diagnosis of neuroirritability.

- Can you tell the difference between your child's cries for attention and cries for pain/discomfort?
  - "No" is consistent with neuroirritability
- Can you localize your child's pain or discomfort?
  - "No" is consistent with neuroirritability
- Do actions known not to be painful (socks, blankets, touching) seem to cause pain or distress?
  - "Yes" is consistent with neuroirritability
- Does your child fuss or cry for no apparent reason?
  - "Yes" is consistent with neuroirritability
- Is the crying difficult to control or prolonged?
  - "Yes" is consistent with neuroirritability

Once diagnosed, treatment with a central neuropathic agent can begin. Gabapentin is often chosen because of its favorable side effect profile as well as its relative lack of interaction with other medications.[44–46] Gabapentin administration is enteral, and is available as a capsule (100 mg, 300 mg, 400 mg), tablet (300 mg, 600 mg, 800 mg), and solution (250 mg/5 mL).

The following advancement protocols are proposed (**Table 2**):

Optimize dosing to relief between the recommended starting dose of 15 mg/kg/d divided 3 times daily up to 45 mg/kg/d. Increases to 60 mg/kg/d may be needed. Doses greater than 60 mg/kg/d are not typically more effective. In the cases in which it is necessary to move to pregabalin (eg, initial benefit but now tolerant to maximum gabapentin dose), use a crossover ratio of 6:1 (gabapentin/pregabalin). There is no need to cross-titrate between gabapentin and pregabalin.[47] In cases in which the gabapentinoids did not provide significant relief, treatment with tricyclic antidepressants or cyproheptadine may be attempted to provide relief.

Table 2
Gabapentin initiation protocols

Days	Morning Dose (mg/kg)	Afternoon Dose (mg/kg)	Evening Dose (mg/kg)
Standard administration			
1–4	0	0	5
5–8	5	0	5
9+	5	5	5
Slower advancement for medication-sensitive children (minimize risk of side effect)			
1–4	0	0	2.5
5–8	2.5	0	2.5
9–12	2.5	2.5	2.5
13–16	2.5	2.5	5
17–20	5	2.5	5
21+	5	5	5
Severe symptoms/rapid titration			
1–2	0	0	5
3–4	5	0	5
5+	5	5	5

Feeding Intolerance

Many children with CCC receive artificial hydration and nutrition (AHN) through a feeding tube.[43] In these children, vigilance is required to identify feeding intolerance and prevent harm.[48]

Feeding intolerance is common among very low birth rate infants, postcardiothoracic surgery patients, patients with serious neurologic injury, technology-dependent children (gastrostomy, gastrojejunostomy, jejunostomy) and as an end-of-life symptom.

Common signs or symptoms of feeding intolerance include early satiety, abdominal bloating and tenderness, cramping, vomiting, diarrhea, fluid retention, general discomfort during feeding, and even respiratory compromise secondary to relative increased abdominal pressure compromising the thoracic cavity, especially of concern in neuromuscular patients, who rely more exclusively on the diaphragm for respiration.[49]

Potentially reversible or transient causes of intolerance include constipation/obstipation, postviral gastroparesis, medication effect, obstruction, and technical malfunction (eg, obstructed jejunostomy port). A detailed history and physical examination should be performed to evaluate for these potentially reversible causes before arriving at the diagnosis of feeding intolerance.

For the child receiving AHN, the protocol proposed in **Box 2** allows the clinician to introduce and advance AHN and to be mindful of introducing further distress.

When feeding intolerance occurs at the end of life, it may be appropriate to focus goals of care on comfort rather than nutrition and forego AHN.[50] In such a scenario, care focuses on measures to promote comfort, rather than intensive, medical measures to provide hydration and nutrition, because they do not benefit the child (eg, providing comfort, dignity) and may cause harm (eg, prolonging the dying process, causing physical pain/discomfort).[51,52] These are delicate conversations and should clearly meet the family and patient where they are, with strong relationships necessary to engage in maintaining focus on what is in the individual child's best interest.

Dysautonomia

Dysautonomia can be a significant challenge when addressing underlying causes of distress. Broadly, dysautonomia can refer to any dysfunction of the autonomic nervous system. These dysfunctions include postural orthostatic tachycardia syndrome, vasovagal syncope, autonomic dysreflexia, neuroleptic malignant syndrome, as well as medication effects such as serotonin syndrome, intrathecal baclofen withdrawal and malignant hyperthermia, and are associated with head injury and periodic autonomic instability with dystonia. Using these known entities as a model, as well as neurophysiologic models including the excitation/inhibition ratio model, a therapeutic plan to address the patient's distressing symptoms can be undertaken.[53]

To aid in diagnosing dysautonomia, it is helpful to note the presence of 4 or 5 of 6 cardinal symptoms without other known physiologic cause (eg, acute pain):

- Tachycardia
- Hypertension
- Thermal regulation (usually hyperthermia, occasionally hypothermia)
- Increased respiratory rate
- Flushing (especially asymmetric) of face/chest
- Sweating

A further aid in diagnosing dysautonomia is the noted presence of the cardinal symptoms in the setting of parasympathetic drive (eg, bowel and bladder dysfunction). In addition to the cardinal symptoms, dysautonomia may also include cool or hot

---

Box 2
Initiating and advancing AHN

Discern child's ideal daily goals for calories and water

- Consider involving a registered dietitian
- Respect past trial and error
- Goal calories and water should be based on patient response; making appropriate amount of wet diapers per day may be a better indicator than receiving 100% of calculated fluid goals

Calculate 24-hour total and administer via feeding pump gradually

- Start 10 mL/h of electrolyte balanced liquid or water
- Increase by 10 mL/h every 4 hours until goal rate achieved
- Adjust based on tolerance, proceeding more rapidly or slowly depending on patient response
- When consistent with family's goals, this may be titrated against intravenous fluid administration for total hourly goal

If tolerating 24-hour fluid volume goal, begin transition to formula

- Start at 25% formula 75% electrolyte solution/water at goal rate for 4 hours
- Advance to 50% formula 50% electrolyte solution/water for 4 hours
- Advance to 75% formula 25% electrolyte solution/water for 4 hours
- Advance to goal 24-hour feeding by formula (free water and formula balance)

Attempt to consolidate feeds to allow time off during the day

- Consider goal nutrition and hydration were at 50 mL/h × 24 h (1200 mL/d)
- Attempt to consolidate this down to 54 mL/h × 22 h (1188 mL/d) and then 60 mL/h × 20 h (1200 mL/d) and further as tolerated
- If a child has a gastrostomy tube, may also attempt boluses or slow boluses throughout the day as tolerated and allow for any remainder to be pump-administered overnight (3 200-mL boluses administered over 1 hour throughout the day, remaining 600 mL pumped overnight at a rate of 60 mL/h × 10 h)
- Children should not receive boluses via jejunostomy

---

hands and feet, red-blue discoloration of the hands or feet, pupillary dilatation, delayed gastric emptying, constipation, and urinary retention.

Triggers include abdominal distention, feeding intolerance, pain, and illness. If 4 or 5 of the cardinal symptoms occur in clusters, this may be identified as dysautonomic storms and warrants specific treatment interventions.[54] These storms may be precipitated by the aforementioned impetuses.

Medication strategies for the treatment of dysautonomia are largely derived from the models of autonomic dysfunction mentioned earlier. The goal is symptom blockade using a theory of controller medications (suppressive therapy) and a breakthrough protocol.[53]

Controller medications to block symptoms and reduce the intensity and frequency of dysautonomic storms include the gabapentinoids[45,46,53,54] (especially with concomitant neuropathic pain or neuroirritability) and cyproheptadine (especially with increased gastrointestinal symptoms). Clonidine has also served as a useful adjunctive medication for dysautonomia. Other avenues for more severe cases include enteral baclofen and even intrathecal baclofen in extreme cases,[54] generally with the guidance of pediatric physiatry.

In addition to a controller medication, protocols for breakthrough symptoms address multiple symptoms in a stepwise fashion, with high-yield/low-risk interventions early in the protocol (**Box 3**).

Over time, the protocol may be tailored for the specific child. For example, if the child receives relief with acetaminophen/ibuprofen approximately 20% of the time but receives relief from diphenhydramine 75% of the time, diphenhydramine should be given before attempting acetaminophen/ibuprofen. In addition, if the diazepam never works, it should be removed from the protocol.

β-Blockers also serve a role in the treatment of dysautonomia. Propranolol may be considered as either a controller medication or on the breakthrough protocol for patients with dysautonomia manifesting as significant tachycardia. Another potential medication for challenging cases is bromocriptine.

Seizures

Within the population of children with CCC, there is a higher incidence of epilepsy when compared with the typical population.[37,43] As a rule, these children should be under the direction of a skilled pediatric neurologist.[55] It is advantageous to be aware of the role that antiepileptics may have on a child, as well as how to manage seizure activity in the child more actively managed by PPC (eg, the actively dying child).

With increased seizure activity in a child with previously controlled seizures, look for a source of the exacerbation. Infection, impaired absorption of the antiepileptics, increased metabolism of the antiepileptics, incorrect dosing of the medication, or advancement of the underlying condition may all affect the seizure frequency. Investigation for potentially reversible causes should be sought (eg, complete blood count,

---

Box 3
Dysautonomia treatment protocol

Controller medication

  Gabapentinoid (gabapentin/pregabalin)

  Cyproheptadine

  Baclofen

  Diazepam

  Clonidine

Sample breakthrough protocol

  Step 1: address nonpharmacologic treatment of distress (changing soiled diaper, repositioning, creating a quiet environment, rocking, holding, playing music, engaging in activities)

  • If no relief

  Step 2: administer acetaminophen/ibuprofen

  • If no relief within 15–20 minutes

  Step 3: administer diphenhydramine

  • If no relief within 15–20 minutes

  Step 4: administer diazepam

  • If no relief within 15–20 minutes

  Step 5: administer enteral morphine

C-reactive protein, drug levels) when consistent with the family's goals and values and the patient's plan of care.

For breakthrough seizures, benzodiazepines continue as a mainstay of first-line treatment, with a wide range of delivery options (**Box 4**).[56]

Careful consideration of the potential adverse effects of antiseizure medications on the child's mood, irritability, and comfort must always be undertaken. Significant gastrointestinal upset, irritability, and agitation may be drug related and are often poorly recognized by both families and treating physicians.

For the actively dying patient, it is crucial to recognize seizures/increased seizure activity as a possible end-of-life symptom. It is important to anticipate this situation and have appropriate medications available. If intravenous access is available, intravenous medications should be readily available. Prophylactic administration of benzodiazepines may also be considered, balancing the goals of therapy using a benefit (decreased seizures) versus burden (sedation) model.

For children approaching end of life, whether currently prescribed antiepileptics are continued should be considered in light of the goals of care. If established antiepileptics are discontinued, it is incumbent to be prepared for breakthrough seizure activity. One may choose to not treat some seizures (eg, eye flutter, blank stare) that the family identifies as nondistressing for the child to experience and the family to witness.

Sleep Disturbance

Children with CCC have an increased risk of sleep disorders when compared with the typical population, with sleep disturbances in more than 67% of children with severe multiple disabilities compared with healthy children (3%–40%).[57,58] This situation has deleterious effects on quality of life. Many children with a complex presentation of distressing symptoms improve dramatically once an exacerbating sleep disorder is effectively treated.

Box 4
Benzodiazepines for breakthrough seizures

Intranasal

- Midazolam

Buccal

- Diazepam
- Lorazepam

Enteral

- Diazepam
- Lorazepam
- Midazolam

Rectal

- Diazepam

Intravenous

- Diazepam
- Lorazepam
- Midazolam

The prevailing sleep disturbances in children with multiple disabilities includes sleep-onset insomnia (25%), sleep-maintenance insomnia (35%), sleep-related breathing disorders (19%), hypersomnia (14%), impaired circadian rhythm (18%), parasomnia (13%), and sleep-related movement disorder (7%).[59]

Addressing sleep disorders provides an opportunity to significantly improve overall quality of life for children with CCC.[60,61] A sleep log is helpful in identifying timing, duration, and frequency of insomnia and consequent daytime napping. Without this tool, exhausted parents often can remember only last night and the worst night.[62]

Average total sleep requirement over a 2-week period is easily calculated from the sleep log: the total number of hours slept is divided by the number of nights. The sleep log can then be used as a guide to improve sleep hygiene by decreasing the hours in bed to approximate the total sleep time. This strategy is known as sleep restriction. Sleep restriction leads to a regularizing of the wake time and bedtime, resulting in improved sleep hygiene. The sleep log also makes the optimal sleep phase obvious. Coordinating bedtime and wake time is easier when the biological clock or circadian rhythm and total sleep requirement are respected (**Fig. 1**).

Nonpharmacologic interventions for sleep disturbances are largely centered on good sleep hygiene: avoiding naps, encouraging appropriate physical activity, addressing disruptive nutrition/medication schedules, and encouraging relaxing bedtime routines.

Pharmacologic treatment options for insomnia include tricyclic antidepressants (amitriptyline, doxepin), trazodone, and benzodiazepines (clonazepam).[63,64] For circadian rhythm disturbances, sleep hygiene and melatonin can provide a useful first-line approach.[65,66]

Sleep-related respiratory problems, particularly obstructive apnea and sleep-related hypoventilation, are common in children with neuromuscular disorders.[67] These children may likely benefit from noninvasive positive pressure ventilation.[68] This intervention alone can have profound effects on several distressing symptoms for this subset of children with CCC, including daytime alertness, increased weight gain (through decreasing metabolic demand of the breathing process), better ability to cope with other distressing symptoms, and overall family and caregiver well-being.[69,70]

In more challenging cases, the involvement of a sleep medicine physician is helpful.

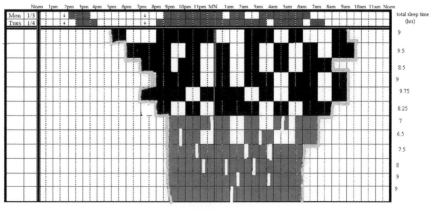

Instructions: The top two rows show a "sample" sleep log. Enter the Days and Dates on the left hand side. The arrows mark "bedtime". Shaded areas mark sleep (note the difference between "bedtime" and actually falling asleep). White/clear areas mark awake periods. Midnight is in the middle of the chart. Dotted lines mark the half-hour. Note the interruptions during the night on the sample—these are night time wakings. Note the shaded areas in the afternoon---these are naps. Feel free to add margin notes or additional information that would be helpful in learning more about your child's sleep.

Fig. 1. Sleep log detailing gradual sleep restriction and consequent sleep consolidation.

Table 3 Tone management strategies		
Tone	Pharmacologic	Interventional
Spasticity	Benzodiazepines Baclofen	Botulinum toxin Phenol Intrathecal baclofen pump Selective dorsal rhizotomy
Dystonia	Levodopa/carbidopa Trihexyphenidyl Diphenhydramine	Botulinum toxin Deep brain stimulation
Choreoathetoid	Benzodiazepines Antipsychotics (risperidone, haloperidol) Tetrabenazine	Botulinum toxin Deep brain stimulation

Tone

Tone is an entity that can be difficult to define but is best understood as unconscious muscle activation and resistance to stretch forces whether such forces are gravity or passive movements. Hypotonic patients often appear floppy, whereas others have high tone, such as is seen in children with cerebral palsy. High tone may negatively affect their quality of life, correlating with their degree of hypertonia.[71] Hypertonia may be perceived as painful, and because of increased muscle activation, nutrition (increased caloric expenditure), positioning, and skin integrity can be a challenge.[41,43] Increased tone from brain damage/dysfunction can be associated with spasticity, dystonia, and choreoathetosis. Such symptoms may also be present in combination, leading to a more accurate description of mixed tone.

Nonpharmacologic therapy should be implemented early and often in children with tone challenges. This therapy includes adaptive equipment (eg, wheelchairs, beds, lifts, props, pillows) as well as skilled physical therapy.[56]

Pharmacologic and procedural interventions are directed by the type of tone present.[72–74] The following is not intended to be exhaustive but to assist the clinician with beginning a treatment plan. Involvement of pediatric neurology and physiatry can also provide subspecialist care for the child with complex tone management issues (**Table 3**).[73,75–77]

Anticipated Forks in the Road: Collaborating with Families to Prepare for and Work Through Decision Points

Many children with CCC have a predictable disease-based pattern (eg, neuromuscular conditions including spinal muscular atrophy type I, Duchenne muscular dystrophy) as well as a specific patient-based pattern (eg, cerebral palsy spastic quadriplegia, neurodegenerative condition). In such children, it is helpful to develop and consider road maps, naturally respecting the individual receiving the benefit and potential burdens of the interventions.

As an example, a boy with Duchenne muscular dystrophy may present to clinic at a relatively young age, well before any overwhelming physical symptoms. It can be anticipated that as he ages and his muscular dystrophy advances, he will reach a point at which continued enteral nutrition may become challenging. His respiratory status will decline because he will no longer have the muscular strength to generate inspiratory force.

Andrew (Andy) was a young Hmong man with Duchenne muscular dystrophy who first met the palliative care team at the age of 12 years, to discuss supplementing his nutrition with a gastrostomy tube. Andy had lost weight over the past 10 months, and was worried. Andy expressed concerns about not being able to eat his mother's traditional Hmong dishes if he had a tube. His family also expressed religious concerns over having an implanted foreign body. In discussion with Andy and his family, it was decided to proceed without the gastrostomy tube, and to work on increasing his caloric intake through supplemental shakes. It was also discussed how the nighttime use of bilevel positive airway pressure (BiPAP) could decrease the metabolic demand of breathing and then increase his weight, because the calories Andy did ingest could be used for anabolic weight gain as opposed to breathing. The family and Andy declined further interventions, because they wanted to minimize the amount of medical technology in the home.

Andy was seen back at the age of 14 years, now with concerns for progressive neuromuscular scoliosis and the recommendation for a posterior spinal fusion. Andy was able to articulate his struggles with pain, requiring him to frequently leave class to lie down in the nurse's office because of his back pain. He also grieved the loss of function, because he found it difficult to draw anymore. He noted progressive breathlessness as well. His weight had remained stable, but he continued to be thin, with many bony prominences, which had caused concerns for pressure ulcers. The family expressed grave concerns about the implanted rods recommended by the orthopedic surgeon, because their religion stated the body cannot go to heaven if there is something in it. Through careful conversations with Andy and his family, they agreed on the philosophy of care of undertaking all meaningful interventions to optimize his quality of life.

Andy remained focused on the surgery, and whether or not he should do it. The benefits (stopping the progressive scoliosis, stopping the progressive restrictive lung disease secondary to the scoliosis, improvement in back pain) and burdens (major surgery with its associated risks, recovery from surgery, respecting family religious background) were discussed, and Andy and his family agreed to the philosophy of the surgery. In the spirit of open communication, his weight and pulmonary status were discussed, and it was pointed out that those were potentially complicating factors to his surgery, which, if addressed before the surgery, could be minimized and improve his chances of a successful surgery. His family once again returned to the religious concern about implanted foreign bodies.

Using the successful surgery as a conversation focus, the conversation was framed on optimizing his nutrition and minimizing his risk of developing pressure ulcers through improved nutrition. After careful thought, Andy and his family agreed to the gastrostomy tube before the surgery (with reassurances that it need not limit his enjoyment of his mother's home cooking).

At the same time, supportive ventilation was discussed, and although it was daunting, Andy was able to recognize the benefit of BiPAP initiation through the immediate improvement in some of his distressing symptoms (fatigue during the day caused by poor sleep at night, headache secondary to carbon dioxide retention) as well as improving his postsurgical pulmonary recovery. After a night in the sleep laboratory to optimize the settings, Andy began using BiPAP at night.

The parents' future concerns were also addressed, because a Hmong funeral home was identified in town that was willing to remove implanted devices at the time of preparation for funeral services, thus allowing the soul to rise unfettered by mortal trappings.

After Andy received the benefit of the supplemental nutrition and BiPAP support, he successfully underwent his posterior spinal fusion. He was seen in follow-up and continued to be a bright and engaging young man. Conversations were had to discuss future decisions down the road (advancing pulmonary care, increased adaptive equipment, and goals for after high school, including potentially moving out of his parents' house), and Andy and his family remained well engaged with the clinic.

In these cases, it is valuable to have the discussion well in advance to address concerns surrounding AHN as well as assistive ventilation.[78,79] When crafting this discussion, the goal is not to be brutally honest, but to have honest conversations, meeting the family where they are in their thinking and understanding of the current situation; gentling pushing a point that may be necessary to voice without harming them with too much information before they are prepared to absorb it.[80]

It is essential to be mindful about the words chosen when discussing these interventions. The underlying condition itself can rarely be cured, and therefore patients rarely need an offered intervention. Discussions around AHN are 1 such example of choosing words carefully (eg, "may benefit from" or "recommend" as opposed to "needs a feeding tube").

Medical/Artificial Nutritional Support

At some point in the life of the child with CCC, the discussion of AHN is likely to arise. This discussion must be carefully balanced with the family's ongoing goals and values and the benefit and burden of the proposed intervention.[81] Current Cochrane reviews[82] continue to highlight the lack of reliable evidence to guide the clinician counseling the family of a child with CCC, thus making the decision truly individualized for the patient and family. The recommendation for AHN may come from either the treatment team or the family.

For example, if the family perceives that mealtimes are no longer pleasing for the child, or if the amount of time required to eat orally becomes burdensome, they may broach the topic of a feeding tube. Likewise, the clinician may recommend AHN with varying levels of strength, including noting progressive dysphagia, difficulty meeting recommended caloric intake, or aspiration of oral nutrition and subsequent pulmonary infections.

If, for example, family mealtime is important, the schedule of the child with AHN should be optimized to coordinate with family mealtime. In addition, if the child finds certain tastes to be pleasurable, advocate for continued pleasure tastes, but still receiving the recommended caloric intake via feeding tube.

CASE VIGNETTE 2: FLORES

Flores was a 7-year-old girl with cerebral palsy gross motor function classification system V, epilepsy, and profound intellectual developmental disability, who was referred to your clinic because "school says she needs a gastrostomy tube." While reviewing her records, it was noted that she had lost 3 kg (15% of her body weight) over the past 4 months without an apparent change in her underlying tone or seizure activity. In discussion with the family, it was learned that Flores had never suffered aspiration pneumonia and tolerated her antiepileptics by mouth well. The family stated that it did take them a while to feed her at mealtime (approximately 45 minutes) and she did require her food to be pureed, but the family also stated the joy that having family mealtime together brought to Flores, her parents, and her 4 brothers. When discussing the concerns for weight loss, Flores's mother described how she has been trying to "eat healthier" because her sons had gained too much weight lately, and by proxy, Flores had had a relative reduction in total calories. After discussion with the family, it was clear that mealtime together was highly important and that the ability to feed Flores by mouth was identified as a caring act of love by her parents. They were counseled to return Flores's diet to full calorie and she thrived with the increased oral calories. The family was counseled that if Flores had challenges tolerating her nutrition by mouth in the future, she began to have challenges with aspiration during feeding, or they were unable to reliably deliver her medications by mouth, they should feel free to contact the team to have another conversation to discuss the possibility of a feeding tube.

Discussions surrounding surgical interventions for AHN also raise the issue for other surgical interventions intended to improve the quality of life of the child at the time of the gastrostomy tube placement. Convincing evidence does not exist regarding the optimal treatment of reflux (fundoplication vs medications) in the child with neurologic impairment at the time of gastrostomy insertion.[83]

Respiratory Support

Although the focus here addresses pulmonary support over the trajectory of an illness, it remains critical to address affecting symptoms of pulmonary support, including secretions, dyspnea, and the underlying medical condition (eg, muscular dystrophy).

The introduction of respiratory technological support, noninvasive positive pressure ventilation, and invasive positive pressure ventilation can be anticipated and discussed. At each of these points, it is essential to note the increase in technological burden and discern how that squares with the family's underlying goals and values. In addition, it is helpful to have these discussions early on to help stave off misinformation, myths, and fears about the interventions (eg, "...if I am trached, I can never leave the hospital"). Further avenues of support include connecting patients and families with a peer network (often facilitated through social work), as well as continued education on the underlying condition and interventions proposed to address the progressive respiratory support.

It is appropriate to chart the anticipated escalations in technological support over time and to reassure the patient and family that their goals and values surrounding escalating treatments will be respected (**Table 4**).

Advancement to the next level of respiratory support is often heralded by consistent increase in the previous. For example, BiPAP initially used only at night and during naps is frequently used throughout the day, or a young man using a sip and puff ventilator can barely speak 2 words in a row before needing a supported breath.

With appropriate recognition of early symptoms, the child with advanced pulmonary care in their home community can be supported through carefully thought out pulmonary protocols for both routine and sick modes.[2] These protocols need to be tailored for the individual child, but the protocol in **Table 5** serves as a sample.

This protocol is not meant to serve as a replacement for appropriate clinician oversight but as a tool to help families avoid acute care visits or hospitalizations and remain

Table 4 Pulmonary interventions	
Pulmonary health	Inhaled medications (albuterol, budesonide) Percussive therapy High-frequency chest wall oscillation (Vest system therapy, The Vest System, Hill-Rom, Batesville, IN, USA) Continuous high-frequency oscillation (MetaNeb, The MetaNeb System, Hill-Rom, Batesville, IN, USA) Cough assist Supplemental oxygen
Noninvasive positive pressure ventilation (NIPPV)	Continuous positive airway pressure BiPAP Sip and puff ventilation Advancement of frequency of NIPPV
Invasive positive pressure ventilation	Tracheostomy Ventilator support

Table 5 Sample home pulmonary protocol	
Routine mode	Budesonide 0.5 mg isoniazid twice a day Albuterol 2.5 mg isoniazidevery 4 h according to shortness of breath Vest therapy twice a day with budesonide Cough assist once daily

Sick mode step 1 (increased respiratory
  distress, cough, cold symptoms)
	Advance budesonide to 4 times a day
	Schedule albuterol 4 times a day and every
	  2 h according to shortness of breath
	Advance Vest therapy to 4 times a day with
	  nebulizations
	Cough assist twice a day and as needed
	BiPAP overnight and as needed

Sick mode step 2 (symptoms not improved, telephone check-in before advancing)	Continue above Add enteral steroids twice a day Add enteral antibiotic
Sick mode step 3 (symptoms not improved, telephone check-in before advancing)	As above Add inhaled tobramycin

within their home community. Close telephone contact is undertaken throughout the escalation process, and changes to the plan of care are initiated when warranted.

Surgical Interventions

Many children with CCC are subject to multiple surgical procedures (eg, gastrostomy, ventriculoperitoneal shunt, tracheostomy, orthopedic procedures, endoscopies). With each offered intervention, attention to goals of care and whether and how the intervention will benefit the child as an individual must be weighed. It is also crucial to ensure that the patient and family understand the goals of the procedure to allow them to engage in the benefit/burden discussion. Often, in the care of the child with CCC, the surgical intervention does not cure the underlying condition. This strategy helps provide a framework for the ongoing benefit/burden discussions.[14]

SPECIAL FOCUS: SPIRITUAL AND PSYCHOSOCIAL CARE

Spiritual and psychosocial care and support for children and families living with CCC are an essential component in palliation of symptoms of distress, anxiety, loss, and bereavement. As a part of the interdisciplinary palliative care team, professional chaplains provide spiritual assessment, active compassion, and support for patient/family values and beliefs that inform decision making about health care and quality of life. The palliative care provider is often confronted with profound spiritual questions in the palliation of suffering. Spiritual care and support seek not only to address spiritual needs but also to respect and affirm the resiliency that individuals and families have nurtured while living with CCC. Bringing a healthy curiosity about the human condition to each encounter of spiritual assessment and care can strengthen the care provider's own resiliency.

Spiritual assessment and palliative psychosocial care address key components of human spirituality:

- Healing and hope[84]
- Grief and loss
- Meaning and values
- Relationships and connections

Spiritual assessment and palliative psychosocial care can be modified to address the unique needs of individuals and families living with CCC. **Box 5** presents some of the ways in palliative care that providers can address spiritual needs and enhance resiliency for individuals and their families.

Spiritual care of individuals and their families living with CCC must take into account the isolation that many feel in relationship to formative religious values and communities. Individuals and families living with CCC are often cut off from conventional

---

Box 5
Spiritual assessment and interventions for those living with CCC

Healing and hope

- Honoring the ways individuals and families have nurtured hope and the transcendent in their lives
- Promoting hope and healing, especially when curative medical treatments are no longer beneficial or present significant risk
- Affirming hopes that center on quality of living that is meaningful for as long as possible (one mother hoped that her son could be wheeled outside to feel the breeze blow through his hair and make pancakes with his personal care attendant, right up until the end of his life)
- Acknowledging the spiritual tensions of living with CCC: acknowledging the dualities of sorrow and joy, hope and despair, praise and lament, solace and pain as daily aspects of living with CCC

Grief and loss

- Exploring anticipatory grieving, chronic loss, and sorrow
- Addressing parental guilt over genetic conditions and birth injuries
- Honoring parental feelings of helplessness in protecting and shielding their child from suffering and pain
- Providing solace for those who are bereaved and struggling with the loss of caring roles

Meaning and values

- Encouraging the recounting of a life story, or family history, as a way to create a context for what is happening now and what is hoped for in the future
- Honoring the beliefs and values of individuals and families, especially in regards to quality of life, the meaning of disease and suffering, and what constitutes a peaceful death

Relationships and connections

- Exploring the ways that individuals and their families have fostered communication and loving connections, even when verbal communication is impaired
- Supporting models of shared decision making that have evolved over time between individuals and their families or between surrogate decision makers
- Promoting the support systems, including faith communities, on which people rely for maintaining spiritual resiliency
- Supporting peer and family connections, which address feelings of isolation and loneliness
- Understanding the conflicts and estrangements that are causing relational pain, addressing issues of forgiveness, and exploring possibilities for reconciliation
- Exploring the contributions and legacy that individuals with CCC wish to leave/are leaving their loved ones; this may include autopsy or postmortem research samples given to enhance understanding of rare medical conditions

religious settings by virtue of the physical barriers to participation in religious services and the life of a faith community.

Many patients and families who live with CCC are exposed to daily suffering and pain, which alienates the spirit from the transcendent, taking a toll on the integrity of a belief system focused on a higher power. Chaplains pay attention to the potential despair that people feel when facing life-limiting situations. Palliative spiritual care promotes hope and assists individuals and families in making new connections or reconnecting to sources of spiritual care and support in the community. Spiritual care and palliative psychosocial support may include advocacy for inclusion of those with CCC in their communities of faith.

CASE VIGNETTE 3: BENJAMIN

Benjamin was a 15-year-old with a congenital myopathy, diagnosed at age 3 years. He had experienced a decline in his medical condition in the past year, requiring multiple hospitalizations for respiratory distress. His mother and maternal grandmother shared care of him in the family home, which included Benjamin's younger sister. Benjamin's father had been minimally involved in his life since he was very young. Benjamin's mother and grandmother lost their son/grandson to the same genetic condition when he was 15 years of age. Even although his mother was his legal surrogate for health care decisions, his mother consulted Benjamin and said she would never consent to treatment he would not view as beneficial. Likewise, she stated she would not limit treatments he would still want. His mother and grandmother were Catholic, but they had not been active in their parish for years and they did not know the priest who currently served the congregation. His grandmother asked, "How can God allow this terrible disease? It's taken so much away from my family!" His mother said that one of the things they loved to do as a family was read aloud. They had read a wide range of books, including the Harry Potter series. This past Halloween, all 4 of their household dressed up in Harry Potter costumes. Benjamin was Harry.

Spiritual assessment and care for Benjamin and his family
Healing and Hope

Benjamin and his family have drawn strength from a modern-day mythologic story of a boy who continues to survive against all odds, even although his survival often leaves him and his companions vulnerable to loss and grief. Spiritual care honors the ways in which the family has created healing and hope by integration of this mythological story into their own family story.

Spiritual care includes encouraging Benjamin and his family to explore what hope and healing might look like as Benjamin's disease progresses. The child life specialist and chaplain may collaborate in offering other stories of hope and healing (eg, Warren Hanson's *Next Place*, C. S. Lewis's *Last Battle*, Katherine Paterson's *Bridge to Terabithia*). Discussions could be fostered with Benjamin and his family about participation in opportunities granted by organizations such as the Make a Wish Foundation. Spiritual care should address whether or not his mother and grandmother wish to reconnect with their local Catholic parish and whether or not they desire assistance to do so.

Grief and Loss

Benjamin's mother, grandmother, and sister find it difficult to talk about the decline or death of Benjamin. They describe both physical and emotional/spiritual symptoms of chronic sorrow and anticipatory grieving. Benjamin plays a central role in their family life, and their family will never be the same without him. Benjamin is worried about his family's well-being, and he is reluctant to speak to them about his own sorrow. He is protective of this family, not wanting to cause them any more pain than they already have. He wonders how they will remember him and how they will be without him.

Spiritual care, in collaboration with social work or psychology, involves offering grief support and counseling, assisting Benjamin and his family in identifying a community resource for these services. Spiritual care offers the opportunity for his mother and grandmother to reflect on the loss of their son/grandson at age 15 years, and what it means for them that Benjamin has reached 15 years of age. Allowing the grandmother to give voice to her lamentation over the injustice of loss in her family promotes healing and allows her to connect to the community of those who lament and grieve. Spiritual care might involve assisting Benjamin in creating an ethical will (ie, a letter, scrapbook, or video for his family that shows the legacy he wishes to leave for them).

Meaning and Values

Benjamin and his mother need professional encouragement and a safe, supportive environment to talk about their values and beliefs in relationship to Benjamin's progressive disease and their goals for his future medical care. The interdisciplinary team benefit from hearing Benjamin's and his mother's values and beliefs to help guide medical decision making.

The palliative care team can assist in approaching Benjamin and his mother about advanced medical planning or a living will. Documents for advanced medical planning are available online or in hard copy to help Benjamin and his mother start these discussions. Interdisciplinary care conferences that create a professionally caring, safe environment for Benjamin, his mother, and family to receive information, share their feelings, and discuss their thoughts and values about his condition, can assist the patient, family, and team in creating an advanced medical plan that upholds the wishes of Benjamin and his family.

Relationships and Connections

Benjamin and his family are devoted to one another. They have reconfigured their conventional family roles to accommodate the needs of their loved one with a life-threatening condition and progressive disabilities. In the absence of a father, the maternal grandmother has assumed a partnership with her daughter in caring for Benjamin and his sister. His mother consults Benjamin in decisions that involve his medical needs and recommended treatment options. Benjamin's sister provides care for Benjamin at home and has accommodated to her older brother's needs for health care in the home setting. The 4 household members are deeply mutual. There is estrangement and pain around the lost relationship with Benjamin's biological father.

The palliative care team encourage exploration of the family's support system and whether or not they want to include others in their inner family circle at this time. Spiritual support addresses the distance from Benjamin's father and how distant or close Benjamin and his family want that relationship to be in the future. As mentioned earlier, spiritual care should address whether or not mother and grandmother wish to reconnect with their local parish and the new priest. Chaplaincy, along with the interdisciplinary team, can offer Benjamin and his family opportunities to network with other patients and families living with a similar condition. The team can offer to help Benjamin and his family set up a controlled Web site through an organization like *CaringBridge*, which enables them to journal updates on their situation and stay connected to a wider community of support.

Palliative Care Conversations with the Bereaved After the Loss of a Child with CCC

Bereavement care begins to move the family and the specialized health care team to a time when the family will receive most support and care from those outside the health care system (it is hoped from their extended family, faith community, and community services). There are many complex losses for families and for the interdisciplinary health care providers who have shared care of a deceased child, teen, or young adult with CCC. Care of a child with CCC often spans years, even a whole lifetime, of mutual and extraordinary care by family members in cooperation with health care professionals, who can seem like a second family to those who rely on them for professional guidance and consultation.

Grief is unique to every individual and relationship. Bereavement can cause one to feel irrational, despairing, relieved, sorrowful, hopeful, angry, inexplicably joyful, and vulnerable. People grieve in ways that are influenced by their culture, age, role, gender, socioeconomic condition, religious heritage, and personal history. Faith can be a strong support or, if too rigid to accommodate lamentation and despair, can become a serious hindrance to the bereaved.

Grief is especially complex if it is protracted. Many children with CCC have lived longer than expected. Advances in medical treatments have allowed individuals who were not expected to survive infancy to live into young adulthood. This lengthening out of their lifespan has also meant expanding the role of caregiver for many parents into their late adulthood. These parents are pioneers. They have done something no one has ever done and no one was prepared to do, providing extraordinary medical care in the home setting for years and years. Many have done so with woefully inadequate societal and financial support. Bereaved parents of children with CCC have a unique wisdom to share with a Western culture that values autonomy and devalues healthy dependency. Bereaved parents of children who died of complications of their CCC offer a poignant reminder to the Western medical world that making the impossible possible has complex ramifications for patients with CCC and for their families.

CASE VIGNETTE 4: BEREAVED FAMILIES: 3 IMPACTFUL CONVERSATIONS

Identity
The bereaved mother of a young adult who died at 17 after living with severe cerebral palsy was struggling with identity and relationships. The question, "Who am I now that she is gone?" was key to exploring and envisioning a new identity and role apart from her former primary role of loving caregiver. Connecting with other (adult) children and grandchildren in new ways could feel both overwhelming and life giving. Redefining family in the absence of the one around whom the family had revolved and around whom family roles were structured was a major shift in family dynamics. Palliative conversations allowed the mother to "sojourn in her grief, speaking the truth of her life without judgment or ready answers."

Meaning
The father of a young man who was dying in hospice from the end stage of his complex medical condition struggled with questions about suffering. He asked, "What is the meaning of my son's years of suffering? What is the meaning of my own suffering?" Palliative conversations with this father allowed him to raise these questions and might offer poetry or the psalms of lamentation as a way to give further voice to these feelings and profound spiritual questions.

Connection
The mother of a young woman who died of end-stage complications from a lifelong complex medical condition sought to integrate her faith into the experience of her daughter's life and her own sense of isolation in mothering a child who had been dependent on her for almost 2 decades for daily care, advocacy, and ministrations. Palliative conversations with this mother allowed her to connect in new ways with resources of comfort, hope, and solidarity to alleviate her feelings of isolation.

SUMMARY

The interdisciplinary skills of an advanced PPC team are ideally suited to children with CCC and their families as they navigate through the complex waters of the modern health care system. Developing a relationship with these families facilitates articulation of their goals and values. Crafting a philosophy of care that can be translated into a medical plan of care for the child is one of the aims of the PPC team. Through close work with the child, family, community, and medical team, PPC can ensure that the child thrives with their life-threatening condition.

ACKNOWLEDGMENTS

Grateful appreciation to John Belew, PhD, Timothy Feyma, MD, Beverly Wical, MD, John Garcia, MD, Samuel Roiko, PhD, Jean Stansbury, CPNP, Neota Moe, LCISW, Melanie Rouse, LCISW, Natalie Kinsky, CCLS, Heather Mason, RN, Nancy He, PharmD, and Christine Eid, JD.

REFERENCES

1. Berry JG, Agrawal R, Kuo DZ, et al. Characteristics of hospitalizations for patients who use a structured clinical care program for children with medical complexity. J Pediatr 2011;159(2):284–90. http://dx.doi.org/10.1016/j.jpeds.2011.02.002.
2. Berry JG, Hall DE, Kuo DZ, et al. Hospital utilization and characteristics of patients experiencing recurrent readmissions within children's hospitals. JAMA 2011;305(7):682–90. http://dx.doi.org/10.1001/jama.2011.122.
3. Burke RT, Alverson B. Impact of children with medically complex conditions. Pediatrics 2010;126(4):789–90. http://dx.doi.org/10.1542/peds.2010-1885.
4. Burns KH, Casey PH, Lyle RE, et al. Increasing prevalence of medically complex children in US hospitals. Pediatrics 2010;126(4):638–46. http://dx.doi.org/10.1542/peds.2009-1658.
5. Cagle WE, Stockwell DC. The complex majority in the pediatric intensive care unit*. Crit Care Med 2012;40(7):2262–3. http://dx.doi.org/10.1097/CCM.0b013e3182536aab.
6. Cohen E, Kuo DZ, Agrawal R, et al. Children with medical complexity: an emerging population for clinical and research initiatives. Pediatrics 2011;127(3):529–38. http://dx.doi.org/10.1542/peds.2010-0910.
7. Cohen E, Berry JG, Camacho X, et al. Patterns and costs of health care use of children with medical complexity. Pediatrics 2012;130(6):e1463–70. http://dx.doi.org/10.1542/peds.2012-0175.
8. Edwards JD, Houtrow AJ, Vasilevskis EE, et al. Chronic conditions among children admitted to U.S. pediatric intensive care units: their prevalence and impact on risk for mortality and prolonged length of stay*. Crit Care Med 2012;40(7):2196–203. http://dx.doi.org/10.1097/CCM.0b013e31824e68cf.
9. Guertin MH, Cote-Brisson L, Major D, et al. Factors associated with death in the emergency department among children dying of complex chronic conditions: population-based study. J Palliat Med 2009;12(9):819–25. http://dx.doi.org/10.1089/jpm.2009.0041.
10. Simon TD, Berry J, Feudtner C, et al. Children with complex chronic conditions in inpatient hospital settings in the United States. Pediatrics 2010;126(4):647–55. http://dx.doi.org/10.1542/peds.2009-3266.
11. Simon TD, Mahant S, Cohen E. Pediatric hospital medicine and children with medical complexity: past, present, and future. Curr Probl Pediatr Adolesc Health Care 2012;42(5):113–9. http://dx.doi.org/10.1016/j.cppeds.2012.01.002.

12. Feudtner C, Feinstein JA, Satchell M, et al. Shifting place of death among children with complex chronic conditions in the United States, 1989-2003. JAMA 2007;297(24):2725–32. http://dx.doi.org/10.1001/jama.297.24.2725.

13. Feudtner C, Kang TI, Hexem KR, et al. Pediatric palliative care patients: a prospective multicenter cohort study. Pediatrics 2011;127(6):1094–101. http://dx.doi.org/10.1542/peds.2010-3225.

14. Ishikawa H, Hashimoto H, Kiuchi T. The evolving concept of "patient-centeredness" in patient-physician communication research. Soc Sci Med 2013;96: 147–53. http://dx.doi.org/10.1016/j.socscimed.2013.07.026.

15. Keele L, Keenan HT, Sheetz J, et al. Differences in characteristics of dying children who receive and do not receive palliative care. Pediatrics 2013;132(1): 72–8. http://dx.doi.org/10.1542/peds.2013-0470.

16. Nageswaran S, Ip EH, Golden SL, et al. Inter-agency collaboration in the care of children with complex chronic conditions. Acad Pediatr 2012;12(3):189–97. http://dx.doi.org/10.1016/j.acap.2012.02.007.

17. Klick JC, Ballantine A. Providing care in chronic disease: the ever-changing balance of integrating palliative and restorative medicine. Pediatr Clin North Am 2007;54(5):799–812. http://dx.doi.org/10.1016/j.pcl.2007.07.003, xii.

18. Graham RJ, Robinson WM. Integrating palliative care into chronic care for children with severe neurodevelopmental disabilities. J Dev Behav Pediatr 2005; 26(5):361–5.

19. Fiks AG, Mayne S, Localio AR, et al. Shared decision making and behavioral impairment: a national study among children with special health care needs. BMC Pediatr 2012;12:153. http://dx.doi.org/10.1186/1471-2431-12-153.

20. Golden SL, Nageswaran S. Caregiver voices: coordinating care for children with complex chronic conditions. Clin Pediatr (Phila) 2012;51(8):723–9. http://dx.doi.org/10.1177/0009922812445920.

21. Hexem KR, Bosk AM, Feudtner C. The dynamic system of parental work of care for children with special health care needs: a conceptual model to guide quality improvement efforts. BMC Pediatr 2011;11:95. http://dx.doi.org/10.1186/1471-2431-11-95.

22. Kuster PA, Merkle CJ. Caregiving stress, immune function, and health: implications for research with parents of medically fragile children. Issues Compr Pediatr Nurs 2004;27(4):257–76. http://dx.doi.org/10.1080/01460860490884165.

23. Raina P, O'Donnell M, Rosenbaum P, et al. The health and well-being of caregivers of children with cerebral palsy. Pediatrics 2005;115(6):e626–36. http://dx.doi.org/10.1542/peds.2004-1689.

24. Carroll JM, Torkildson C, Winsness JS. Issues related to providing quality pediatric palliative care in the community. Pediatr Clin North Am 2007;54(5):813–27. http://dx.doi.org/10.1016/j.pcl.2007.06.002, xiii.

25. Hall DE. The care of children with medically complex chronic disease. J Pediatr 2011;159(2):178–80. http://dx.doi.org/10.1016/j.jpeds.2011.03.031.

26. Okumura MJ, Heisler M, Davis MM, et al. Comfort of general internists and general pediatricians in providing care for young adults with chronic illnesses of childhood. J Gen Intern Med 2008;23(10):1621–7. http://dx.doi.org/10.1007/s11606-008-0716-8.

27. Feudtner C, Hays RM, Haynes G, et al. Deaths attributed to pediatric complex chronic conditions: national trends and implications for supportive care services. Pediatrics 2001;107(6):E99.

28. Kitazumi E. Medical care and support in school and community life to very severe neurologically-impaired children–advance and problems in medical,

educational and social management for improvement of QOL. No To Hattatsu 2003;35(3):200–5.

29. Miller EG, Laragione G, Kang TI, et al. Concurrent care for the medically complex child: lessons of implementation. J Palliat Med 2012;15(11):1281–3. http://dx.doi.org/10.1089/jpm.2011.0346.

30. Rahi JS, Manaras I, Tuomainen H, et al. Meeting the needs of parents around the time of diagnosis of disability among their children: evaluation of a novel program for information, support, and liaison by key workers. Pediatrics 2004; 114(4):e477–82. http://dx.doi.org/10.1542/peds.2004-0240.

31. Wang C, Guttmann A, To T, et al. Neighborhood income and health outcomes in infants: how do those with complex chronic conditions fare? Arch Pediatr Adolesc Med 2009;163(7):608–15. http://dx.doi.org/10.1001/archpediatrics.2009.36.

32. McCluggage HL. Symptoms suffered by life-limited children that cause anxiety to UK children's hospice staff. Int J Palliat Nurs 2006;12(6):254–8.

33. Breau LM, McGrath PJ, Camfield CS, et al. Psychometric properties of the non-communicating children's pain checklist-revised. Pain 2002;99(1-2): 349–57.

34. Malviya S, Voepel-Lewis T, Burke C, et al. The revised FLACC observational pain tool: improved reliability and validity for pain assessment in children with cognitive impairment. Paediatr Anaesth 2006;16(3):258–65. http://dx.doi.org/10.1111/j.1460-9592.2005.01773.x.

35. Regnard C, Reynolds J, Watson B, et al. Understanding distress in people with severe communication difficulties: developing and assessing the disability distress assessment tool (DisDAT). J Intellect Disabil Res 2007;51(Pt 4): 277–92. http://dx.doi.org/10.1111/j.1365-2788.2006.00875.x.

36. Stone BL, Boehme S, Mundorff MB, et al. Hospital admission medication reconciliation in medically complex children: an observational study. Arch Dis Child 2010;95(4):250–5. http://dx.doi.org/10.1136/adc.2009.167528.

37. Baxter P. Comorbidities of cerebral palsy need more emphasis–especially pain. Dev Med Child Neurol 2013;55(5):396. http://dx.doi.org/10.1111/dmcn.12137.

38. Belew J. Unraveling the sources of chronic pain in cerebral palsy. Dev Med Child Neurol 2012;54(9):779. http://dx.doi.org/10.1111/j.1469-8749.2012.04374.x.

39. Breau LM, Camfield CS, McGrath PJ, et al. The incidence of pain in children with severe cognitive impairments. Arch Pediatr Adolesc Med 2003;157(12): 1219–26. http://dx.doi.org/10.1001/archpedi.157.12.1219.

40. Parkinson KN, Dickinson HO, Arnaud C, et al, SPARCLE Group. Pain in young people aged 13 to 17 years with cerebral palsy: cross-sectional, multicentre European study. Arch Dis Child 2013;98(6):434–40. http://dx.doi.org/10.1136/archdischild-2012-303482.

41. Penner M, Xie WY, Binepal N, et al. Characteristics of pain in children and youth with cerebral palsy. Pediatrics 2013;132(2):e407–13. http://dx.doi.org/10.1542/peds.2013-0224.

42. Yamaguchi R, Nicholson Perry K, Hines M. Pain, pain anxiety and emotional and behavioural problems in children with cerebral palsy. Disabil Rehabil 2013. http://dx.doi.org/10.3109/09638288.2013.782356.

43. Novak I, Hines M, Goldsmith S, et al. Clinical prognostic messages from a systematic review on cerebral palsy. Pediatrics 2012;130(5):e1285–312. http://dx.doi.org/10.1542/peds.2012-0924.

44. Hauer JM, Wical BS, Charnas L. Gabapentin successfully manages chronic unexplained irritability in children with severe neurologic impairment. Pediatrics 2007;119(2):e519–22. http://dx.doi.org/10.1542/peds.2006-1609.

45. Rabchevsky AG, Patel SP, Duale H, et al. Gabapentin for spasticity and autonomic dysreflexia after severe spinal cord injury. Spinal Cord 2011;49(1): 99–105. http://dx.doi.org/10.1038/sc.2010.67.

46. Tuchman M, Barrett JA, Donevan S, et al. Central sensitization and ca(V) alpha(2)delta ligands in chronic pain syndromes: pathologic processes and pharmacologic effect. J Pain 2010;11(12):1241–9. http://dx.doi.org/10.1016/j.jpain.2010.02.024.

47. Bockbrader HN, Budhwani MN, Wesche DL. Gabapentin to pregabalin therapy transition: a pharmacokinetic simulation. Am J Ther 2013;20(1):32–6. http://dx.doi.org/10.1097/MJT.0b013e318250f80e.

48. Sullivan PB. Gastrointestinal problems in the neurologically impaired child. Baillieres Clin Gastroenterol 1997;11(3):529–46.

49. Good P, Cavenagh J, Mather M, et al. Medically assisted hydration for palliative care patients. Cochrane Database Syst Rev 2008;(2):CD006273. http://dx.doi.org/10.1002/14651858.CD006273.pub2.

50. Rapoport A, Shaheed J, Newman C, et al. Parental perceptions of forgoing artificial nutrition and hydration during end-of-life care. Pediatrics 2013;131(5): 861–9. http://dx.doi.org/10.1542/peds.2012-1916.

51. Canfield KN, Frader JE. Forgoing artificial nutrition and hydration: what to make of parents' views. Pediatrics 2013;131(5):993–4. http://dx.doi.org/10.1542/peds.2013-0380.

52. van der Riet P, Good P, Higgins I, et al. Palliative care professionals' perceptions of nutrition and hydration at the end of life. Int J Palliat Nurs 2008;14(3): 145–51.

53. Baguley IJ, Heriseanu RE, Cameron ID, et al. A critical review of the pathophysiology of dysautonomia following traumatic brain injury. Neurocrit Care 2008; 8(2):293–300. http://dx.doi.org/10.1007/s12028-007-9021-3.

54. Baguley IJ, Heriseanu RE, Gurka JA, et al. Gabapentin in the management of dysautonomia following severe traumatic brain injury: a case series. J Neurol Neurosurg Psychiatry 2007;78(5):539–41. http://dx.doi.org/10.1136/jnnp.2006.096388.

55. Hussain S, Sankar R. Pharmacologic treatment of intractable epilepsy in children: a syndrome-based approach. Semin Pediatr Neurol 2011;18(3):171–8. http://dx.doi.org/10.1016/j.spen.2011.06.003.

56. Wusthoff CJ, Shellhaas RA, Licht DJ. Management of common neurologic symptoms in pediatric palliative care: seizures, agitation, and spasticity. Pediatr Clin North Am 2007;54(5):709–33. http://dx.doi.org/10.1016/j.pcl.2007.06.004, xi.

57. Jan JE, Owens JA, Weiss MD, et al. Sleep hygiene for children with neurodevelopmental disabilities. Pediatrics 2008;122(6):1343–50. http://dx.doi.org/10.1542/peds.2007-3308.

58. Wiggs L. Behavioural aspects of children's sleep. Arch Dis Child 2009;94(1): 59–62. http://dx.doi.org/10.1136/adc.2007.125278.

59. Tietze AL, Blankenburg M, Hechler T, et al. Sleep disturbances in children with multiple disabilities. Sleep Med Rev 2012;16(2):117–27. http://dx.doi.org/10.1016/j.smrv.2011.03.006.

60. Hart CN, Palermo TM, Rosen CL. Health-related quality of life among children presenting to a pediatric sleep disorders clinic. Behav Sleep Med 2005;3(1): 4–17. http://dx.doi.org/10.1207/s15402010bsm0301_3.

61. Sandella DE, O'Brien LM, Shank LK, et al. Sleep and quality of life in children with cerebral palsy. Sleep Med 2011;12(3):252–6. http://dx.doi.org/10.1016/j.sleep.2010.07.019.

62. Iglowstein I, Jenni OG, Molinari L, et al. Sleep duration from infancy to adolescence: reference values and generational trends. Pediatrics 2003;111(2): 302–7.

63. Kotagal S, Broomall E. Sleep in children with autism spectrum disorder. Pediatr Neurol 2012;47(4):242–51. http://dx.doi.org/10.1016/j.pediatrneurol.2012. 05.007.

64. Owens JA, Babcock D, Blumer J, et al. The use of pharmacotherapy in the treatment of pediatric insomnia in primary care: rational approaches. A consensus meeting summary. J Clin Sleep Med 2005;1(1):49–59.

65. Leu RM, Beyderman L, Botzolakis EJ, et al. Relation of melatonin to sleep architecture in children with autism. J Autism Dev Disord 2011;41(4):427–33. http:// dx.doi.org/10.1007/s10803-010-1072-1.

66. De Leersnyder H, Zisapel N, Laudon M. Prolonged-release melatonin for children with neurodevelopmental disorders. Pediatr Neurol 2011;45(1):23–6. http://dx.doi.org/10.1016/j.pediatrneurol.2011.02.001.

67. Simard-Tremblay E, Constantin E, Gruber R, et al. Sleep in children with cerebral palsy: a review. J Child Neurol 2011;26(10):1303–10. http://dx.doi.org/10.1177/ 0883073811408902.

68. Berry RB, Chediak A, Brown LK, et al. Best clinical practices for the sleep center adjustment of noninvasive positive pressure ventilation (NPPV) in stable chronic alveolar hypoventilation syndromes. J Clin Sleep Med 2010;6(5):491–509.

69. Mellies U, Ragette R, Schwake C, et al. Daytime predictors of sleep disordered breathing in children and adolescents with neuromuscular disorders. Neuromuscul Disord 2003;13(2):123–8.

70. Suresh S, Wales P, Dakin C, et al. Sleep-related breathing disorder in Duchenne muscular dystrophy: disease spectrum in the paediatric population. J Paediatr Child Health 2005;41(9–10):500–3. http://dx.doi.org/10.1111/j.1440-1754.2005. 00691.x.

71. Geister TL, Quintanar-Solares M, Martin M, et al. Qualitative development of the 'questionnaire on pain caused by spasticity (QPS),' a pediatric patient-reported outcome for spasticity-related pain in cerebral palsy. Qual Life Res 2013. http:// dx.doi.org/10.1007/s11136-013-0526-2.

72. Tilton A. Management of spasticity in children with cerebral palsy. Semin Pediatr Neurol 2009;16(2):82–9. http://dx.doi.org/10.1016/j.spen.2009.03.006.

73. Vidailhet M. Treatment of movement disorders in dystonia-choreoathtosis cerebral palsy. Handb Clin Neurol 2013;111:197–202. http://dx.doi.org/10.1016/ B978-0-444-52891-9.00019-1.

74. Allen NM, Lin JP, Lynch T, et al. Status dystonicus: a practice guide. Dev Med Child Neurol 2014;56(2):105–12. http://dx.doi.org/10.1111/dmcn.12339.

75. Bonouvrie LA, Becher JG, Vles JS, et al. Intrathecal baclofen treatment in dystonic cerebral palsy: a randomized clinical trial: The IDYS trial. BMC Pediatr 2013;13(1):175. http://dx.doi.org/10.1186/1471-2431-13-175.

76. Pin TW, Elmasry J, Lewis J. Efficacy of botulinum toxin A in children with cerebral palsy in gross motor function classification system levels IV and V: a systematic review. Dev Med Child Neurol 2013;55(4):304–13. http://dx.doi.org/10.1111/j. 1469-8749.2012.04438.x.

77. Thorley M, Donaghey S, Edwards P, et al. Evaluation of the effects of botulinum toxin A injections when used to improve ease of care and comfort in children with cerebral palsy whom are non-ambulant: a double blind randomized controlled trial. BMC Pediatr 2012;12:120. http://dx.doi.org/10.1186/1471-2431- 12-120.

78. Del Rio MI, Shand B, Bonati P, et al. Hydration and nutrition at the end of life: a systematic review of emotional impact, perceptions, and decision-making among patients, family, and health care staff. Psychooncology 2012;21(9): 913–21. http://dx.doi.org/10.1002/pon.2099.

79. Erby LH, Rushton C, Geller G. "My son is still walking": stages of receptivity to discussions of advance care planning among parents of sons with Duchenne muscular dystrophy. Semin Pediatr Neurol 2006;13(2):132–40. http://dx.doi.org/10.1016/j.spen.2006.06.009.

80. Tan JS, Docherty SL, Barfield R, et al. Addressing parental bereavement support needs at the end of life for infants with complex chronic conditions. J Palliat Med 2012;15(5):579–84. http://dx.doi.org/10.1089/jpm.2011.0357.

81. Mahant S, Friedman JN, Connolly B, et al. Tube feeding and quality of life in children with severe neurological impairment. Arch Dis Child 2009;94(9):668–73. http://dx.doi.org/10.1136/adc.2008.149542.

82. Gantasala S, Sullivan PB, Thomas AG. Gastrostomy feeding versus oral feeding alone for children with cerebral palsy. Cochrane Database Syst Rev 2013;(7):CD003943. http://dx.doi.org/10.1002/14651858.CD003943.pub3.

83. Vernon-Roberts A, Sullivan PB. Fundoplication versus postoperative medication for gastro-oesophageal reflux in children with neurological impairment undergoing gastrostomy. Cochrane Database Syst Rev 2013;(8):CD006151. http://dx.doi.org/10.1002/14651858.CD006151.pub3.

84. Liben S, Papadatou D, Wolfe J. Paediatric palliative care: challenges and emerging ideas. Lancet 2008;371(9615):852–64. http://dx.doi.org/10.1016/S0140-6736(07)61203-3.

Interdisciplinary Care
Using Your Team

 CrossMark

Monica Ogelby, MSN, APRN, CPNP[a], Richard D. Goldstein, MD[b],*

KEYWORDS

- Interdisciplinary • Pediatric palliative care
- Children and youth with special health care needs • Medical home
- Continuity of care

KEY POINTS

- The importance of interdisciplinary care and its basis as the composition of a mature team is broadly embraced.
- There is a growing body of evidence to support positive outcomes of inpatient/hospital-based pediatric palliative care involvement.
- With increased and earlier use of pediatric palliative care, the interdisciplinary pediatric palliative care team has a responsibility to broaden collaboration with outpatient and community-based supports so as to provide optimal care throughout life.
- Embracing team meetings to ensure shared understanding and a unified approach among disciplines can bridge challenges in the care team and improve the child's care process.
- Challenges within the interdisciplinary team itself, as part of the larger care team, can be anticipated and improved with a clear team philosophy and understanding of roles.

CASE VIGNETTE

Justin's cancer has recently relapsed. With cure seeming unlikely, the focus of his care is more deliberately supporting quality of life. Despite incredible fatigue and intermittent pain, every day he gets up and goes to school on the bus with his friends, wanting no special treatment from his teachers. His symptoms, however, require diligent assessment and intervention. Justin's home care nurse is able to provide on-going consultation with the school nurse, his teacher, and principal with the back-up of Justin's oncologist, primary care pediatrician, and the palliative care team, so that he can finish the school year with his classmates. During an inpatient admission, his palliative care team is consulted to review his symptom management and supports. How can the team best work to ensure that Justin's care is consistent and optimal across all settings?

---

[a] Pediatric Palliative Care Program, Department of Vermont Health Access, State of Vermont, 312 Hurricane Lane, Suite 201, Williston, VT 05495, USA; [b] Pediatric Advanced Care Team, Boston Children's Hospital, Dana-Farber Cancer Institute, Harvard Medical School, 450 Brookline Avenue, Boston, MA 02215, USA
* Corresponding author.
E-mail address: Richard_Goldstein@dfci.harvard.edu

Pediatr Clin N Am 61 (2014) 823–834
http://dx.doi.org/10.1016/j.pcl.2014.04.009
0031-3955/14/$ – see front matter © 2014 Elsevier Inc. All rights reserved.
pediatric.theclinics.com

INTRODUCTION

Interdisciplinary care is a core value in palliative care and a foundation of quality practice.[1,2] It is an essential part of the team-based practice of palliative care, although the form it takes will vary based on limitations in available resources and local preferences. On another organizational level, interdisciplinary care is also an important part of caring for those children with complex conditions[3] and treatment courses receiving pediatric palliative care, where the palliative care team may be one of several involved, to ensure and optimize care in the many settings in which children may find themselves. Limitations to the evidence base with regard to outcomes from this approach stand in contrast to the fundamental confidence in its advantages.

Palliative care is appropriate and beneficial for most children with life-threatening illness for months, years, or their entire lifetime. The vast majority of children do not spend their entire lives inpatient, where robust palliative care services more typically exist. Therefore, pediatric palliative care as a medical subspecialty must confront its responsibility to expand its services and attitudes, and to meet the needs of children earlier and regardless of location. Based on best practice and trends, it should be recognized that with earlier implementation of interdisciplinary palliative care in a child's illness trajectory, interdisciplinary teamwork will expand and encompass more key players than just the traditional inpatient palliative care team.

To effect earlier involvement, a palliative care team may need to contribute to the environment of interdisciplinary collaboration by providing education about the communication needs of families with ill children, the symptom burden of potential patients, the nature of suffering, or improved outcomes with earlier involvement.[4] Another critical issue is promoting an understanding that cure-directed and palliative care are not mutually exclusive[5] in any of the settings in which a child might receive care, particularly with the assurances of concurrent care provided by the Patient Protection and Affordable Care Act of 2010 (discussed in the article by Sheetz and colleagues, elsewhere in this issue). The increasing incorporation of palliative care in the treatment of children who will benefit promises earlier conversations about goals of care, and the feeling among families of having more choices sooner in their child's care, in many settings.

COMPOSITION OF THE INTERDISCIPLINARY TEAM

Virtually all literature related to palliative care standards stresses the importance of an interdisciplinary palliative care team structured around the child and family, equipped to address physical, psychosocial, emotional, practical, and spiritual needs of the child and family.[6] A truly holistic interdisciplinary approach will provide genuine coordination of care, starting at the time of diagnosis, across the continuum, during transitions, and facilitated by effective communication and case management.[7] Research on health care teams has concluded that diversity of participants predicts better discussions, adjustment to developments, and service delivery.[8]

The American Academy of Pediatrics recommends that mature palliative care teams include physicians, nurses, social workers, case managers, spiritual care providers, bereavement specialists, and child life specialists, and that all hospitals that frequently care for children with palliative care needs should have dedicated interdisciplinary teams for the provision of palliative care.[6] Simple distinctions between the expertise available on a palliative care team is outlined in **Table 1**. Although these roles may seem separate, interdisciplinary collaboration by its nature may lead to overlap and the adoption of common methodologies so as to provide unified care, as is discussed later in this article.

Table 1 Distinctions between palliative care professionals	
Discipline	**Expertise**
Medicine	• Address medical needs, such as pain and symptom management, as well as speaking to the implications of medical interventions. • Take the lead on framing the illness trajectory and prognosis, as well as having a special role in interacting with other medical specialties.
Nursing	• Clinical support and hands-on care while teaching families how to best provide care for their children. • Support other staff at bedside.
Social work	• Address broad spectrum of factors that influence families, such as housing, transportation,[41] family dynamics. • Provide psychosocial/emotional and bereavement supports.
Child life	• Provide psychosocially driven interventions that promote coping through play, preparation, education, and self-expression activities[48] for both patient and siblings.
Pastoral care	• Support spiritual needs of child and family. • Access supports specific to a family's religious beliefs and values. • Communicate spiritual needs of family to care team for consideration in care plan.

Such well-established teams are most often found in hospital settings in which these disciplines are readily available. Of 226 hospitals identified by the National Association of Children's Hospitals and Related Institutions, almost 50% have a pediatric palliative care program, with continued growth likely.[9] These teams continue to be strengthened by professional advancement opportunities. Since 2006, the American Board of Medical Subspecialties has recognized Hospice and Palliative Medicine as a subspecialty requiring board certification. Nurse practitioners have newly established Advanced Certification in Hospice and Palliative Nursing by the National Board for Certification of Hospice and Palliative Nurses. Advanced practice nurses who hold this certification are regarded as experts in their field. With consideration for the relative newness of the specialty, it is understood that teams may be led by a variety of disciplines, changing as needs evolve.

Even in the last year of life, most children will spend significantly more time at home than inpatient,[10] which raises consideration of how children can access palliative care services outside hospital walls. Beyond the core inpatient palliative care team, valuable supports may be available from community-based providers and services. **Table 2** illustrates examples of the wide variety of both inpatient and outpatient providers and services, whose involvement may positively impact any given child's and family's quality of life and therefore should be integrated more fully in the plan of care. Both the medical home model and community-based pediatric palliative care programs offer encouraging opportunities for support of palliative care principles across care settings.

The Family-Centered Medical Home

Medical care has long been associated with fragmentation, high costs, high utilization, reduced value, and ultimately poor quality of life. In particular, children with complex medical problems and/or multiple chronic conditions may receive less than optimal care through the traditional, physician-centered model.[11] As an alternative, a patient-centered approach places an emphasis on coordinated care and

Table 2	
Interdisciplinary team members	
Inpatient	**Outpatient**
Attending medical team	Primary care provider or medical home
Continuing subspecialty providers	Community pediatric palliative care service
Bedside nurse	Home health agency
Case manager	Hospice (when appropriate)
Rehabilitation therapies	Care coordinator/case management
Palliative care team	School/school-based services
• Nurse practitioner	Faith-based community
• Palliative care nurse	Durable medical equipment providers
• Social worker	Early intervention
• Pastoral care	Infusion company
• Child life specialist	Rehabilitation therapies
	School-based services
	Creative arts or expressive therapy
	Pharmacy
	Integrative medicine
	Mental health providers
	Emergency medical services

communication, and has been shown to lead to improved patient outcomes, satisfaction, and associated reductions in health care costs.[12] The medical home framework of accessible, continuous, family-centered, coordinated, and culturally effective care is an especially helpful model of care for those children with complex conditions and special health care needs.[13]

Undeniably, much of the literature related to successful efforts in pediatric palliative care also stresses the value of care coordination as a critical element,[14] and there is strong accord in the values set forth in the family-centered medical home and pediatric palliative care teams. This congruence in patient-care values makes the medical home a natural but underutilized extension of a child's palliative care team. The most recent American Academy of Pediatrics palliative care policy statement[6] reinforces the importance of all general pediatricians, subspecialists, and family providers being comfortable with palliative care principles and having knowledge specific to the basic provision of palliative care. If the medical home and palliative care model were integrated, and children were able to receive this basic palliative care as part of primary care, this would positively support the growing capacity issue of palliative care specialists available for the highest-need patients.[15,16] There is tremendous opportunity for the medical home model and palliative care to collaborate and support the family-centered mission of care moving forward.

Community-Based Pediatric Palliative Care Programs

The evidence base supporting satisfaction with home-based pediatric palliative care is growing as delivery models develop. In a recent study, improvement in patient quality of life and provider communication was found after pediatric palliative care was introduced, as well as decreased parental distress.[17] The implications of the Patient Protection and Affordable Care Act of 2010 have altered the landscape of community-based palliative and hospice supports for children who would not previously have had access to services. In addition, community-based pediatric palliative care programs are multiplying throughout the United States via various funding streams, waivers, and initiatives. This expansion demands training and workforce development, as the existing hospice community lacks available pediatric palliative care experience. This is further complicated by the decrease in number of hospices willing to care for children despite increasing acceptance of hospice care.[18] A recent study of hospital-based pediatric palliative care programs found that only 10% provide home-based palliative care services, with most staffed only during work-week days,[9] despite continuous access to a palliative care clinician being highly valued by families.[19] There is tremendous opportunity to capitalize on the growth of these community-based programs as collaborative extensions of hospital-based teams, as they continue to multiply. Such a partnership would provide community-based teams with access to resources through more well-established inpatient teams, while supporting the home-based, around-the-clock, level of care that provides the added layer of support so valued by families.

No single provider or team can adequately manage the holistic care of a child and family. Programs should explore beyond themselves and partner with others who may be significant participants in the child's and family's life, be they clergy, teachers, or complementary and alternative providers, and provide leadership for this collaboration (**Fig. 1**). Just as a child's health may wax and wane, the interdisciplinary care team must remodel itself to ensure that key figures are central and available, with the entire team remaining closely informed. Ultimately it is the responsibility of the entire team,

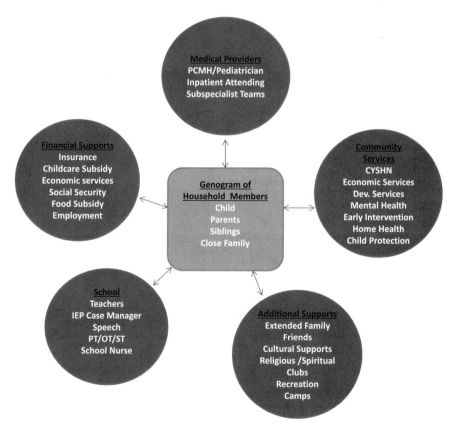

Fig. 1. An example eco map for a child and family, symbolizing the wide variety of providers, services, and supports that may be involved at any given point. CYSHN, children and youth with special health needs; IEP, individualized education plan; PCMH, patient-centered medical home; PT/OT/ST, physical therapy, occupational therapy, speech therapy.

both inpatient and outpatient, to collaboratively care for a child and family, whether it is the community pediatrician having a basic understanding of palliative care principles, or the inpatient team supporting adoption of the medical home model.

INTERDISCIPLINARY PRACTICE

Palliative care teams are fluid in priorities and focus. There may be adopted recommendations and standards for the composition of such teams, but certainly there are not established formulas. In addition to understanding *who* best ought to be involved, it is important to understand *how* they may be best involved. An important feature of palliative care is that different team members may take the lead in a child's care based on the goals of the family and the needs of the team at any given time. As a result, palliative care teams can be tremendously effective for patients, and rewarding for participating providers. This is not to ignore that the flexible nature of palliative care teams can be challenging as they distinguish themselves from the traditional medical model, with physicians at the top of the hierarchy.[20] Nonetheless, benefits to families and clinician teams far outweigh the inevitable challenges that accompany the dynamics of collaboration. To this end, it is essential to make the distinction between multidisciplinary and interdisciplinary care.

Multidisciplinary care is delivered by a variety of unique disciplines, each identified by their own specialty and methodology. At the multidisciplinary level, providers may operate with an awareness of other involved professionals, but do not integrate among each other. Multidisciplinary care can be considered to operate in a mode of coexistence, where care is delivered by a variety of unique disciplines, each identified by their own specialty and methodology, each interfacing with the child and family, but not necessarily integrating with one another.[21] Interdisciplinary care also involves multiple professionals, but with a shared philosophy, common goals, and integrated practice among disciplines. This allows providers to work dynamically and collaboratively together in service of the child's and family's goals of care.

Perhaps the greatest distinction between the 2 models of care is in methods of communication. Communication among a multidisciplinary team is commonly through electronic medical records, charting, or via the child and family. There is very little, if any, face-to-face communication between disciplines. Although this care may be collaborative in intent, treatment plans are typically not integrative of each other. There are fewer opportunities for involved caregivers to augment each other's expertise and perspective and, in the dynamic process of illness evolution, such an approach is at a disadvantage with regard to adapting to unexpected changes. Although the terms are often used interchangeably, it is *inter*disciplinary teamwork at the heart of a functioning pediatric palliative care team.

When caring for children with complex medical needs, many disciplines are likely involved, which only enhances the importance of an interdisciplinary approach. To better understand interdisciplinary, as opposed to multidisciplinary care,[4] it is helpful to consider the impact of each approach from the receiving end, specifically from the perspective of the child and family. The multidisciplinary model holds the child and family as central, with a variety of input from various disciplines (**Fig. 2**A). Elements of care (eg, information, direct care delivery, diagnostics, prognostics) all flows directly to the child and family, but not among the disciplines. This can leave a family to interpret and balance information from various individual sources. Despite a multidisciplinary team of very well-intentioned providers, there is inevitably an increased burden on the child and family as the keepers and distributers of all information.

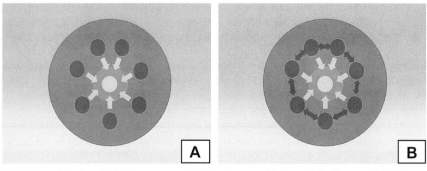

Fig. 2. A model of multidisciplinary care (*A*) involves multiple contributions with little coordination between their sources. Interdisciplinary care (*B*) involves coordination and collaboration between involved professionals. (*Adapted from* Freibert S, Chrastek J, Brown MR. Team relationships. In: Wolfe J, Hinds PS, Sourkes BM, editors. Textbook of Interdisciplinary Pediatric Palliative Care. Philadelphia: Elsevier Saunders; 2011.)

Interdisciplinary care adds communication across the continuum and development of a common approach among providers while families remain central (see **Fig. 2**B). The family's burden of having to communicate information to providers and coordinate care is reduced or eliminated. With a clearly unified approach by the care team, treatment decisions have a greater likelihood of being framed in common terms and delicate decision-making is less likely to be abruptly undermined by an uncoordinated caregiver's opinion.

Instead of each individual specialty feeding information directly to the family independent of one another, a different care environment occurs when providers communicate directly with one another. During an interview about palliative care teamwork, one physician put this into such simple, clear perspective: "If I go to a patient for 5 minutes, of course I have an impression, but if a psychotherapist, an occupational therapist, a nurse, and a social worker all spend 5 minutes each with the patient, you get a completely different picture."[22] With an understanding of the impressions and recommendations of the treatment team as a whole, communication with the child and family is delivered in a coordinated manner.

INPATIENT AND OUTPATIENT COLLABORATION

Appreciating the strengths of each care provider creates opportunities to minimize gaps and weaknesses. The climate for hospitalized children is changing as steadily as the medical technology that is prolonging and sustaining their lives. The rate of childhood mortality is decreasing while the frequency and lengths of hospitalizations and interventions are increasing.[23] The combination of increased life expectancy and hospitalization frequency, coupled with the understanding that decision-making is suboptimal in the face of acute hospitalizations, has been an important factor in the development of inpatient pediatric palliative care teams. The introduction of a palliative care team does not replace the interdisciplinary approach necessary by the larger care team as a whole, but can certainly assist in ongoing collaborative communication. Each provider, not just the palliative care team, has a critical role in supporting ongoing conversations about the family's goals and philosophy of care.

Hospitals were historically intended to diagnose illness, treat the condition, and discharge a patient when they were "well."[24] Hospital-based providers, be they subspecialists or intensivists, are experts in their area, but may not be well-positioned to provide holistic care of a child and family. Because of their regular exposure, they are, however, most familiar and well-versed in both caring for children with significant complex medical needs and with their disease trajectories. This knowledge is a critical piece to the puzzle when supporting a family in developing goals of care, but only a piece. Inpatient providers also are more likely to be caring for a child in an acute crisis, and conduct difficult conversations with parents related to urgent decision-making regularly. Many times, especially during emergencies, there is no alternative than to talk directly and frankly about health care decisions. This may not be, however, the best time for the family to fully digest the impact of decisions being made for the long term.

Conversely, providers who are caring for a child during an acute hospitalization may be less likely to have the extensive history and knowledge that comes with caring for a child in the community in the absence of a crisis. Primary care pediatricians have built a relationship over time, sometimes across generations, and may have a critical understanding of a family's strengths, weaknesses, and ability to cope with adversity. With the exception of children who have never left the hospital, parents may view their child's pediatrician as their primary doctor, regardless of whether there are multiple specialists closely involved. Primary pediatricians often have knowledge about how a family functions and communicates and therefore may be a resource for the inpatient treatment team when there are misunderstandings or knowledge deficits. Parents may feel more comfortable confiding in their child's "regular" provider about fears, worries, and doubts. A routine visit to the pediatrician and being in the community setting adds to a family's sense of normalcy, more likely seen as part of "life." Community providers are likely to have familiarity with the community- and home-based services necessary to support the outcomes of decisions made in the hospital. The general pediatrician may have an ongoing relationship with a family in caring for a child's siblings, an especially crucial role in the event that a child dies. It is a relationship that cannot be overlooked in caring for a child, even in the midst of a prolonged hospitalization.

Evidence suggests improvement in quality of life[25] and hopeful parental thinking[26] when there is early establishment of care goals. There may be advantages when these conversations are started with a trusted pediatrician as an anticipatory support measure, appreciating that goals of care conversations are preferable outside of a crisis, when families may take their time, ask questions, and be most thoughtful. For example, what is the best way to introduce limited or no nursing services available for home-based support into the decision to undergo surgery that will leave a child ventilator dependent? This is not an uncommon scenario in the face of a national nursing shortage where there are even fewer qualified pediatric nurses.[27] When possible, conversations in anticipation of these moments and collaborative communication between the inpatient and outpatient world can illuminate valuable information in considering implications of complex health care decisions.

However, many general pediatricians lack experience with palliative care in their professional setting.[28] Many leave residency with little training in palliative care or confidence in their abilities,[29–31] and do not feel equipped to confidently weigh the benefits and burdens of certain medical interventions, a critical component when outlining goals of care. Who holds responsibility if goals-of-care conversations are best had before a crisis, but pediatricians are not well-versed in having these discussions with families? This is an important concern to the interdisciplinary care of seriously ill children. Palliative care teams can have a great effect in this realm.

INTERDISCIPLINARY COMMUNICATION

There is value in clear communication within and across the different professional disciplines before approaching patients and families so that information and recommendations are broadly encompassing rather than discipline-specific or misaligned with the overall goals of care. The practice of interdisciplinary care is better achieved when interdisciplinary team meetings are incorporated into the treatment plan. These meetings are typically, but not exclusively, held before a family meeting. The "team meeting" may focus on developing a coordinated update of medical information or clarifying the treatment-related priorities of involved teams. It also may be held to sharpen the need for particular decision-making related to interventions, technologies, or the goals of care. There is little research available on pediatric family meetings, and there does not appear to be any pediatric-specific research related to interdisciplinary team meetings. However, there is little reason to think that advantages found in the care of adults do not apply.

Research suggests that when interdisciplinary teams share their perspectives and assessments, the advantages are greater than additive.[32] Staff interaction and coordination have been shown to be a critical factor in reduced mortality, controlling for patient severity.[33] Advantages have been demonstrated in oncology and critical care settings.[34–40] One study of adult patients with lung cancer found that team meetings predicted greater palliative care involvement in addition to treatment decisions prioritizing greater attention to symptom management and quality of life. This may be more true when the environment allows for "role-blurring," where collective ownership by the professionals involved is encouraged and roles are encouraged to change as the priorities and needs of the patient and family change.[41]

Consider the common content of family meetings including palliative care teams held in the pediatric intensive care unit (PICU). A recent review of family conferences for children admitted to the PICU[22] were found to address length of stay, palliative care involvement, initiation of chronic ventilation, extracorporeal membrane oxygenation use, orders for life-sustaining treatment, death, and transition of care.[42] The impact on families of each situation is tremendous, and the input needed from various providers expansive. Team meetings before these discussions allow for understanding and appreciating all the available treatment options across disciplines, and avoids conflicting information shared with the family. Additionally, team meetings also may provide a forum for care providers to introduce critical elements to be discussed in subsequent family meetings. Parenthetically, this review found goals-of-care discussions were documented in only 23% of family meetings, perhaps too low a percentage given the well-understood value of early, frequent, and ongoing goals-of-care conversations.

Such a dynamic approach is not without its difficulties, however. Interdisciplinary team meetings and an interdisciplinary approach within the palliative care team involve attention and skill. Time and resource allocation, a collaborative environment, and a clear appreciation for leadership are important factors in success. Knowledge and trust of the many members of the care team improves outcomes but, conversely, when interdependence is not acknowledged by all team members, collaboration is undermined. An insufficient amount of time allowed for a meeting or incomplete participation of involved caregivers leads to a focus on solving immediate problems at the expense of understanding and supporting broader goals, preventing suffering, or other interpersonal factors,[22] and that limited focus may in itself undermine the collaborative environment.[43] Overall, an ineffective interdisciplinary team meeting can leave some team members feeling incompetent, less important when compared with other team members, and in a diminished role within the process of care.[44] In fact, several studies of the ICU environment have found that a medical ICU nurse's sense of their collaboration better predicts patient outcomes than that of physicians, including mortality and readmission rates.[39,40] Finally, for patients and families, an inclusive and

---

Box 1
Strategies for improved interdisciplinary teamwork

- Clearly defined leadership
- Ongoing formal communication in addition to informal information sharing
- Shared documentation using standardized language
- Collaborative approach
- Balanced teams by discipline
- Interprofessional education
- Clarification of roles
- Regular and constructive performance feedback

---

timely process of interdisciplinary meetings may reduce the many conversations that occur without the knowledge of others on the interdisciplinary team, those frank bedside conversations that can leave patients and families overloaded and burdened by many different messages and gaps.[45,46] Strategies to prevent common barriers in interdisciplinary teamwork are outlined in **Box 1**.

One critical aspect of the interdisciplinary environment is the importance of leadership at these meetings. Within the palliative care team, it is important to ensure clarity and close, positive exchange among team members.[47] Mutual respect and common, family-centered purpose are key. Among various care teams, palliative care team leaders may not be asked to lead the meetings in many areas in a hospital or community, but they typically are afforded a special status in balancing the team's perspective to include parent or patient priorities.

SUMMARY

Interdisciplinary care is a strength of palliative care teams and an important ingredient to improved care for patients in palliative care. There is complexity to delivering care that is interdisciplinary, and collaborating with other involved teams in an interdisciplinary fashion. Leadership and the recognition of the many strengths each involved professional has to offer in the care of patients needing palliative care is key. Successful models of palliative care will use the strengths of the available caregivers in each setting in a coordinated, consistent fashion.

REFERENCES

1. American Academy of Pediatrics. Committee on Bioethics and Committee on Hospital Care. Palliative care for children. Pediatrics 2000;106(2 Pt 1):351–7.
2. National consensus project for quality palliative care. Clinical practice guidelines for quality palliative care. 3rd edition. Pittsburgh (PA): National consensus project for quality palliative care; 2013.
3. Chen AY, Schrager SM, Mangione-Smith R. Quality measures for primary care of complex pediatric patients. Pediatrics 2012;129(3):433–45.
4. Wolfe J, Hinds P, Sourkes B. Textbook of interdisciplinary pediatric palliative care. Philadelphia: Elsevier; 2011.
5. Mack JW, Wolfe J. Early integration of pediatric palliative care: for some children, palliative care starts at diagnosis. Curr Opin Pediatr 2006;18(1):10–4.

6. American Academy of Pediatrics. Policy statement: pediatric palliative care and hospice care commitments, guidelines, and recommendations. Pediatrics 2013; 132(5):966–72.

7. Levine D, Lam CG, Cunningham MJ, et al. Best practices for pediatric palliative cancer care: a primer for clinical providers. J Support Oncol 2013;11(3):114–25.

8. Haward R, Amir Z, Borrill C, et al. Breast cancer teams: the impact of constitution, new cancer workload, and methods of operation on their effectiveness. Br J Cancer 2003;89(1):15–22.

9. Feudtner C, Womer J, Augustin R, et al. Pediatric palliative care programs in children's hospitals: a cross-sectional national survey. Pediatrics 2013;132(6): 1063–70.

10. Miller EG, Laragione G, Kang TI, et al. Concurrent care for the medically complex child: lessons of implementation. J Palliat Med 2012;15(11):1281–3.

11. Bodenheimer T, Wagner EH, Grumbach K. Improving primary care for patients with chronic illness. JAMA 2002;288(14):1775–9.

12. Craig C, Eby D, Whittington J. Care coordination model: better care at lower cost for people with multiple health and social needs. IHI innovation series white paper. Cambridge (MA): Institute for Healthcare Improvement; 2011.

13. Medical Home Initiatives for Children With Special Needs Project Advisory Committee, American Academy of Pediatrics. The medical home. Pediatrics 2002; 110(1 Pt 1):184–6.

14. Carroll JM, Torkildson C, Winsness JS. Issues related to providing quality pediatric palliative care in the community. Pediatr Clin North Am 2007;54(5):813–27, xiii.

15. Knapp C, Baker K, Cunningham C, et al. Pediatric palliative care and the medical home. J Palliat Med 2012;15(6):643–5.

16. Quill TE, Abernethy AP. Generalist plus specialist palliative care—creating a more sustainable model. N Engl J Med 2013;368(13):1173–5.

17. Vollenbroich R, Duroux A, Grasser M, et al. Effectiveness of a pediatric palliative home care team as experienced by parents and health care professionals. J Palliat Med 2012;15(3):294–300.

18. Lindley LC, Mark BA, Daniel Lee SY, et al. Factors associated with the provision of hospice care for children. J Pain Symptom Manage 2013;45(4):701–11.

19. Groh G, Borasio GD, Nickolay C, et al. Specialized pediatric palliative home care: a prospective evaluation. J Palliat Med 2013;16(12):1588–94.

20. Porter-O'Grady T. Teams and teamwork: the critical elements. Semin Nurse Manag 1998;6(4):176.

21. Papadatou D, Bluebond-Langer M, Goldman A. The team. In: Wolfe J, Hinds PS, Sourkes BM, editors. Textbook of interdisciplinary pediatric palliative care. Philadelphia: Elsevier Saunders; 2011. p. 55–63.

22. Klarare A, Hagelin CL, Furst CJ, et al. Team interactions in specialized palliative care teams: a qualitative study. J Palliat Med 2013;16(9):1062–9.

23. Feudtner C, Kang TI, Hexem KR, et al. Pediatric palliative care patients: a prospective multicenter cohort study. Pediatrics 2011;127(6):1094–101.

24. Schrader SL, Horner A, Eidsness L, et al. A team approach in palliative care: enhancing outcomes. S D J Med 2002;55(7):269–78.

25. Hui D, Con A, Christie G, et al. Goals of care and end-of-life decision making for hospitalized patients at a Canadian tertiary care cancer center. J Pain Symptom Manage 2009;38(6):871–81.

26. Feudtner C, Carroll KW, Hexem KR, et al. Parental hopeful patterns of thinking, emotions, and pediatric palliative care decision making: a prospective cohort study. Arch Pediatr Adolesc Med 2010;164(9):831–9.

27. Buerhaus PI. Current and future state of the US nursing workforce. JAMA 2008; 300(20):2422–4.
28. Junger S, Vedder AE, Milde S, et al. Paediatric palliative home care by general paediatricians: a multimethod study on perceived barriers and incentives. BMC Palliat Care 2010;9:11.
29. Baker JN, Torkildson C, Baillargeon JG, et al. National survey of pediatric residency program directors and residents regarding education in palliative medicine and end-of-life care. J Palliat Med 2007;10(2):420–9.
30. Khaneja S, Milrod B. Educational needs among pediatricians regarding caring for terminally ill children. Arch Pediatr Adolesc Med 1998;152(9):909–14.
31. Kolarik RC, Walker G, Arnold RM. Pediatric resident education in palliative care: a needs assessment. Pediatrics 2006;117(6):1949–54.
32. Porter-Williamson K, Parker M, Babbott S, et al. A model to improve value: the interdisciplinary palliative care services agreement. J Palliat Med 2009;12(7):609–15.
33. Knaus WA, Draper EA, Wagner DP, et al. An evaluation of outcome from intensive care in major medical centers. Ann Intern Med 1986;104(3):410–8.
34. Boxer MM, Vinod SK, Shafiq J, et al. Do multidisciplinary team meetings make a difference in the management of lung cancer? Cancer 2011;117(22):5112–20.
35. Gabel M, Hilton NE, Nathanson SD. Multidisciplinary breast cancer clinics. Do they work? Cancer 1997;79(12):2380–4.
36. Burton S, Brown G, Daniels IR, et al. MRI directed multidisciplinary team preoperative treatment strategy: the way to eliminate positive circumferential margins? Br J Cancer 2006;94(3):351–7.
37. Birchall M, Bailey D, King P. Effect of process standards on survival of patients with head and neck cancer in the south and west of England. Br J Cancer 2004;91(8):1477–81.
38. Forrest LM, McMillan DC, McArdle CS, et al. An evaluation of the impact of a multidisciplinary team, in a single centre, on treatment and survival in patients with inoperable non-small-cell lung cancer. Br J Cancer 2005;93(9):977–8.
39. Baggs JG, Ryan SA, Phelps CE, et al. The association between interdisciplinary collaboration and patient outcomes in a medical intensive care unit. Heart Lung 1992;21(1):18–24.
40. Baggs JG, Schmitt MH, Mushlin AI, et al. Association between nurse-physician collaboration and patient outcomes in three intensive care units. Crit Care Med 1999;27(9):1991–8.
41. Bronstein LR. A model for interdisciplinary collaboration. Soc Work 2003;48(3): 297–306.
42. Michelson KN, Clayman ML, Haber-Barker N, et al. The use of family conferences in the pediatric intensive care unit. J Palliat Med 2013;16(12):1595–601.
43. Wittenberg-Lyles EM. Information sharing in interdisciplinary team meetings: an evaluation of hospice goals. Qual Health Res 2005;15(10):1377–91.
44. Sabur S. Creating an optimal culture and structure for the IDT. Hospice Palliative Insights 2003;4:22–3.
45. Jenkins VA, Fallowfield LJ, Poole K. Are members of multidisciplinary teams in breast cancer aware of each other's informational roles? Qual Health Care 2001;10(2):70–5.
46. Jensen HI, Ammentorp J, Johannessen H, et al. Challenges in end-of-life decisions in the intensive care unit: an ethical perspective. J Bioeth Inq 2013;10(1):93–101.
47. Junger S, Pestinger M, Elsner F, et al. Criteria for successful multiprofessional cooperation in palliative care teams. Palliat Med 2007;21(4):347–54.
48. Gursky B. The effect of educational interventions with siblings of hospitalized children. J Dev Behav Pediatr 2007;28(5):392–8.

End-of-Life Care for Hospitalized Children

Liza-Marie Johnson, MD, MPH, MSB*, Jennifer M. Snaman, MD,
Margaret C. Cupit, BA, Justin N. Baker, MD

KEYWORDS

- End-of-life care • Children • Palliative care • Hospital

KEY POINTS

- Caring for hospitalized children at the end of life (EOL) requires an interdisciplinary approach to address the complex physical, psychosocial, and spiritual needs of patients and families.
- Using a standard operating procedure at EOL can help ensure that children who die in the hospital and their families receive high-quality care that addresses their physical, psychosocial, and spiritual needs.
- Using a checklist to address these areas and assigning tasks to members of the interdisciplinary team can facilitate the delivery of comprehensive EOL care.
- Ethics consultation is advisable to resolve refractory conflict over goals of care, ethical or moral distress, or considerations of uncommon medical pathways at EOL.
- The religious and spiritual needs of families are diverse, and these needs should not be overlooked when children die in the inpatient setting.

INTRODUCTION

Pediatric palliative medicine[1–3] can be thought of as "the art and science of patient- and family-centered care aimed at enhancing quality of life, promoting healing and attending to suffering."[4] The National Quality Forum (NQF), Institute of Medicine, and the National Institutes of Health have identified palliative and end-of-life (EOL) care as a national priority and proposed that palliative care should be a key component of high-quality medical care for children with advanced illness. The NQF has outlined preferred practices to ensure the provision of high-quality palliative care,[5] with the role of the palliative care clinician including anticipatory counseling for EOL symptoms; symptom control; and emotional, social, spiritual, and bereavement care. This NQF-recommended interdisciplinary approach needs to be integrated early so that the interdisciplinary palliative care team can support families and patients in defining

St. Jude Children's Research Hospital, 262 Danny Thomas Place, MS 260, Memphis, TN 38105, USA
* Corresponding author. Department of Pediatrics, St. Jude Children's Research Hospital, 262 Danny Thomas Place, MS 260, Memphis, TN 38105.
E-mail address: Liza.johnson@stjude.org

Pediatr Clin N Am 61 (2014) 835–854
http://dx.doi.org/10.1016/j.pcl.2014.04.012
0031-3955/14/$ – see front matter © 2014 Elsevier Inc. All rights reserved.
pediatric.theclinics.com

goals of care near the EOL and in determining what type of care can best meet these goals. Designing a palliative care treatment plan that is transferable across all medical settings allows for a smooth transition between different care settings, with the goal of maximizing symptom management and psychosocial support.

CLINICAL PRACTICES AT THE EOL
Medical Decision Making at the EOL

When it is anticipated that a child or infant will die in the inpatient setting, it is helpful to engage in advance care–planning discussions to facilitate decision making about issues that commonly arise at the EOL. The issues that should be addressed include preferences for limiting the scope of treatment from advanced life-sustaining therapies (eg, dialysis or mechanical ventilation) to basic noninvasive therapies (eg, antibiotics, artificial nutrient, or hydration); preferences for organ donation (when applicable); autopsy; and after-death or funeral planning.[6] For families choosing to discontinue an artificial life-sustaining technology, such as mechanical ventilation, it is recommended that family preferences about the process be solicited and a plan be developed to meet their goals. Considerations around the discontinuation of ventilatory support can include the location for extubation (perhaps outside of the hospital room [eg, in the hospital garden or at home]), family members to be present, and preferences for holding and comforting the infant or child.[6]

Children have an evolving ability to form opinions about their health care, particularly if they have a significant illness history; their opinions should be included and valued in the discussion. Whenever possible, caregivers should make an effort to invite children to participate in medical decision making and honor their EOL care wishes. Inclusion is particularly important for any child, regardless of age, who can understand his or her medical condition, communicate his or her preferences, and can reach a reasonable decision and understand its consequences.[7] For children and adolescents with life-threatening illness, developmentally appropriate advance care–planning documents can provide the opportunity to express their preferences for how they want to be treated should a time come when they cannot speak for themselves. Similar to the "Five Wishes" document for adults (http://www.agingwithdignity.org/five-wishes. php), the "My Thoughts, My Wishes, My Voice" documents can be used with adolescents and young adults,[8] and "My Wishes" can be used with younger patients to facilitate discussions about EOL care and preferences. These tools can facilitate communication in families who may be uncertain about how to engage their child in discussion around preferences about their care.

Inpatient Care Coordination at the EOL

The individualized care planning and coordination (ICPC) model outlined in **Fig. 1** was designed to facilitate the integration of a cancer-directed goal of cure with a comfort-related goal of reducing suffering[4,9] but can be extrapolated to EOL care for children with a nonmalignant condition, particularly those in the hospital setting. The goal of individualized care planning is to value patient and family experiences and to use a patient- and family centered approach to information delivery and needs assessment, thus enhancing communication about difficult issues by discerning patient and family values and priorities before crisis occurs or critical decision points are reached. Application of the ICPC model helps patients, families, and clinicians negotiate care options under uncertain conditions by assessing the patients' and families' understanding of prognosis, elucidating their goals of care, and allowing them to choose from available goal-directed treatment alternatives.

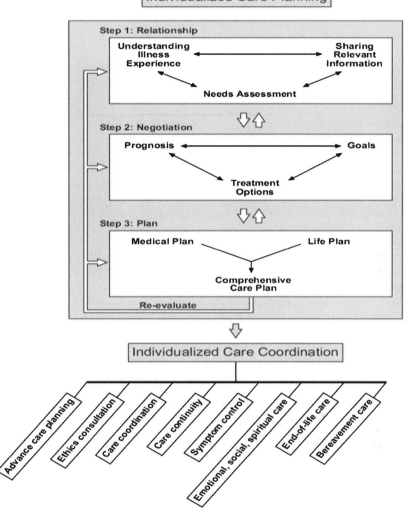

Fig. 1. Individual care coordination model. This model outlines a process to facilitate decision making and improve care coordination for hospitalized children with life-limiting or life-threatening illness. (*From* Kane JR, Himelstein BP. Palliative care for children. In: Berger AM, Shuster JL, Von Roenn JH, editors. Principles and practice of palliative medicine and supportive oncology. 3rd edition. Philadelphia: Lippincott Williams & Wilkins; 2007. p. 225; with permission.)

At no time is use of the ICPC model more important than at the EOL, when clear goals of care are needed to provide quality care. The negative effects of poor communication and insensitive delivery of bad news on the parents' long-term emotional and psychological well-being are well documented.[10] In a qualitative study of parents of children who died of cancer, doctor-patient communication and continuity of care were characterized as markers of high-quality physician care.[11] Continuity of care was defined as proof that the health care professionals knew the child well enough to provide the best care, that they cared about the child, and that the child felt like an active part of the decision-making process.[12] Because of the large number of providers who care for hospitalized children approaching the EOL, inpatient care requires good communication that clearly conveys the patients' and families' goals to the entire care team. The end of this review presents a sample ICPC: an interdisciplinary checklist and communication tool that incorporates clinical practice strategies, psychosocial concerns, and ethical issues for hospitalized children approaching the EOL.

Symptoms at the EOL

The National Consensus Project for Quality Palliative Care outlines a care team structure for the EOL. It is recommended that the interdisciplinary team (IDT) identifies, communicates, and manages the signs and symptoms of patients at the EOL to meet the physical, psychosocial, spiritual, social, and culture needs of patients and families.[13] Providers are responsible for educating the family and other care providers about the symptoms of imminent death in a culturally and developmentally appropriate way. The IDT members should routinely assess patients for sources of distress (physical or psychosocial) and develop, document, and implement care plans to initiate preventative and immediate treatment of actual or potential sources of distress. This process should incorporate the patients' and families' preferences, including any unique needs that arise during the dying process or after the child's death.

Children who are hospitalized at the EOL may receive intensive treatment aimed at cure or extending life and are at risk for experiencing significant suffering related to new or worsening symptoms.[14] Fatigue, pain, dyspnea, and poor appetite are among the most commonly reported symptoms of pediatric patients with cancer at the time of death. Symptoms for patients without cancer may vary based on disease and clinician situation but commonly include pain and dyspnea. The National Comprehensive Cancer Network (although largely focused on care for adults with cancer) and various pediatric palliative care experts have developed clinical practice guidelines and symptom algorithms to manage emesis, anemia, fatigue, distress, and pain in patients with cancer, which may be used in pediatric patients and those without cancer who have similar symptoms.[6,15–18] Teams caring for children at EOL should integrate symptom assessment tools into patient care that facilitate the identification of sources of suffering. Symptom control practices should be quickly and properly implemented and continually reassessed in patients. Symptom management should include effective stepwise pharmacologic and nonpharmacologic (eg, hypnosis, acupuncture, relaxation techniques) approaches. Institutional guidelines for accessing palliative care consultation, if this has not already occurred, can facilitate early detection and proactive management of symptoms at their outset.

Physicians or other members of the IDT should allow time to discuss other possibly concerning symptoms, such as changes in behavior, changes in appearance, pain, weakness and fatigue, and breathing changes.[19,20] The most useful techniques in managing these symptoms have been identified in patients with cancer but are broadly applicable: appropriately treating pain and anxiety, spending time with patients and their families, providing competent care, and giving advice or providing anticipatory guidance. Preparing families and staff members during the dying process may contribute to the family's sense of control during this tumultuous time.

Management of Pain and Nonpain Symptoms

Age-adapted tools and principles as well as specific therapeutic parameters guide the assessment and management of symptoms.[21,22] **Tables 1** and **2** summarize the most commonly used medications to manage pain and other common symptoms at EOL as well as dosing information for children.[6,16,23–25]

Pain assessment should be age appropriate and include a careful history and physical examination, determination of the primary causes of pain, and evaluation of secondary causes or modulating features. Pain concerns should always be taken seriously, with severe pain treated as a medical emergency. In general, pain

Table 1
Symptom management (nonpain) in pediatric palliative care

Symptom	Medication	Common Pediatric Dosage (<60 kg)	Maximum Daily Dosage[a]
Agitation and/or delirium	Nonpharmacologic	Familiar objects, low lighting, soothing tones, music	—
	Lorazepam[b]	0.05 mg/kg/dose PO, SL (preferred for seizure), or PR every 4–6 h	2 mg per dose
	Chloral hydrate	25–50 mg/kg/d PO/PR divided ever 6–8 h	1 g/d for infants 2 g/d for children
	Haloperidol	0.01–0.02 mg/kg per dose PO, SL, or PR every 8–12 h	0.15 mg/kg/d
Constipation/opioid induced (refractory)	Lactulose (can be diluted in water, juice, milk)	<12 y 7.5 mL PO/d, may be repeated after 2 h >12 y 15–30 mL PO/d, may be repeated after 2 h	60 mL/d
	Polyethylene glycol	Half to 1 packet (17 g) PO every day up to TID	3 packets per day
	Docusate/senna	2–6 y: half tab daily, 1 tab BID 6–12 y: 1 tab daily 2 tabs BID ≥12 y: 2 tabs daily	1 tab BID 2 tabs BID 4 tabs BID
	Methylnaltrexone	<38 kg: 0.15 mg/kg (round up to nearest 0.1 mL of volume) SQ QOD prn 38–62 kg: 8 mg SQ QOD prn	1 dose per 24 h
Dyspnea	Nonpharmacologic	Elevate head of bed, fluid restriction, suctioning (gentle), bedside fan, flowing air (oxygen no benefit over flowing air) prn comfort	—
	Morphine	0.15 mg/kg PO/SL q 2 h prn (titrate to effect)	—
With associated anxiety	Lorazepam[b]	0.05 mg/kg PO/SL q 4-6 h prn (titrate to effect)	2 mg per dose

(*continued on next page*)

Table 1
(continued)

Symptom	Medication	Common Pediatric Dosage (<60 kg)	Maximum Daily Dosage[a]
Nausea/dysmotility	Nonpharmacologic	Avoid irritating foods or smells, relaxation, biofeedback, acupuncture, aromatherapy	—
	Ondansetron	0.15 mg/kg/dose PO/IV q 8 h prn	8 mg per dose
	Promethazine	>2 y: 0.25 mg/kg per dose PO or IV q 6–8 h prn	1 mg/kg/24 h
	Scopolamine (transdermal)	8–15 kg: half patch TD q 3 d, >15 kg: 1 patch TD q 3 d	1 patch every 3 d
	Metoclopramide	0.01–0.02 mg/kg per dose IV q 4 h	—
Pruritus/opioid associated	Nonpharmacologic	Distraction, topical emollients, oatmeal baths, relaxation; when applicable, consider opioid rotation	—
	Diphenhydramine[b]	0.5–1.0 mg/kg per dose PO/IV q 6–8 h	5 mg/kg/24 h or 400 mg/24 h
	Hydroxyzine	<6 y: 50 mg/d PO divided q 6–8 h	4 mg/kg/24 h
		>6 y: 50–100 mg/d PO divided q 6–8 h	—
	Naloxone (low dose)	0.5–1 mcg/kg/h infusion	—
Secretions	Nonpharmacologic	Fluid restriction, gentle suctioning	—
	Glycopyrrolate	0.04–0.1 mg/kg per dose PO q 4–8 h 0.01–0.02 mg/kg IV q 4–6 h	1–2 mg per dose or 8 mg/d
Seizures	Lorazepam[b]	0.05 mg/kg per dose PO, SL (preferred for seizure), or PR every 4–6 h	2 mg per dose

Abbreviations: IV, intravenous; PR, per rectum; QOD, every other day; SL, sub-lingual; SQ, subcutaneous; tab, tablet.

[a] Common maximum dosage; however, dose escalation may be necessary at the EOL to relieve patient suffering.

[b] Lorazepam may also be used to help manage nausea.

management should follow the World Health Organization's revised 2-step approach of administering low doses of a strong opioid for moderate pain.[26] Note that codeine is no longer recommended in children because of genetic differences in metabolism of this agent.[26,27] Medications for pain should be administered according to a regular schedule, with rescue doses provided for intermittent or severe breakthrough pain. A subset of patients may require rapid dose escalation of opioids to achieve adequate control of refractory pain. The goal of increasing opioid therapy is to relieve distressing pain symptoms and not to hasten death; therefore, under the principle of double effect, opioid escalation is not contraindicated. Used correctly, opioids are safe,

Table 2
Pharmacologic and nonpharmacologic management of pain in pediatric palliative care

Nonpharmacologic	Deep Breathing (blowing bubbles), Progressive Relaxation, Biofeedback, Hypnosis
	Touch therapy (massage, physical therapy, heat/cold, acupuncture/pressure)
	Distraction (art/music/play therapy, imagery)

Drug	Initial Dose (mg/kg per Dose Unless Noted Otherwise)	Route	Interval	Maximum Dose	Formulation
Acetaminophen	10–16	PO/PR/IV	q 4 h	1 g/dose; 4 g/d	T, CT, L, D, S, I
Ibuprofen	5–10	PO	q 6 h	2.4 g/d; 3.4 g/d (adults)	T, CT, L, D
Choline magnesium trisalicylate	7.5–20.0	PO	BID–TID	1.5 g/dose	T, L
Naproxen	5–7	PO	q 8–12 h	1 g/dose; 4 g/d	T, L
Ketorolac	0.5	PO, IV	q 6 h	30 mg/dose iv, 10 mg/dose PO	I, T
Tramadol	1–2	PO	q 6 h	100 mg/dose, 400 mg/d	T
Morphine	0.2–0.5	PO, SL, PR	q 3–4 h	Titrate	T, L, D, S
	0.1	IV, SQ	q 2–4 h	Titrate	I, T
	0.3–0.6 (long acting)	PO	q 8–12 h	Titrate	SRT
Hydromorphone	0.03–0.08	PO, PR	q 3–4 h	Titrate	T, L, S
	0.015	IV, SQ	q 2–4 h	Titrate	I, T
Methadone	0.2	PO	q 8–12 h	Titrate	T, L
	0.1	IV, SQ	q 8–12 h	Titrate	I, T
Fentanyl	0.5–1 μg/kg/h	Transdermal	q 48–72 h	Titrate	P
	5–15 μg/kg (sedative)	TM	q 4–6 h	Titrate	LO
	1–2 μg/kg	IV, SQ	q 1–2 h	Titrate	I, T
Oxycodone	0.05–0.15	PO	q 6 h	Titrate	T, L
	0.1–0.3 (long acting)	PO	q 12 h	Titrate	SRT

Abbreviations: CT, chewable tablet; D, drops; I, injection; IV, intravenous; L, liquid; LO, lozenge; P, patch; PR, per rectum; S, suppository; SL, sub-lingual; SQ, subcutaneous; SRT, sustained-release tablet; T, tablet or capsule; TM, trans-mucosal.

effective medications for pain that do not hasten death. Imminently dying children should not be allowed to experience suffering, and judicious dose escalation is appropriate for these children along with the consideration of an alternative opioid. If a pediatric palliative care team is not involved in the care of a patient, consultation with a pain team (or pediatric anesthesia if team if there is no formal pain team) is advisable.

Palliative Sedation

Unfortunately, some children experience intractable physical or psychological suffering at EOL that is refractory to usual interventions, such as rapid escalations in the dose of analgesics and sedatives or opioid rotation; these children may continue to experience highly distressing symptoms. In such situations, an interdisciplinary approach is particularly important in ensuring that all potentially contributing sources of distress are addressed. In these rare circumstances, palliative sedation therapy (PST) with medications (eg, propofol) to achieve a continuous deep sedation may be necessary to provide adequate symptom relief and allow the child to die without pain or distress.[28] The goal of PST is not to hasten death but to relieve distress from refractory physical symptoms. The use of PST for existential suffering in children is rare.[28] Rather than being granted, requests for euthanasia, assisted suicide, or the deliberate hastening of death should be acknowledged and used as a starting point to identify the physical or emotional suffering that is underlying the patients' expressed desire to hasten death. Given the rarity of PST in pediatric populations, extensive education of clinical staff and clinical ethics consultation may be useful to ameliorate concerns about hastening death. **Fig. 2** provides a guideline for clinicians considering PST in imminently dying patients.[28]

PSYCHOSOCIAL CONCERNS AT THE EOL
Cultural, Spiritual, and Religious Concerns

In the ideal setting, the end of a child's life occurs in the most comfortable manner possible, allowing the family and child to be together in their chosen place. More commonly, this ideal scenario is complicated by continuing advances in medical regimens that, although introduced with the hope of restoring function, may ultimately expose a child to overly intensive treatments or interventions aiming to extend life within the last days or weeks of life. Such treatment often occurs in the inpatient setting. Despite this, the medical team should strive to provide EOL care that is inclusive of a family's personal, cultural, religious, or spiritual beliefs. Although commonly

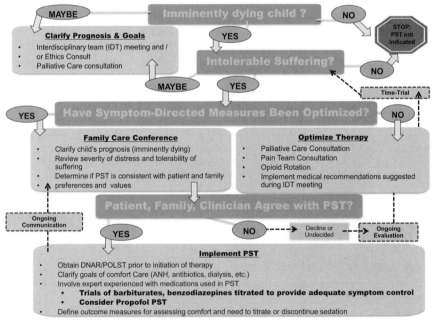

Fig. 2. Algorithm for initiation of palliative sedation. ANH, artificial nutrition and hydration; DNAR/POLST, do not attempt resuscitation/physician orders for life-sustaining treatment.

thought to be important, the role of these needs of families at the end of a child's life is understudied in pediatric populations. Facilitating the expression of a family's religious or spiritual beliefs as a child approaches EOL may provide comfort and a sense of meaning by supporting a sense of connection to a higher power. Therefore, the IDT should include a trained and certified chaplain to address the religious and spiritual needs of dying children and their families.

The growing diversity throughout the world brings a wealth of different religious and spiritual preferences and practices[29] to the hospital setting. However, such religious and spiritual preferences and practices are rarely incorporated into clinical care, especially in the inpatient setting at the end of life. Health professionals should become conscious of and open to the many religious, spiritual, and secular views and needs of their patients and family members, with an eye toward reduction of spiritual suffering. Various spiritual assessment tools are available to assist health care providers with this task: FICA, HOPE, the Spiritual Well-Being Scale, the Index of Core Spiritual Experiences, and Internet-based sources about beliefs according to geography or culture.[30,31] Chaplaincy services may be consulted to assist with assessing the religious and spiritual needs of a child and family.[29] Additionally, discussions with community-based religious leaders, interpreters, or other members of the cultural group can be informative. Parents often identify community religious figures and important members of their support system.[30] A community clergy person is typically more grounded in specific religious traditions and may already have an existing long-term relationship with the family; however, a hospital chaplain has more experience with counseling individuals through illness and death, so the most ideal combination of resources may result from partnerships between the two.[29]

After the death of a child, parents are often asked to make decisions about funeral, burial, or cremation plans. Families of children with complex chronic conditions or life-threatening illness may have already thought about the child's funeral and plans before the death as a part of "anticipatory grief."[32] However, families who experience the unexpected death of a child may need more assistance to plan a funeral or memorial service. Various members of the IDT, especially social workers and chaplains, may be helpful in supporting families and helping to make arrangements.

Legacy and Memory Building

For children and adolescents with life-threatening illnesses, efforts to build memories and confirm that they will be remembered are important.[32] During this time, children and adolescents may wish to attend to unfinished business, such as delegating who will receive certain belongings after their death, writing letters, drawing pictures, or talking with significant people.[33,34] Legacy building can be defined as doing or saying something that is remembered, including creating items that are both intentional and serendipitous.[35] Legacy-making activities include memory books, hand molds, songwriting, artwork, photographs, and videos. Most children's hospitals throughout the United States offer legacy-making activities to patients or to their families, including siblings,[36] usually through child-life specialists (health care professionals who focus on helping children and families cope with the stressors of illness, hospitalization, and treatment). By building a therapeutic relationship with the patients, child-life specialists can help families create a legacy together that starts before, continues through, and endures beyond the illness and its treatment.

Few studies have evaluated the efficacy of legacy building. However, a recent study suggests that legacy making may have positive effects for ill children and their family members, such as giving ill children opportunities to do or say something to be remembered, creating opportunities for ill children to communicate about death, providing a coping strategy for patients and family members (before and after the death), and offering tangible memories for families.[36] This study also suggests benefits for staff members, particularly nurses, who may contribute to legacy-making activities with or for ill children and their families, a phenomenon not yet explored.

Legacy making may have a greater effect if initiated much sooner in the illness trajectory (ie, at diagnosis of a life-threatening illness). However, in cases of traumatic or unexpected death, these activities will need to be modified appropriately to the clinical situation. Therefore, standardized EOL practices within a hospital can be important in helping provide keepsake articles to the family. These articles may include a lock of hair, a handprint or footprint mold, pictures, or other legacy items. Although offered in a standardized way, these legacy items can be individualized according to the patients' and families' needs, preferences, and coping styles.

Grief and Bereavement

Bereavement is the objective situation of losing someone significant through death and the adjustment that follows.[37] Grief refers to the distress resulting from bereavement and includes complex cognitive, emotional, and social difficulties. Together, these constitute the grief process. The death of a child is one of the most intense and painful events that a parent can experience, and parental grief is more intense and longer lasting than other types of grief and is associated with increased risk of psychological and physical illness.[38–43] A chaplain or psychosocial clinician on the IDT can help the family during the immediate period after a child's death as well as throughout the bereavement process.

Bereaved parents may experience severe personal guilt in the years after their child's death, particularly if they did not expect their child to die during the week before their death.[44] When death is anticipated, it is important that the attending staff and other members of the IDT clearly discuss the child's condition with the parents. Families who have access to and use psychological support during the last month of their child's life are more likely to work through grief, particularly if they have the opportunity to discuss their child's condition with the team.[45] Health care professionals should display empathy and remain attentive to familial needs in a manner that is open and culturally sensitive. Families should be informed that there is no right way to feel or act at the time of death, and their privacy should be respected. Families should be allowed to spend as much time with their child as they need after death, and accommodations should be made to allow for personal, cultural, or spiritual needs within the hospital setting.

After the death of a child, the health care team should not immediately withdraw from the parents, as they are essential in aiding the family during bereavement. Parents appreciate efforts by staff members to support them and commemorate the deceased child and notice when, in contrast, they do not see familiar faces or receive condolence cards.[46] Parental grieving evolves over time, and sharing emotional burdens with others throughout the grieving process is extremely helpful in their integration of their grief experience.[45]

For children and adolescents, the death of a sibling is a "serious life crisis," made more severe because it occurs when the sibling is "forming their view of the world and their own identity."[47] Emotional responses may include sadness, fear, anger, rejection, pain, grief, confusion, and loneliness as well as more complicated feelings.[47] For example, siblings may feel guilt about being alive, about having argued with the deceased, or about being jealous of the deceased getting the parents' attention during the grief process.[47] Health care providers should be attentive to the needs of the sibling before and after the death of patients. Children have found the following to be particularly helpful after a sibling's death[33]:

- Spending time with their mother
- Spending time with family friends
- Support groups
- Keeping possessions of the dying or dead sibling
- Reading
- Writing
- Participation in sports
- Focusing on school activities
- Drawing on religious faith
- Attending services for the deceased

Traumatic Deaths

Unintentional injuries are the leading cause of death in children and adolescents older than 1 year.[48] Not only is the sudden traumatic death of a child in the hospital catastrophic for the family but these events can also test the personal and professional boundaries of the medical staff, who may feel angry and powerless about the event, particularly when placing it in the context of their own children. **Table 3** provides suggestions to help health care providers to communicate with families of a child who has sustained a sudden, unexpected, and life-threatening injury.[49–51] Many of the principles can also be applied to other challenging conversations with families, such as the delivery of bad news.

Support for Clinical Staff

Physicians, nurses, and other clinical support staff on the inpatient units at pediatric hospitals can have various levels of experience in providing inpatient EOL care. Caring for children at EOL and supporting their families can be emotionally challenging for even the most-experienced member of the care team. Team health is an important component of a successful inpatient IDT. Without appropriate informational support, role identification, open communication, and time for self-care, members of the team are at risk for compassion fatigue or emotional burnout, which can negatively affect the caregiver's personal life and job performance and impair team dynamics. **Table 4** provides the sources of distress among nurses working in the acute care setting, with interventions that can be used to minimize this stress.[52–54] These strategies would likely be useful for any member of the IDT.

Moral Distress

Moral distress is the emotional reaction that occurs when individuals think that they know the right thing to do but do not do it because of internal (personal) constraints, external constraints, or both.[55,56] This distress can be common in nurses or other clinical staff who work with critically or chronically ill patients but have limited input into medical decision making because of a hierarchical power structure of the clinical team or unit environment. The lack of a voice in medical decision making can result in feelings of powerlessness, sadness, anger, and frustration. Unfortunately, this problem is not uncommon. In a study of clinicians providing care in the pediatric intensive care unit, several respondents indicated that they had "acted against their consciences in providing treatment to the children in their care.[57]" These distressing clinical experiences can result in cumulative moral distress and lead to depression, compassion fatigue, and ultimately burnout (**Box 1**).

Table 3
Communicating with families after the serious traumatic injury or unexpected death of a child

	Interpersonal Actions	Interdisciplinary Actions
Prepare	Clarify the facts before meeting with the family. Locate the parents and assist with the notification of other potentially vulnerable family members (siblings, grandparents). Identify potential strengths, vulnerabilities, and coping styles of the family for responding to this trauma. Prepare for fluctuations in emotion (ie, sadness, guilt, anger, blame, self-blame).	Facilitate a timely discussion between the family and clinical staff after an event. Alert the clinical staff to emerging problems or conflicts within the family. Misunderstanding of prognosis Conflicts about treatment options Identify psychosocial red flags. Intentional or nonaccidental event Perception of preventable event Concurrent family stress (ie, divorce)
Support	Convey compassion and empathy. Avoid blunt or overly technical jargon. Use clear, simple language. Avoid euphemisms. Remember to convey emotion. Establish trust. Allow extra time to communicate with the family; avoid appearing rushed. Answer parents' questions in detail, and prepare them for the events to unfold in the days ahead. Reassure the parents of the child's treatment and care.	Provide a quiet, private, or semiprivate area for the family. Access social worker, chaplains, child-life specialists, and any other referrals requested by family. Provide guidance related to communication with siblings or other family members. Help the family to maximize final visits with the child whose death is imminent or who has recently died while receiving acute medical care. Engage in legacy-building tasks. Provide guidance on the final decisions, such as withdrawal of life-sustaining technologies, organ donation, autopsy, and preparation for funeral services.
Follow-up	Plan formal and informal debriefing with staff. Acknowledge the need for and make time to engage in self-care.	Make a follow-up telephone call to assess grief. Provide information on resources for community support and reinforce the availability of resources.

Moral distress can be ameliorated through improved communication among members of the IDT, wherein sharing of divergent opinions are encouraged and differing perspectives are respected. It is important to raise awareness among clinical staff that health care professionals can and do hold different points of view. Education focused on published academic guidelines, institutional policies, and ethics literature can allow team members to develop well-informed opinions and familiarity with alternative viewpoints. Improved communication among IDT members can reduce staff perceptions of inappropriateness of care, improve shared decision making, reduce burnout and moral distress among the clinical team, and improve the quality of care delivered to patients and families.[55,56] Additionally, a team debriefing after difficult or unexpected deaths may prove to be helpful and ameliorate staff distress by providing a venue for sharing feelings and concerns about the loss.

Table 4
Identifying and ameliorating stress of nurses providing in-hospital EOL care

Stressors	Support Mechanisms
Systems-Based Stressors	**Systems-Based Interventions**
Not understanding the difference between palliative and EOL care Lack of a plan relating to medical care or uncertainty surrounding goals of therapy	Shadow senior staff member experienced in palliative care to facilitate clinical experience in caring for dying children and their families
Not knowing what to do with an imminently dying child and their family Discontinuing basic nursing interventions (laboratory test results, vital signs, and so forth)	Standard operating procedures to support children and families approaching EOL
Symptom-Based Stressors	**Symptom-Based Interventions**

Lack of education and hands-on training in palliative care
• Not knowing what to expect as new symptoms develop at EOL
• Not being able to control pain or other distressing symptoms
• Feeling helpless in helping to achieve patient and family comfort
	• Educational courses and modules in palliative care
	  ○ Expected trajectories of various diseases
	  ○ Managing complex pain and other symptoms
	• Access to specialist in palliative care or pain management who can assist with symptom management

Interpersonal Stressors	**Interpersonal Interventions**
Not knowing what to say to family or having trouble identifying family needs and wants	Courses to facilitate communication skills of pediatric nurses providing inpatient palliative care
Managing attachments to child and family	Clinical scenarios and education on professional boundaries and managing emotional attachments
Dealing with personal emotions and lack of time to debrief with others	Access to supervisor or support staff to whom they may speak freely about feelings and emotions

Box 1
Sources of moral distress encountered by clinical staff

Overly intensive treatment

    Unnecessary tests and treatments (burdensome care)

Incomplete information provided to patients or families

    Inadequate informed consent

    Withholding information from patients or families

    Patients' (families') preferences disregarded by a physician

Disparate goals

    Among family members

    Between the care team and family

Intraprofessional conflict

Inappropriate use of health care resources

ETHICAL ISSUES AT THE EOL
Ethics Consultation

Despite the earlier integration of palliative care and emphasis on advance care planning, the process of caring for children at EOL is not always without conflict. Occasionally, conflict may occur between family members, between staff, or between family members and staff about the goals of care or which treatments are in the best interest of the child. Conflicts may be highly emotional and result in moral distress. Often these conflicts are the result of a breakdown in communication rather than a true ethical dilemma. Palliative care teams, with their expertise in family communication and shared decision making, can often meet with individual family members or hold family care conferences and work through perceived conflicts about the goals of care. Clinical ethics consultation may be helpful for difficult cases in which IDT meetings or family care conferences have not resolved disagreements or in which a true ethical dilemma is thought to exist (Johnson LM, Church CL, Metzger M, et al. Clinical ethics consultation in pediatrics: long-term experience from a pediatric oncology center. Submitted for publication.) When conflicts over goals of care occur within the care team and result in moral distress among clinical staff, ethics consultation can facilitate communication among the IDT. This consultation may be particularly helpful when the conflict involves ancillary staff who may feel excluded from primary decision making. Clinical ethics consultations can help resolve conflicts, educate clinical staff on ethical issues, and provide a forum to discuss hospital policies (Johnson LM, Church CL, Metzger M, et al. Clinical ethics consultation in pediatrics: long-term experience from a pediatric oncology center. Submitted for publication.) Ethics consultations can often be used for curbside advice and can offer an opinion on the utility of a formal consultation. An ethics consultation may provide some reassurance for the family and staff when a medical decision involves a rarely used intervention (eg, palliative sedation, discontinuation of artificial nutrition and hydration after a severe traumatic brain injury).

Life-Sustaining Medical Treatments

Life-sustaining medical treatments include all interventions that may prolong the life of patients and can range from technologically complex treatments (eg, ventilator, dialysis, or vasoactive drugs) to less-complex measures (eg, antibiotics, insulin, or artificial nutrition and hydration).[7,58] The decision to initiate, continue, or discontinue life-sustaining medical treatment most commonly involves a consideration of the benefits and burdens of the therapy in the context of the preferences and goals of the child and family. The *ability* to provide life-sustaining medical treatments (such as artificial nutrition and hydration) is not an *obligation* to do so, especially if the burdens of therapy are greater than the perceived benefits. It may be appropriate to limit or stop the life-sustaining medical treatment if it only preserves biologic existence or if the goals of care have shifted from life prolongation to comfort-directed care.[7] When the risk/benefit ratio of an intervention is unclear, then a timed trial of the intervention may be beneficial. The life-sustaining medical treatment can be discontinued later if it fails to achieve the desired outcome. Discontinuation of a life-sustaining medical treatment is ethically equivalent to not starting the treatment and is permissible if the treatment is not compatible with the goals of care, even if discontinuation results in death. The discontinuation of nonbeneficial life-sustaining medical treatments is within the scope of parental decision-making authority and should not be viewed as inconsistent with a child's best interests. Clinicians who cannot participate in forgoing life-sustaining medical treatments may recuse themselves and arrange for the transfer of care to another physician or care provider.[7] Overriding family wishes should only be considered when these wishes are in conflict with the best interests of the child. Clinical ethics consultation and input from other clinicians, such as palliative care specialists, are advisable in cases of conflict.

RECOMMENDATIONS

Integrating the clinical, psychosocial, and spiritual concerns at the EOL into a standard operating procedure (SOP), which is based on quality standards established by the NQF,[5] can help ensure that all of these domains are addressed during inpatient deaths. At the time of imminent death, the medical staff should first recognize that the child is dying. The following automatic triggers can help identify when the SOP should be activated:

- Admittance to the hospital for symptom management at the EOL
- Patient identified by the care team as likely to die during this admission
- Any patient having physician orders for scope of treatment or life-sustaining treatment that indicate a do-not-resuscitate status, comfort care only, or limited interventions
- Any patient for whom the primary attending physician thinks that there is no further disease-directed therapy
- Patients with advanced-stage disease for whom the care team considers the need for IDT meetings
- Situations in which not starting or discontinuing life-sustaining therapies might be in the best interest of the child
- Patients having limited life expectancy and marked physical and functional decline, increased hospitalizations, or high symptom burdens

Once a patient is identified as needing EOL care, the care team should schedule an IDT meeting to prepare and discuss the Care Planning and Coordination checklist (**Fig. 3**). The IDT should include the attending physician; fellow; nurse practitioner; resident; nurses; pharmacists; social workers; child-life specialists; nutritionists; spiritual care professionals/chaplain; quality-of-life/palliative care specialist; and other support staff, such as psychologists, rehabilitation service specialists, and the nursing coordinator.

During the IDT meeting, participants can address decision making; advance care planning; symptom control; emotional, social, and spiritual needs; care coordination and continuity; and bereavement care. The meeting can also address staff bereavement, moral distress, compassion fatigue, and follow-up. In addition, a list of care team members who want to be contacted in the event of a patient's death can be compiled and kept with this document.

In partnership with the family, an individualized care plan should be developed for each patient and reviewed for accuracy by the team before it is uploaded into the electronic medical record. The plan of care should delineate the goals of care for the patients, list tasks that need to be completed and the members who will be completing them, and list plans for the follow-up. Members of the care team will be required to document the interventions they completed in response to the meeting, with plans to reconvene the full IDT every 2 weeks for a brief discussion about the follow-up and address new needs. A debriefing session should occur following an inpatient death to reflect on the family's and the team's experience with the patient's EOL care. This session can explore both the areas that were successful during the care period and the areas for improvement and can identify ongoing opportunities for supporting the bereaved family. Staff members should be encouraged to express their feelings about the patient's course and to remember the patient and provide support to the family. Staff members who experience emotional distress should also be provided appropriate support.

Checklist of Individualized Care Planning and Coordination processes[1]

Individualized Care planning and Coordination
☐ Comprehensive encounter completed and place in medical record

Advanced Care Planning[2]

☐ Participation of child and family in decision making
☐ Negotiation with family regarding plan of care
    ☐ Prognosis and goal-directed treatment options☐ Use of artificial hydration and nutrition
    ☐ Use of artificial life-prolonging measures☐ Use of transfusion therapies (platelets, RBCs, etc.)
    ☐ Use of antibiotics☐ Use of cancer-directed therapies (chemotherapy, radiation, surgery)
    ☐ Admission to the critical care unit or transfer to the floor
☐ POLST/DNaR signed and available in the medical record
☐ Advanced Care Plan/5 wishes/My wishes in chart, if applicable
☐ Unique patient/family requests identified and distributed to staff
☐ Appointment of health care agent in chart, if applicable
☐ Family conference offered to share the gravity of the patient's status with family members designated by primary care givers.
☐ Family notified that patient is imminently dying and medical decisions regarding care noted.
    ☐ Medication Review☐ Need for vital signs
    ☐ Discussed need for further diagnostic tests, invasive/painful procedures, and labs
☐ Non-essential equipment reviewed (e.g., monitors)
☐ Discussion complete on preferences of where death will occur
    Hospice Care at Home____ Inpatient Hospice____ Hospital____ Home Hospital_____ ICU____ Other
☐ Ethical issues identified, Ethics Committee consulted (as needed)
☐ Autopsy discussion☐ Organ Donation
☐ Consent Completed (Autopsy or Organ Donation, when applicable)
By whom?____

Symptom control

☐ Comfort optimized
    ☐ Physical symptoms addressed☐ Psychological symptoms addressed
    ☐ Pain team notified of admission via pager, if applicable
    ☐ Quality-of-Life Service notified of admission or via pager, if applicable
☐ Function optimized
    ☐ Rehabilitation service notified of admission or via pager if applicable
☐ Signs and symptoms of imminently dying discussed with family (i.e., changes in vital signs, respiration, skin, neurological response)
☐ Educational/resource materials provided

Emotional, Social and Spiritual Care

☐ Assessments reviewed by family member
    ☐ Child's needs☐ Siblings' needs☐ Parents' needs
☐ Assessments reviewed by discipline
    ☐ Emotional needs☐ Social needs☐ Spiritual needs☐ Cultural needs
☐ Sibling and patient relationship needs addressed (i.e., expressions of love, gratitude, forgiveness, and farewell)
☐ Family presence facilitated (e.g.,Red Cross, military)
☐ Accommodations arranged for family gathering on unit (i.e., larger, quieter room)
☐ The need for calling cards addressed☐ Family members contacted about status ___Yes ___ No ____N/A
    Contact Made by:____
☐ End-of-life cultural concerns addressed
☐ Financial burdens assessed☐ Discussion of St. Jude's financial assistance complete
☐ Financial support optimized (i.e., Clayton Dabney)
☐ Services/Funeral Arrangements☐ Funeral Home Notified (name):
    Arrangements made by____

Fig. 3. Sample care planning and coordination checklist.

Funeral Home Contact Person:_____

Burial Options -☐Cremation☐Burial

☐ Transportation Home arranged____Yes____No____ N/A

Mode of transportation_____family car_____ambulance_____air ambulance

☐ Housing Rule addressed_____N/A☐ Extension given for housing____

☐ Make A Wish or other wish agency contacted____Yes____No____N/A

Care Coordination and Continuity

☐ Room flagged with Symbol

☐ Social worker notified of admission via pager☐ Child Life notified of admission via pager

☐ Chaplain notified of admission via pager☐ Psychology notified of admission via pager____N/A

☐ Primary Care Team emailed of admission for end-of-life care

☐ Plan for contacts at the time of death completed Plan:_____

☐ Identification of key health care member to contact in urgent situations

☐ Patient and family requesting notifications to ___ Family & Friends____ Schools____ Church____ Other

☐ Notifications at time of death

    ☐Other Service Providers

    ☐ Primary Care Physician_____

    ☐ Home hospital _____

    ☐Referring physician _____

    ☐Family members _____

    _____

    _____

☐ Postmortem packet stamped and placed in nursing binder

☐ Planned follow-up interdisciplinary care team meeting

Bereavement care

☐ Anticipatory needs for bereavement process applied (i.e., assist family and staff with staying connected to the child, facilitated communication between child and family, addressed decisional regret, facilitated memorial objects/legacy items, educational/resource materials provided)

☐ Bereavement care of surviving family members

    ☐ Risk assessment for complicated bereavement

    ☐ Bereavement materials provided

☐ Sympathy Booklet in Nursing Binder for Staff to sign

☐ Sympathy Booklet Mailed

☐ Bereavement care of staff

    ☐ Debriefing scheduled

Signature/Initial:

FORMS:(Initial When completed)

_____ Record of Death

_____ Final Disposition

_____ Death Certificate

_____ Autopsy Consent

1. This checklist has been adapted from the checklist used by the Quality-of-Life/Palliative Care Service at St. Jude Children's Research Hospital in Memphis, TN, USA (2013).

2. The goal is to obtain items before the child enters the imminently dying phase of illness.

3. A Column may be added to identify which staff members are assigned to follow-up on an individual task

Fig. 3. (continued)

REFERENCES

1. Vickers JL, Carlisle C. Choices and control: parental experiences in pediatric terminal home care. J Pediatr Oncol Nurs 2000;17:12–21.

2. Davies B, Deveau E, deVeber B, et al. Experiences of mothers in five countries whose child died of cancer. Cancer Nurs 1998;21:301–11.

3. Field MJ, Behrman RE, editors. When children die: improving palliative and end-of-life care for children and their families. Institute of Medicine (U. S. Committee on Palliative and End-of-Life Care for Children). Washington, DC: National Academies Press; 2003.

4. Kane JR, Himelstein BP. Palliative care for children. In: Berger AM, Shuster JL, Von Roenn JH, editors. Principles and practice of palliative medicine and supportive oncology. 3rd edition. Philadelphia: Lippincott Williams & Wilkins; 2007. p. 1044–61.

5. A national framework and preferred practices for palliative and hospice care quality. National Quality Forum. 2006. Available at: www.qualityforum.org. Accessed November 15, 2013.

6. Johnson LM, DeLario M, Baker J, et al. Chapter 63: palliative care in pediatrics. In: Berger AM, Shuster JL, Von Roenn JH, editors. Principles and practice of supportive care and supportive oncology. 4th edition. Philadelphia: Lippincott Williams & Wilkins; 2013. p. 819–38.

7. Committee on Bioethics (American Academy of Pediatrics). Guidelines on foregoing life-sustaining medical treatment. Pediatrics 1994;93(3):532–6.

8. Wienr L, Zadeh S, Battles H, et al. Allowing adolescent and young adults to plan their end-of-life care. Pediatrics 2012;130(5):897–905.

9. Baker JN, Barfield R, Hinds PS, et al. A process to facilitate decision making in pediatric stem cell transplantation: the individualized care planning and coordination model. Biol Blood Marrow Transplant 2007;13(3):245–54.

10. Contro N, Larson J, Scofield S, et al. Family perspectives on the quality of pediatric palliative care. Arch Pediatr Adolesc Med 2002;156:14–9.

11. Mack JW, Hilden JM, Watterson J, et al. Parent and physician perspective on quality of care at the end of life in children with cancer. J Clin Oncol 2005; 23(36):9155–61.

12. Goldman A, Hain R, Liben S. Palliative care for children. New York: Oxford University Press; 2012.

13. Clinical practice guidelines for quality palliative care. 3rd edition. Pittsburgh (PA): National Consensus Project for Quality Palliative Care; 2013. Available at: http://www.nationalconsensusproject.org/NCP_Clinical_Practice_Guidelines_3rd_Edition.pdf.

14. Hinds PS, Schum L, Baker JN, et al. Key factors affecting dying children and their families. J Palliat Med 2005;8(Suppl 1):S70–8.

15. National Comprehensive Cancer Network guidelines for supportive care. Available at: http://www.nccn.org/professionals/physician_gls/f_guidelines.asp#supportive. Accessed December 15, 2013.

16. Levine D, Lam CG, Cunningham MJ, et al. Best practices for pediatric palliative cancer care: a primer for clinical providers. J Support Oncol 2013;11:114–25.

17. Wrede-Seaman L, editor. Pediatric pain and symptom management algorithms for palliative care. Cape Town (South Africa): Intellicard; 2005.

18. Wolfe J, Hinds P, Sourkes B, editors. Textbook of interdisciplinary pediatric palliative care. Philadelphia: Saunders; 2011.

19. Pritchard MP, Burghen E, Srivastava DK, et al. Cancer-related symptoms most concerning to parents during the last week and last day of their child's life. Pediatrics 2008;121(5):e1301–9.

20. Wolfe J, Grier HE, Klar N, et al. Symptoms and suffering at the end of life in children with cancer. N Engl J Med 2000;342(5):326–33.

21. Goldman A, Hewitt M, Collins GS, et al. Symptoms in children/young people with progressive malignant disease: United Kingdom Children's Cancer Study Group/Paediatric Oncology Nurses Forum survey. Pediatrics 2006;117(6): e1179–86.

22. Klick JC, Hauer J. Pediatric palliative care. Curr Probl Pediatr Adolesc Health Care 2010;40(6):120–51.

23. Srouji R, Ratnapalan S, Schneeweiss S. Pain in children: assessment and non-pharmacological management. Int J Pediatr 2010;2010:1–11.

24. Berde CB, Sethna NF. Analgesics for the treatment of pain in children. N Engl J Med 2002;347(14):1094–103.

25. Anghelescu DL, Oakes L, Hinds PS. Palliative care and pediatrics. Anesthesiol Clin 2006;24(1):145–61.
26. WHO guidelines on the pharmacological treatment of persisting pain in children with medical illnesses. 2014. Available at: http://whqlibdoc.who.int/publications/2012/9789241548120_Guidelines.pdf?ua=1. Accessed January 15, 2014.
27. Tremlett M, Anderson BJ, Wolf A. Pro-con debate: is codeine a drug that still has a useful role in pediatric practice? Paediatr Anaesth 2010;20:183–94.
28. Anghelescu DL, Hamilton H, Faughnan LG, et al. Pediatric palliative sedation therapy with propofol: recommendations based on experience in children with terminal cancer. J Palliat Med 2012;15(10):1082–90.
29. Nelson-Becker H, Ai A, Hopp F, et al. Spirituality and religion in end-of-life care ethics: the challenge of interfaith and cross-generational matters. Br J Soc Work 2013. [Epub ahead of print].
30. Robinson MR, Thiel MM, Backus MM, et al. Matters of spirituality at the end of life in the pediatric intensive care unit. Pediatrics 2006;118(3):718–29.
31. Pierce B. The introduction and evaluation of a spiritual assessment tool in a palliative care unit. Scottish Journal of Healthcare Chaplaincy 2004;7(2):39–43.
32. Levetown M, Liben S, Audet M. Palliative care in the pediatric intensive care unit. In: Carter BS, Levetown M, editors. Palliative care for infants, children, and adolescents: a practical handbook. Baltimore (MD): John Hopkins University Press; 2004. p. 273–91.
33. Walker A. Adolescent bereavement and traumatic deaths. In: Balk D, Corr C, editors. Adolescent encounters with death, bereavement, and coping, Chapter 14. New York: Springer Publishing Company; 2009. p. 253–70.
34. Foster TL, Gilmer MJ, Davies B, et al. Bereaved parents' and siblings' reports of legacies created by children with cancer. J Pediatr Oncol Nurs 2009;26(6):369–76.
35. Foster TL, Dietrich MS, Friedman DL, et al. National survey of children's hospitals on legacy-making activities. J Palliat Med 2012;15(5):573–8.
36. Allen RS, Hilgeman MM, Ege MA, et al. Legacy activities as interventions approaching the end of life. J Palliat Med 2008;11(7):1029–38.
37. Bruce CA. Helping patients, families, caregiver, and physicians, in the grieving process. J Am Osteopath Assoc 2007;107(7):33–40.
38. Middleton W, Raphael B, Burnett P, et al. A longitudinal study comparing bereavement phenomena in recently bereaved spouses, adult children, and parents. Aust N Z J Psychiatry 1998;32:235–41.
39. Kissane DW, Bloch SB, Onghena P, et al. The Melbourne family grief study I: perceptions of family functioning in bereavement. Am J Psychiatry 1996;153:650–8.
40. Kreicbergs U, Valdimarsdóttir U, Onelöv E, et al. Anxiety and depression in parents 4-9 years after the loss of a child owing to a malignancy: a population-based follow-up. Psychol Med 2004;34(8):1431–41.
41. Harper M, O'Connor RE, O'Carroll RC. Increased mortality in parents bereaved in their first year of their child's life. BMJ Support Palliat Care 2011. http://dx.doi.org/10.1136/bmjspcare-2011-000025.
42. Li J, Hansen D, Mortensen P, et al. Myocardial infarction in parents who lost a child: a nationwide prospective cohort study in Denmark. Circulation 2002;106:1634–9.
43. Kersting A, Brahler E, Glaesmer H, et al. Prevalence of complicated grief in a representative population-based sample. J Affect Disord 2011;131(1–3):339–43.

44. Surkan P, Kreicbergs U, Valdimarsdottir U, et al. Perceptions of inadequate health care and feelings of guilt in parents after the death of a child to a malignancy: a population-based long-term follow-up. J Palliat Med 2006;9(2):317–31.

45. Kreicbergs U, Lannen P, Onelov E, et al. Parental grief after losing a child to cancer: impact of professional and social support on long-term outcomes. J Clin Oncol 2007;25:3307–12.

46. Macdonald ME, Liben S, Carnevale FA, et al. Parental perspectives on hospital staff members' acts of kindness and commemoration after a child's death. Pediatrics 2005;116(4):884–90.

47. Forward DR, Garlie N. Search for new meaning: adolescent bereavement after the sudden death of a sibling. Can J Sch Psychol 2003;18(23):23–53.

48. Hamilton BE, Hoyert DL, Martin JA, et al. Annual summary of vital statistics. Pediatrics 2013;131(3):548–58.

49. Truog RD, Christ G, Browning DM, et al. Sudden traumatic death in children – "We did everything, but your child didn't survive". JAMA 2006;295(22):2646–54.

50. Parker-Raley J, Jones BL, Maxson RT. Communicating the death of a child in the emergency department: managing dialectical tensions. J Healthc Qual 2008; 30(5):20–31.

51. Meert KL, Eggly S, Pollack M, et al. Parents' perspectives on physician-parent communication near the time of a child's death in the pediatric intensive care unit. Pediatr Crit Care Med 2008;9(1):2–7.

52. Joinson C. Coping with compassion fatigue. Nursing 1992;22(4):118–9.

53. Figley CR. Compassion fatigue: toward a new understanding of the costs of caring in secondary traumatic stress: self-care issues for clinicians, researchers, and educators. London: Sidran Press; 1995.

54. Pearson HN. You've only got one chance to get it right: children's cancer nurses' experiences of providing palliative care in the acute hospital setting. Issues Compr Pediatr Nurs 2013;36(3):188–211.

55. Austin W, Kelecevic J, Goble E, et al. An overview of moral distress and the pediatric intensive care team. Nurs Ethics 2009;16(1):57–68.

56. Rushton CH, Kaszniak AW, Halifax JS. Addressing moral distress: application of a framework to palliative care practice. J Palliat Med 2013;16(9):1080–8.

57. Solomon MZ, Sellers DE, Heller KS, et al. New and lingering controversies in pediatric end-of-life care. Pediatrics 2005;116(4):872–83.

58. Diekema DS, Botkin JR. Committee on Bioethics (American Academy of Pediatrics). Clinical report – forgoing medically provided nutrition and hydration in children. Pediatrics 2009;124(2):813–22.

Index

Note: Page numbers of article titles are in **boldface** type.

Moving?

Make sure your subscription moves with you!

To notify us of your new address, find your **Clinics Account Number** (located on your mailing label above your name), and contact customer service at:

Email: journalscustomerservice-usa@elsevier.com

800-654-2452 (subscribers in the U.S. & Canada)
314-447-8871 (subscribers outside of the U.S. & Canada)

Fax number: 314-447-8029

Elsevier Health Sciences Division
Subscription Customer Service
3251 Riverport Lane
Maryland Heights, MO 63043

*To ensure uninterrupted delivery of your subscription, please notify us at least 4 weeks in advance of move.